Systems Population Health

Past and Present

For access to digital chapters,
visit the APHA Press bookstore (APHA.org).

Systems That Impact Population Health
Past and Present

Ivory Clarke, MS • Donald Warne, MD, MPH
Mienah Zulfacar Sharif, PhD, MPH • Micere Keels, PhD
Ruth Enid Zambrana, PhD, MSW • Antonia M. Villarruel, PhD, RN
Kristine J. Ajrouch, PhD • Laufou Jacob Fitisemanu Jr., MPH
Erika Blacksher, PhD • Matt Wray, PhD, MA • Marshall H. Chin, MD, MPH

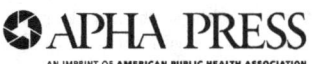

American Public Health Association
800 I Street, NW
Washington, DC 20001-3710
www.apha.org

© 2025 by the American Public Health Association

All rights reserved. No part of this publication may be reproduced, stored in a retrieval system, or transmitted in any form or by any means, electronic, mechanical, photocopying, recording, scanning, or otherwise, except as permitted under Sections 107 and 108 of the 1976 United States Copyright Act, without either the prior written permission of the Publisher or authorization through payment of the appropriate per-copy fee to the Copyright Clearance Center [222 Rosewood Drive, Danvers, MA 01923, (978) 750-8400, fax (978) 646-8600, www.copyright.com]. Requests to the Publisher for permission should be addressed to the Permissions Department, American Public Health Association, 800 I Street, NW, Washington, DC 20001-3710; fax (202) 777-2531.

DISCLAIMER: Any discussion of medical or legal issues in this publication is being provided for informational purposes only. Nothing in this publication is intended to constitute medical or legal advice, and it should not be construed as such. This book is not intended to be and should not be used as a substitute for specific medical or legal advice, since medical and legal opinions may only be given in response to inquiries regarding specific factual situations. If medical or legal advice is desired by the reader of this book, a medical doctor or attorney should be consulted. The use of trade names and commercial sources in this book does not imply endorsement by the American Public Health Association. The views expressed in the publications of the American Public Health Association are those of the contributors and do not necessarily reflect the views of the American Public Health Association, or its staff, advisory panels, officers, or members of the Association's Executive Board. While the publisher and contributors have used their best efforts in preparing this book, they make no representations with respect to the accuracy or completeness of the content. The findings and conclusions in this book are those of the contributors and do not necessarily represent the official positions of the institutions with which they are affiliated.

Georges C. Benjamin, MD, MACP, Executive Director

Printed and bound in the United States of America
Book Production Editor: Keira McCarthy
Typesetting: The Charlesworth Group
Cover Design: Katie Avelar
Cover Art: Bobby C. Martin
Printing and Binding: Sheridan Books

Library of Congress Cataloging-in-Publication Data

Names: Clarke, Ivory author | Warne, Donald author | Sharif, Mienah
   Zulfacar author | Keels, Micere author | Zambrana, Ruth E. author |
   Villarruel, Antonia M. author
Title: Systems that impact population health : past and present / by Ivory
   Clarke, MS, Donald Warne, MD, MPH, Mienah Zulfacar Sharif, PhD, MPH,
   Micere Keels, PhD, Ruth Enid Zambrana, PhD, MSW, Antonia M. Villarruel,
   PhD, RN, Kristine Ajrouch, PhD, Jacob Fitisemanu Jr., MPH, Erika
   Blacksher, PhD, Matt Wray, PhD, MA, and Marshall H. Chin, MD, MPH.
Description: Washington, DC : American Public Health Association Press,
   [2025] | Includes bibliographical references and index. | Summary: "This
   book adopts both a historical and contemporary lens to understand the
   origins of the current health inequities crisis and underscore the
   urgent need to address the effects of systemic and structural racism on
   health. Evidence shows that interrelated social determinants of health,
   including voting rights, reproductive rights, legal reform, and health
   care access, individually and collectively impact health, underscoring
   the critical need for comprehensive frameworks, policies, and programs
   to address the root causes of health inequities"-- Provided by publisher.
Identifiers: LCCN 2025037475 (print) | LCCN 2025037476 (ebook) | ISBN
   9780875533629 paperback | ISBN 9780875533636 adobe pdf
Subjects: LCSH: Population--Health aspects | Public health--Social aspects
   | Public health--Political aspects | Social medicine
Classification: LCC RA418 .C6325 2025 (print) | LCC RA418 (ebook)
LC record available at https://lccn.loc.gov/2025037475
LC ebook record available at https://lccn.loc.gov/2025037476

Contents

Foreword: Confronting Systemic Barriers and Building Equity Into the Future of Health   vii
Richard E. Besser, MD

Foreword: Strengthening Systems to Create Healthier Communities for All   xi
Victor J. Dzau, MD

Preface   xv
Amy Gyau-Moyer, MS, MBA, MSW, and Shaneah Taylor, MPH

Introduction   1
Ivory Clarke, MS, Gilbert C. Gee, PhD, Tina Kauh, PhD, MS, Dwayne Proctor, PhD, Julie Morita, MD, Alonzo Plough, PhD, MPH, and Antonia M. Villarruel, PhD, RN

1. Systemic Racism and the Health of American Indians and Alaska Natives   11
   Donald Warne, MD, MPH, Melanie Nadeau, PhD, MPH, Stacy A. Bohlen, Emily A. Haozous, PhD, RN, Benjamin A. Jacuk, ThM, MDiv, Maria Christina Crouch, PhD, Stephen Long, Loretta Grey Cloud, Michelle Johnson-Jennings, PhD, Tipiziwin Tolman, MEd, Abigail Echo-Hawk, MA, Brinda Sivaramakrishnan, MPH, and Allison Kelliher, MD

2. Structural Racism, Asian American Communities, and Health Equity: A Historical, Transnational, and Intersectional Perspective   49
   Mienah Zulfacar Sharif, PhD, MPH, Marshall H. Chin, MD, MPH, Ignatius Bau, JD, Melissa Borja, PhD, Nadia Islam, PhD, Nadia Kim, PhD, LeiLani Nishime, PhD, Paul M. Ong, PhD, MUP, and Gilbert C. Gee, PhD

   Appendix 2A   92

3. Strengthening the Health of Black People in the United States Through Systemic and Structural Change 97
   Micere Keels, PhD, Velma McBride Murry, PhD, MS, Robynn Cox, PhD, MA, Tyson H. Brown, PhD, Wendy Ellis, DrPH, MPH, Chelsea Dorsey, MD, Angela Diaz, MD, PhD, MPH, and Eliseo J. Pérez-Stable, MD

4. Examining the Impacts of the Interrelated Systems of Education, Employment, and Health Care on the Life Course and Well-Being of Latino Populations 129
   Ruth Enid Zambrana, PhD, MSW, José E. Rodríguez, MD, José A. Pagán, PhD, Angela Diaz, MD, PhD, MPH, Lenny López, MD, MPH, MDiv, and Antonia M. Villaruel, PhD, RN

   Appendix 4A 169

5. Structural Inequities and Middle Eastern and North African American Health 179
   Kristine J. Ajrouch, PhD, Nadia N. Abuelezam, ScD, Niaz Kasravi, PhD, Jen'nan G. Read, PhD, and Muniba Saleem, PhD

6. We Are the Ocean 211
   Laufou Jacob Fitisemanu Jr., MPH, Maile Tauali'i, PhD, MPH, Yvette C. Paulino, PhD, and Fuimaono Nia Aitaoto, PhD, MPH, MS

7. Health Inequities in White European Americans: Key Systems, Root Causes, and the Legacies of Whiteness 245
   Erika Blacksher, PhD, Matt Wray, PhD, MA, and Steven H. Woolf, MD, MPH

8. Cross-Cutting Solutions to Address Structural Racism to Advance Health Equity 281
   Marshall H. Chin, MD, MPH, Tyson H. Brown, PhD, and Anna Ricklin, MHS

Contributors 309

Index 325

Foreword: Confronting Systemic Barriers and Building Equity Into the Future of Health

In 2020, the disproportionate harms that people of color endured in the COVID-19 pandemic, alongside the tragic murder of George Floyd at the hands of police officers that summer, prompted a long-overdue, though short-lived, societal reckoning with systemic and structural racism. For the health field, it was an inflection point. The convergence of those events brought to light the connections between health inequity and other racial and social inequities and illustrated in stark terms the ways in which they close off opportunities for millions of people and families.

In response, health practitioners, medical researchers, policymakers, nonprofits, and others began to rethink their missions, priorities, and actions. Many took steps to meet the urgency of the moment and lay the groundwork for a better future. At the Robert Wood Johnson Foundation (RWJF), where I serve as president and CEO, we began to undertake a deep reexamination of our priorities and strategy and initiated new investments, including $90 million to support community power in 2020. After continued reflection, in 2024 we pledged to put the dismantling of structural racism at the center of our work to build a future where health is not a privilege, but a right. This commitment to dismantling structural racism marked a transition in the more than 50-year history of RWJF—one that, looking back, we wish had begun far sooner, for it is impossible to see a future where health is a right for all without eliminating this most entrenched and pernicious barrier. This is the beginning of a long-term change, and we will continue to learn from our partners and evolve as we advocate for health equity in the years to come.

For communities, public health officials, researchers, and others including RWJF, the last five years were initially defined by bold ambitions and growing momentum as we sought to eliminate structural and systemic racism in health. But progress has been impeded by retrenchment: an ideologically driven caricature of equity and diversity approaches and efforts to eliminate any consideration of racial equity in research or government policies and practices.

The publication of *Systems That Impact Population Health: Past and Present* is a product of our time, when the backlash to equity dominates our politics, government, and culture. Stakeholders involved in developing the studies here—in particular, our partners at the National Academy of Medicine, which relies on federal funding support—felt the chilling effects of government-led attacks on the concepts outlined in the chapters ahead.

It should not be controversial to identify factors that affect health and well-being and provide evidence-based studies of the different and often disproportionate ways those factors affect certain groups. But at a time when political and government leaders have put ideology and hostility ahead of evidence and equity, the publication of this book amounts to an act of resistance.

Moments like this require us to raise our voices. We cannot sit idly by while vital data sources that doctors use to guide treatment decisions and researchers use to advance medical knowledge are erased from public view. We cannot stay quiet as the government defunds important research because it references certain words and topics now deemed off-limits. We cannot be silent when systemic and structural racism remain life-and-death issues in our health systems and communities.

By providing an in-depth historical examination of health inequity and a chapter-by-chapter articulation of its impacts on a range of different population groups, this book fortifies the robust scientific basis for acknowledging and addressing racial disparities in health. It builds a vital evidence base that stands in contrast to emotionally charged, unscientific criticisms that often arise in the discourse among opponents of health equity. By tackling those topics with rigorous study and analysis, this book also serves as a response to the larger dismantling of trust in health expertise. Major institutions today are struggling under agendas that run counter to sound science and public service, while decisions around lifesaving medical innovations are informed by unfounded and even discredited claims. At the same time, scientists, health experts, and researchers—not to mention doctors and nurses interacting directly with patients—confront a steady flow of misinformation and disinformation. This book helps remove many charged issues from the arena of polarized debate and viral social media posts and grounds them in science, data, history, and lived experiences.

The evidence base presented in these chapters is an important contribution as medical innovations take hold in the years to come. Take artificial intelligence (AI), for example. Researchers believe it can revolutionize the pace and impact of medical breakthroughs and future treatments. But AI is built on the existing body of medical information and data, which has historically overlooked or dismissed the inequities that too many people face in our health system. We already see innovations like algorithmic dermatology scans that are ineffective on darker skin. It is imperative that further AI-driven advances don't suffer from similar shortcomings. The evidence base AI needs is incomplete without robust studies of structural and systemic racism, social determinants of health, and health equity. A deeper understanding of the interactions between health and housing, health and education, health and environmental quality, and health and myriad other factors will be a powerful asset in this new frontier of medical exploration. This is yet another area where this book provides a timely and necessary contribution and can help strengthen the effectiveness and accessibility of future advances.

Finally, this book should serve as a valuable resource for communities, health advocates, policymakers, and philanthropic leaders who continue to fight for health equity. As a former pediatrician who spent 30 years working in community clinics, served more than a decade at the Centers for Disease Control and Prevention, and now leads a foundation focused on health equity, I have had firsthand experience with nearly every facet of our health system. I know how significant today's disruptions are, from the systemic to the individual level. But I also believe they present opportunities for the dedicated and brilliant people in this field to open new pathways to progress and ultimately build a system that finally serves all communities.

This is a time to reimagine the slate of possible solutions ahead of us and ensure that what comes next is far better than the pre-pandemic status quo. In that regard, the chapters ahead are a call to action. Policymakers should use the expanded evidence base on health equity as the foundation for policy innovations. Funders should mine the insights here to explore new avenues for driving change. Communities should look to the experiences of individual groups outlined here to enhance their own power-building efforts. Many of the health systems that exist today were deliberately constructed to exclude certain people. Rather than just being a cause for despair, that should give us hope. An intentionally built system can be intentionally rebuilt. We can remove and replace the unfair structures that exist today. This book improves our chances of success by expanding our knowledge of the past and present health inequities and systemic challenges we must overcome.

Those who have worked to portray equity, systemic racism, and other concepts as divisive often claim that acknowledging the realities of our past—and present—is about villainizing perpetrators of injustices, casting a shadow over history, and deepening divisions. But the truth is, this work is about healing. Every health practitioner knows that we must look at history if we hope to diagnose the challenges of the present and determine a course toward a better future.

Systems That Impact Population Health: Past and Present arrives as we are once again called upon to meet a dark and challenging moment. I am grateful to the individuals and organizations who helped shepherd this important work along its winding journey to publication, especially National Academy of Medicine President Dr. Victor J. Dzau, who was steadfast in his commitment to finding a home for this vital work. I also thank the contributors who have provided resources, insights, and inspiration for the necessary and lifesaving work ahead.

Richard E. Besser, MD
President and CEO
Robert Wood Johnson Foundation

Foreword: Strengthening Systems to Create Healthier Communities for All

As a child in post–World War II Shanghai, and later in Hong Kong, I saw what scarcity and illness meant in the lives of families and communities. Infectious diseases were common. Medical care was limited. For many, survival depended less on science than on circumstance—where you lived, whether food was available, whether a doctor could be reached in time. These early experiences left an indelible mark. They taught me that health is shaped as much by the systems around us (housing, education, work, community) as by what happens in a clinic or hospital. They also impressed upon me an enduring belief: Leadership and science must serve people in every community, not just the fortunate few.

Health outcomes in the United States are profoundly shaped by many interlocking social and structural systems. These systems are shaped not only by resources and infrastructure but also by systemic forces such as racism, economic inequality, and policy environments that influence whether opportunities for health are widely shared or withheld. The alignment of housing, schools, jobs, community networks, and health care creates the foundation for better outcomes. When misaligned, they create and reinforce inequities that result in preventable illness, premature death, and inequities that persist across generations. Research has shown consistently that the conditions of daily life exert a powerful influence on health and that they can be improved through purposeful action.

The urgency is clear. The United States spends more on health care than peer nations, yet life expectancy lags and progress remains uneven. This gap is not inevitable. It reflects choices about how care is organized and paid for, how information is collected and used, and how leaders across sectors coordinate to strengthen the conditions that allow people and places to thrive.

In response to these pressing challenges, *Systems That Impact Population Health: Past and Present* offers a timely contribution to that work. The book brings historical perspective and lived experience into conversation and highlights priorities that emerge across many different population groups. Its value is orientation, not prescription. It points leaders toward strategies with promise for improving health, especially in places where progress has been uneven. It is a companion for policymakers, practitioners, and community partners who want steadier gains that reach every community.

Four themes stand out as especially important:

1. **Measure what matters and make it trustworthy.** Better decisions depend on timely, accurate, and appropriately detailed information. Yet many institutions still lack a full picture of need and progress. Data must be shared responsibly, linked when appropriate, and analyzed in ways that support action by health care, public health, and community partners. When results are visible, trust grows, and resources can be directed where they have the greatest effect.
2. **Design care and payment around outcomes that matter to people.** Access to strong primary care, continuity of services, and coverage are essential foundations. Equally important is ensuring that incentives encourage prevention, coordination, and results that families can feel in their daily lives. Across the nation, health systems and communities are testing new approaches to value-based care that emphasize person-centered outcomes rather than volume of services. The details will vary by place and population, but the principle is clear: primary care should be the front door to the system, behavioral health and social support must be integrated when they shape outcomes, and measurement should reflect what matters to people. When financing and delivery systems move in this direction, clinicians and organizations can focus more squarely on improving health and well-being, not just delivering more care.
3. **Build durable multisectoral partnerships.** No sector can deliver population-level improvement alone. Public health, health care, education, employers, civic leaders, and community organizations each hold part in the solution, and their work is most effective when it addresses the systemic barriers that cut across these sectors. Effective collaboration requires clear roles, shared accountability, and respect for local knowledge. A strong practice base exists. *Communities in Action: Pathways to Health Equity*, for example, focuses on what communities can do to promote health equity and what actions are needed by the many and varied stakeholders that are part of communities or support them.[1]
4. **Address systemic factors that shape opportunities for health.** Durable gains come from improving everyday conditions: housing, transportation, safe environments, quality education, and worker protections. Because policies and investment have differed across places and over time, some populations face greater exposure to risk and less access to protective resources due to systemic factors. Progress means aligning policy across sectors, simplifying rules, ensuring language access, and making public services easy to use. Health systems can be effective partners by supporting housing stability, connecting patients to civil legal help when appropriate, collaborating with schools and early childhood programs, and investing in local workforce pipelines. Keep goals universal, tailor approaches by population and place, and track results so improvements are both broad and felt where needs are greatest.

These themes connect to the country's broader challenge. The United States spends at historic levels, yet too many people still experience avoidable illness, shortened lives, and barriers to basic care. There is also wide variation by place and income, which tells us that policy and practice matter. In some communities, people with fewer financial resources live markedly longer than counterparts elsewhere, a signal that local systems and supports can bend the curve. Identifying what those communities do differently and adapting those lessons responsibly is a practical path forward.

The chapters in this book reflect thoughtful contributions and strong connections with communities. They offer perspectives on where public health attention can make a broad difference: improving the data we rely on and using it to illuminate both need and progress; strengthening primary care and aligning payment with outcomes that families value; and inviting missing partners to the table and working with them in ways that build trust and momentum. None of these require a single program or a universal template. They require commitment, follow-through, and the discipline to learn from what works.

The National Academy of Medicine is committed to advancing science that informs real-world decisions, elevates diverse perspectives into open dialogue, and broadens the reach of better health for every community. The priorities that surface in this book align with that aim. They also align with what many local leaders already know: Improvement is possible, but it is not automatic. It depends on choices about how we invest, how we measure, and how we partner.

I have a few suggestions for how readers should use this book. Begin with the outcomes that matter most in your setting. Identify what you can measure reliably today and what you will improve next. Consider how payment and delivery in your system encourage prevention, continuity, and coordination. Invite partners who are not yet at your table and agree on a small number of shared metrics that reflect local priorities.

Progress does not come from a single intervention. It comes from consistent attention to a clear set of aims, transparent measurement, and partnerships that persist.

Books do not change health on their own. People do. Policymakers who align incentives with better results, researchers who expand and share the evidence base, clinicians and health system leaders who redesign care with patients and communities, and public health practitioners, educators, employers, and civic leaders who confront systemic barriers and strengthen the conditions for health all play a role.

I'd like to extend my sincere thanks to Dr. Richard E. Besser and the Robert Wood Johnson Foundation for their commitment to health equity and for standing alongside those working tirelessly to bring it to life. Their leadership is truly valued and appreciated. To all contributors, I am most grateful. Their insight and dedication shaped this work into something truly meaningful.

Systems That Impact Population Health: Past and Present offers leaders a shared point of reference, drawing on scholarship and experience that can help the nation move from recognition to real progress.

Victor J. Dzau, MD
President
National Academy of Medicine

REFERENCES

1. Baciu A, Negussie Y, Geller A, Weinstein JN, eds; National Academies of Sciences, Engineering, and Medicine. *Communities in Action: Pathways to Health Equity.* National Academies Press; 2017.

Preface

The book *Systems That Impact Population Health: Past and Present* is the product of an extraordinary collective effort that originated within the Culture of Health Program at the National Academy of Medicine, funded by the Robert Wood Johnson Foundation. What began as a series of individually authored papers has evolved into a full-length book through partnership with the American Public Health Association—a reflection of the urgency, depth, and national relevance this work holds in addressing structural barriers that impact health and well-being during these pivotal times. Representing over 40 authors, including voices from community leadership, academia, public health, advocacy, and lived experience, this book stands as both a scholarly contribution and a testament to relational rigor, cocreation, and shared purpose.

Grounded in the belief that systemic transformation must begin with those most affected by inequity, the contributors engaged in an intentional process of dialogue, reflection, and synthesis. Rather than producing isolated chapters, this work unfolded as a braided conversation—one that wove together a broad spectrum of solid research, ancestral knowledge, policy critique, and visionary practice. Each chapter embodies a commitment to community agency, truth-telling, and the urgent necessity of structural accountability in our nation.

The staff of the Culture of Health Program extend their deep gratitude to every contributor for the generosity of spirit, intellectual clarity, and vulnerability they brought to this endeavor. This publication is not simply a resource—it is a living archive of resistance, resilience, and possibility. We invite readers to engage with its insights as both compass and catalyst and to carry forward the commitment to equity, healing, and justice that animates every page.

Amy Gyau-Moyer, MS, MBA, MSW, Director, Culture of Health Program
Shaneah Taylor, MPH, Acting Director of Programs, National Academy of Medicine

Introduction

Ivory Clarke, MS, Gilbert C. Gee, PhD, Tina Kauh, PhD, MS,
Dwayne Proctor, PhD, Julie Morita, MD, Alonzo Plough, PhD, MPH, and
Antonia M. Villarruel, PhD, RN

The pursuit of health equity, where everyone has the opportunity to attain their full health potential, is both a global and domestic challenge.[1] *Health inequities*—the systematic and unjust differences in health outcomes between groups—continue to remain prevalent, and many are shaped by factors amenable to policy change.[2] These inequities are deeply rooted in the *social determinants of health*—the conditions in which people are born, grow, work, live, and age.[3,4] While our nation holds diverse opinions about the nature of social inequities, the scientific literature has been steadily building an evidence base on the important role that racism plays in generating these inequities. Systemic and structural racism in the United States are deeply ingrained in the nation's history and societal fabric, influencing health outcomes for all. The insidious nature of racism manifests through formal systems and structures, creating pathways for inequities to persist.[5,6] Rather than shy away from discussing these issues, it is important that we examine the research base and engage in constructive dialogue. This book aims to do just that. It seeks to illuminate how systems of inequity, particularly racism, relate to health equity. Braveman et al. define *systemic racism* as involving whole systems, including political, legal, economic, health care, education, and criminal legal systems, and *structural racism* as the laws, policies, institutional practices, and entrenched norms that uphold these systems.[7] The interconnectedness of these two manifestations of racism creates a complex web where discrimination, marginalization, and oppression are sustained and thrive.

    The development of this book did not occur in a vacuum. It began when the role of racism and its impact on systems affecting health was gaining attention well over a decade ago. Our work grew in urgency and was related to discourse surrounding violence against Black individuals and communities of color, anti-Asian violence related to COVID-19 politicization, and "anti-DEI" legislation banning diversity, equity, and inclusion funding, offices, trainings, and programs. In 2025, anti-immigrant, anti-DEI executive orders and other federal and state policies are beginning to adversely affect vulnerable communities. The debate and polarization of these issues continues to leave the opportunity to live a healthy life out of reach for many. This book embarks on a comprehensive examination of the historical and contemporary factors perpetuating systemic and structural racism and aims to elucidate the deep-seated influences that have shaped health inequities. Complex interactions of societal influences are navigated, shedding light on the pathways and mechanisms by which systemic and structural racism, inclusive of discrimination and oppression, harm health and create health disparities. Individual chapters delve into the salient issues for specific populations, providing both insights and solutions for dismantling entrenched inequities. The collective goal of the authors of this book—to achieve health equity for all—drives this work.

Research and scholarship on health equity and approaches to combat systemic and structural racism are not new.[8-10] This book builds on reports by the National Academies of Sciences, Engineering, and Medicine (NASEM) exploring health equity; establishing the evidence base, relevance, and value of health equity approaches; detailing perspectives of communities affected by inequities; demonstrating how changes in systems affecting the social determinants of health can support health and well-being; and showing how federal policies can advance health equity. For example, the seminal report *Unequal Treatment: Confronting Racial and Ethnic Disparities in Health Care* was updated to reflect new knowledge of health disparities and the benefits of health equity.[11,12] Additionally, NASEM outlines how health equity approaches in biomedical sciences have challenged and changed adverse race-based beliefs and practices.[13] In the realm of science, technology, engineering, mathematics, and medicine, organizations are examining structural inequities in recruitment, retention, and mobility of scientists of color, exploring paths for removing barriers and attracting creative talent.[14] Of course, other influential reports have built this scholarship, such as the *Report of the Secretary's Task Force on Black and Minority Health*.[15] This book draws from this body of work and seeks to further enrich the evidence base and promote actionable solutions to achieve health equity.

THE NEED FOR BOTH A HISTORICAL AND CONTEMPORARY DISCUSSION OF SYSTEMIC AND STRUCTURAL RACISM

This book adopts both a historical and a contemporary lens to understand the origins of the current health inequities crisis and underscore the urgent need to address the effects of systemic and structural racism on health. Efforts to dismantle safety net programs (e.g., Medicaid, SNAP, WIC, financial assistance to schools serving low-income families) at the federal and state level will exacerbate profound and persistent inequalities within our societal structures. Evidence shows that interrelated social determinants of health, including voting rights, reproductive rights, legal reform, and health care

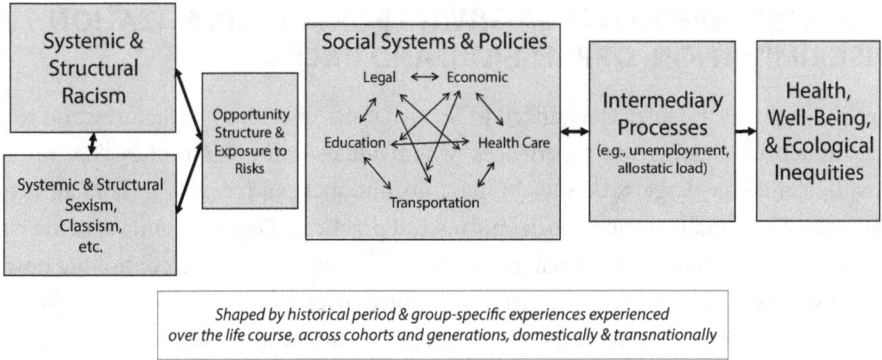

Figure 1. Conceptual Framework

access, individually and collectively impact health, underscoring the critical need for comprehensive frameworks, policies, and programs to address the root causes of health inequities.

Racism occurs at multiple levels.[16,17] Individual racism involves prejudicial attitudes and discriminatory behaviors by persons. Institutional racism relates to discriminatory policies and actions from social institutions such as banks, hospitals, courts, and police.[5,18] Although both are important, this book focuses on structural and systemic racism and health. It highlights how specific institutions perpetuate health inequities and discusses how these institutions may work together to do so. We adopt a conceptual framework (Figure 1) emphasizing structural connections, with the premise that racism permeates all aspects of US society. Systemic and structural racism interact with other forms of oppression, such as sexism and classism. Systems that perpetuate racial inequality are further modified by systems that perpetuate gendered and economic inequality. These forces shape social systems, driving policies, practices, and efforts to reinforce beliefs that uphold inequity and white supremacy. These forces affect diverse systems related to economics, housing, education, and medical care, among others. Due to spatial constraints, the individual chapters focus on specific systems, but they all recognize that the list of systems is not exhaustive.

Our conceptual framework acknowledges a life course perspective, recognizing the importance of historical context, generations, aging, and time itself.[5,19,20] Human development is shaped by generational cohort, historical moments, and social institutions. For example, the 2020 murder of George Floyd (a historic event) may have been experienced differently by a 15-year-old compared with an 80-year-old person. Indigenous scholarship notes that historical trauma in one generation can affect up to seven generations later.[21] It is crucial to explore historical antecedents that shape the policies impacting institutions today, particularly regarding health inequities.

A SYSTEMS APPROACH: PATHWAYS FOR MARGINALIZATION, DISCRIMINATION, OPPRESSION, AND RACISM

Health inequities are intricately linked to the dynamics of systems, structures, and societal influences, shaping the experiences of individuals and communities. *Systems* are broadly defined as large-scale social forces, institutionalized formally in laws and regulations or informally through social norms and practices. These dynamic systems play a significant role in resource distribution, creating opportunities, and controlling power within society. The interaction of these social forces over time results in the production and reproduction of social inequities, creating an environment where certain groups face systemic disadvantages.[22] These forces become embedded in societal institutions, impacting access to education, employment, housing, and health care.

Addressing inequities requires a holistic understanding of how these systems operate and intersect, laying the groundwork for dismantling entrenched hierarchies that perpetuate inequitable health outcomes. Although our focus is at broader levels of analysis, research shows that racism affects individuals at multiple levels, via mechanisms such as diminished access to quality health care, employment, and healthy food; chronic stress resulting in increased allostatic load and accelerated aging; unhealthy coping behaviors like substance use; and physical and mental trauma from hate crimes and microaggressions. These assaults result in poor health outcomes across the lifespan, including infant mortality, shortened adult life expectancy, heart disease, depression, sleep disturbances, and obesity. Clinical biomarkers such as C-reactive protein, increased carotid intima-media thickness, shortened telomere lengths, and dysregulation of the brain-gut microbiome are associated with poor health and experiences of discrimination.[23–26]

AN INDIVIDUAL POPULATION APPROACH: INDIVIDUAL THREADS, A COLLECTIVE TAPESTRY

Addressing structural inequities and their effects on populations and subgroups is complex. This book acknowledges the historical and contemporary categorization of population groups, recognizing the complexities and implications of such classifications. For decades, racial and ethnic classifications in the United States have been guided by the Office of Management and Budget Race and Ethnic Standards for Federal Statistics contained in Statistical Policy Directive No. 15.[27] These standards were established to create uniformity in federal reporting for the census, population standards, and requirements associated with civil rights monitoring and reporting. However, racial and ethnic categories have changed over the years, and were most recently revised in March 2024.[28] Research shows that racial categories are not biological "truths" but rather, social constructs. Although these categories are often contested (as they should be), they are nonetheless useful for documenting social inequities.

This book describes the unique history and context of seven major racial and ethnic population categories in the United States, consistent with the 2024 revised Office of Management and Budget classifications: Asian, Black or African American, American Indian or Alaska Native, Hispanic or Latino, Middle Eastern or North African, Native Hawaiian or Pacific Islander, and white (European). Each chapter is written and edited by teams of researchers, scholars, and community members representative of the focus population, ensuring the content is informed by both expertise and lived experiences. The approach aims to (1) explore manifestations of racism, oppression, marginalization, and discrimination for each population group and (2) identify systems approaches that address both unique and common aspects across groups to advance health equity.

Each population chapter includes the following:

- Background and defining the population
- Data on population-specific health inequities
- Systemic barriers to health equity
- Key events and policies linked to health inequities
- Discussion of three specific systems perpetuating health inequities
- Identification of actionable solutions to catalyze change
- Guidance for further research, policy, and programming

While common elements are present in all chapters, there is purposeful variation to honor each group's preference for presenting their history, issues, strengths, and solutions. Additionally, each population chapter includes "community voices"—perspectives of people affected by inequities. Approaches vary across chapters and include case studies, consultations with community members, or integration of community members in writing or review groups.

Chapter 1, "Systemic Racism and the Health of American Indians and Alaska Natives," describes the impact of historical trauma and systemic racism on health outcomes for Indigenous peoples of the continental United States, advocating for a biopsychosocial-spiritual approach spanning all life stages. The authors call for a holistic understanding of how health, education, workforce development, and economic systems uniquely affect Indigenous communities, highlighting the need for a comprehensive framework to address these inequities.

Chapter 2, "Structural Racism, Asian American Communities, and Health Equity: A Historical, Transnational and Intersectional Perspective," addresses direct discrimination from government policies and the damaging "model minority" stereotype, revealing hidden layers of racism in legal, economic, media, and health care frameworks. The authors propose a transnational, intersectional approach, acknowledging historical and contemporary nuances among Asian Americans.

Chapter 3, "Strengthening the Health of Black People in the United States Through Systemic and Structural Change," emphasizes shifting focus from individual-level interventions to systemic changes, detailing how racism inhibits health opportunities and disproportionately harms Black communities. The authors advocate for repair(ations) to address deep-rooted health disparities.

Chapter 4, "Examining the Impacts of the Interrelated Systems of Education, Employment, and Health Care on the Life Course and Well-Being of Latino Populations," explores how systemic racism embeds itself within education, employment, and health care systems. The authors call for implementing fair and inclusive systems of economic justice, immigration policies, access, and institutional representation to achieve health equity for Latino populations.

Chapter 5, "Structural Inequities and Middle Eastern and North African American Health," exposes how systemic racism in foreign policy and immigration impacts health care and legal systems, perpetuating marginalization. The authors underscore the importance of a unique identifier for Middle Eastern and North African individuals, often misclassified as "white," to enhance data collection and better address population needs.

Chapter 6, "We Are the Ocean," provides a narrative of the rich history and advanced sociopolitical structures of Oceanian people and discusses how colonial legacies steeped in systemic racism distort housing, economic, and health systems in the Pacific Islands. The authors advocate for integrating Indigenous knowledge and governance systems to revitalize health and ensure equity.

Chapter 7, "Health Inequities in White European Americans: Key Systems, Root Causes, and the Legacies of Whiteness," explores how systemic racism impacts even those presumed to benefit from it. The authors document the origins and consequences of whiteness in shaping labor markets, social safety nets, and health outcomes.

Chapter 8, "Cross-Cutting Solutions to Address Structural Racism to Advance Health Equity," summarizes potential strategies that benefit multiple populations and illustrates how a systems approach can support health equity for all.

As the intricate tapestry of systemic and structural racism across population groups is explored, it becomes clear that the challenges and solutions are diverse and interconnected. This examination underscores the necessity of moving beyond individual or group experiences to broader systemic issues. Engaging in both historical and contemporary analysis of these structures is paramount. Further, this implies that interventions cannot focus on individual systems in isolation, but rather, on multiple systems simultaneously. It is also important to recognize that simply adopting "best practices" is not enough; interventions need to be tailored to the needs of communities and their contexts. Systemic and structural racism are not only relics of the past but also present forces shaping the lives and health outcomes of millions today.

CONCLUSION

Throughout the book, a clear consensus emerges on the need to make the invisible visible, consider both historical and contemporary contexts, recognize and value the heterogeneity within groups, and apply a structural lens to all solutions. Exploring the deep roots of systemic and structural racism in historical, legal, and policy frameworks has allowed the authors to highlight the potential within these structures and propose transformative policies aimed at achieving health equity. This dual perspective underscores the complexity of addressing health disparities, requiring both a critical understanding of their origins and strategic interventions to reform the systems that maintain them.

The book confronts painful histories and truths, yet it is also optimistic, suggesting that a thorough understanding of both unique and shared experiences can foster hope. It aims to spotlight critical issues for the nation, offering solutions grounded in scholarly research, practical strategies, and lived experiences. These solutions are crafted to inform and transform policies and systems effectively, promoting substantial and enduring changes in health equity. In the following chapters, this book seeks to increase the dialogue on interventions and policy solutions that are informed by science and engaged with communities.

REFERENCES

1. Tangcharoensathien V, Lekagul A, Teo YY. Global health inequities: More challenges, some solutions. *Bull World Health Organ*. 2024;102(2):86–86A. doi:10.2471/BLT.24.291326
2. Blacksher E. Redistribution and recognition—Pursuing social justice in public health. *Camb Q Health Ethics*. 2012;21:320–331. doi:10.1017/S0963180112000047
3. Marmot M. 2005. Social determinants of health inequalities. *Lancet*. 2005;365(9464):1099–1104. doi:10.1016/S0140-6736(05)71146-6
4. Lavizzo-Mourey RJ, Besser RE, Williams DR. Understanding and mitigating health inequities—Past, current, and future directions. *N Engl J Med*. 2021;384(18):1681–1684. doi:10.1056/NEJMp2008628
5. Gee GC, Ford CL. Structural racism and health inequities: Old issues, new directions. *Du Bois Rev*. 2011;8(1):115–132. doi:10.1017/S1742058X11000130
6. Bailey ZD, Krieger N, Agénor M, Graves J, Linos N, Bassett MT. Structural racism and health inequities in the USA: Evidence and interventions. *Lancet*. 2017;389(10077):1453–1463. doi:10.1016/S0140-6736(17)30569-X
7. Braveman PA, Arkin E, Proctor D, Kauh T, Holm N. Systemic and structural racism: Definitions, examples, health damages, and approaches to dismantling. *Health Aff (Millwood)*. 2022;41(2):171–178. doi:10.1377/hlthaff.2021.01394
8. Krieger N, Sidney S, Coakley E. Racial discrimination and skin color in the CARDIA study: Implications for public health research. Coronary Artery Risk Development in Young Adults. *Am J Public Health*. 1998;88(9):1308–1313. doi:10.2105/ajph.88.9.1308

9. Williams DR, Yan Yu, Jackson JS, Anderson NB. Racial differences in physical and mental health: Socio-economic status, stress and discrimination. *J Health Psychol*. 1997;2(3):335–351. doi:10.1177/135910539700200305
10. Noh S, Beiser M, Kaspar V, Hou F, Rummens J. Perceived racial discrimination, depression, and coping: A study of Southeast Asian refugees in Canada. *J Health Soc Behav*. 1999;40(3):193–207. doi:10.2307/2676348
11. (US) Institute of Medicine. *Unequal Treatment: Confronting Racial and Ethnic Disparities in Health Care*. National Academies Press; 2003.
12. National Academies of Sciences, Engineering, and Medicine; Nass SJ, Amankwah FK, DeVoe JE, Benjamin GC, eds. 2024. *Ending Unequal Treatment: Strategies to Achieve Equitable Health Care and Optimal Health for All*. National Academies Press; 2024.
13. National Academies of Sciences, Engineering, and Medicine. *Using Population Descriptors in Genetics and Genomics Research: A New Framework for an Evolving Field*. National Academies Press; 2023.
14. National Academies of Sciences, Engineering, and Medicine; Barabino GA, Fiske ST, Scherer LA, Vargas EA, eds. *Advancing Antiracism, Diversity, Equity, And Inclusion In STEMM Organizations: Beyond Broadening Participation*. National Academies Press; 2023.
15. Heckler M. *Report of the Secretary's Task Force on Black and Minority Health*. Vol 1. US Dept of Health and Human Services; 1986.
16. Carmichael S, Hamilton CV. *Black Power: The Politics of Liberation*. Vintage Books; 1967.
17. Jones CP. Levels of racism: A theoretic framework and a gardener's tale. *Am J Public Health*. 2000;90(8):1212–1215. doi:10.2105/ajph.90.8.1212
18. Bonilla-Silva E. What makes systemic racism systemic? *Sociol Inq*. 2021;91(3):513–533. doi:10.1111/soin.12420
19. Gee GC, Hing A, Mohammed S, Tabor DC, Williams DR. Racism and the life course: Taking time seriously. *Am J Public Health*. 2019;109(suppl 1):S43–S47. doi:10.2105/AJPH.2018.304766
20. Chatters LM, Taylor HO, Taylor RJ. Racism and the life course: Social and health equity for Black American older adults. *Public Policy Aging Rep*. 2021;31(4):113–118. doi:10.1093/ppar/prab018
21. Nutton J, Fast E. Historical trauma, substance use, and Indigenous peoples: Seven generations of harm from a "big event". *Subst Use Misuse*. 2015;50(7):839–847. doi:10.3109/10826084.2015.1018155
22. Krieger N. *Epidemiology and the People's Health: Theory and Context*. Oxford University Press; 2011.
23. Dong TS, Gee GC, Beltran-Sanchez H, et al. How discrimination gets under the skin: Biological determinants of discrimination associated with dysregulation of the brain-gut microbiome system and psychological symptoms. *Biol Psychiatry*. 2023;94(3):203–214. doi:10.1016/j.biopsych.2022.10.011
24. Lewis TT, Aiello AE, Leurgans S, Kelly J, Barnes LL. Self-reported experiences of everyday discrimination are associated with elevated C-reactive protein levels in older African-American adults. *Brain Behav Immun*. 2010;24(3):438–443. doi:10.1016/j.bbi.2009.11.011

25. Lewis TT, Everson-Rose SA, Powell LH, et al. Chronic exposure to everyday discrimination and coronary artery calcification in African-American women: The SWAN Heart Study. *Psychosom Med*. 2006;68(3):362–368. doi:10.1097/01.psy.0000221360.94700.16
26. Chae DH, Nuru-Jeter AM, Adler NE, et al. Discrimination, racial bias, and telomere length in African-American men. *Am J Prev Med*. 2014;46(2):103–111. doi:10.1016/j.amepre.2013.10.020
27. US Office of Management and Budget. 1997 Standards for Maintaining, Collecting, and Presenting Federal Data on Race and Ethnicity. 1997. Accessed April 14, 2025. https://spd15revision.gov/content/spd15revision/en/history/1997-standards.html
28. US Office of Management and Budget. Revisions to OMB's Statistical Policy Directive No. 15: Standards for maintaining, collecting, and presenting federal data on race and ethnicity. March 29, 2024. Accessed April 14, 2025. https://www.federalregister.gov/documents/2024/03/29/2024-06469/revisions-to-ombs-statistical-policy-directive-no-15-standards-for-maintaining-collecting-and

Systemic Racism and the Health of American Indians and Alaska Natives

Donald Warne, MD, MPH, Melanie Nadeau, PhD, MPH, Stacy A. Bohlen,
Emily A. Haozous, PhD, RN, Benjamin A. Jacuk, ThM, MDiv,
Maria Christina Crouch, PhD, Stephen Long, Loretta Grey Cloud,
Michelle Johnson-Jennings, PhD, Tipiziwin Tolman, MEd, Abigail Echo-Hawk,
MA, Brinda Sivaramakrishnan, MPH, and Allison Kelliher, MD

INTRODUCTION

American Indian and Alaska Native (AI/AN) populations in the United States have been subjected to systemic and structural racism, impacting all aspects of life since contact with European explorers. Despite centuries of oppression and deliberate genocide, the original inhabitants of North America have persisted to the present day, although not without health inequities. This chapter will provide a brief overview of the historical context for the social milieu surrounding AI/AN populations in the United States. It will also present three systems that illustrate the unequal conditions, including health care, education, and economic development. The chapter will conclude with proposed solutions providing Indigenous-centered ways forward.

DEFINING THE POPULATIONS

Defining this population includes a semantic deconstruction of terminology. The Latin word, *Indigena*, translated to mean "sprung from the land," provides the most accurate representation of who is meant when discussing AI/AN peoples. At a more general level, *Indigenous populations* are the original inhabitants of a region, and have served as stewards of the lands, seas, and waterways.[1,2] This chapter focuses on the AI/AN populations in the United States. A separate chapter (Chapter 6) will address Native Hawaiian and Pacific Islander populations, who by some definitions are also considered Native American.

Politicization of American Indian/Alaska Native Identity

Race is a social and political construct that influences behaviors, policies, ideologies, identities, and power dynamics.[3] Races and ethnicities in the United States are described by the Office of Management and Budget (OMB). For the 2020 census, the racial categories included White; Black or African American; Asian; Native Hawaiian or Other Pacific Islander; and American Indian or Alaska Native. OMB defines *AI/AN* as a "person having origins in any of the original peoples of North and South America (including Central America) and who maintains Tribal affiliation or community attachment."[4]

Within the United States, the designation of *federally recognized Tribe* indicates an AI/AN population that has a legal and historic relationship with the federal government. Similarly, a *state-recognized Tribe* is established within a state but does not have the same legal relationship with the federal government. In census data, an individual can self-identify as AI/AN. However, enrollment in a federally recognized Tribe is a political designation determined by the enrollment rules of that sovereign Tribe. There are 574 federally recognized Tribes in the United States, of which 228 are in Alaska and 109 are in California.[5] Each Tribe is diverse in terms of culture, language, history, number of members, and size of land base. In Alaska, there is additional complexity. The Tribes are also arranged into Alaska Native Corporations and are organized under the laws of the state of Alaska in compliance with the Alaska Native Claims Settlement Act (ANCSA) signed into law December 18, 1971.[6] There are unique cultural and political circumstances that differentiate Alaska Native Indigenous peoples, which supports the differentiation in terminology through the term *American Indian or Alaska Native* in demographic data.

To further illustrate the complexity of AI/AN status in the United States, it is useful to understand the implications associated with citizenship as an AI/AN individual. Although OMB classifies *AI/AN* as a race, Tribal citizenship is not a racial category. Instead, an *Enrolled Tribal Member* is considered a citizen of a Tribal Nation. Therefore, it is a political status, and many AI/AN peoples have "tri-citizenship" as citizens of the United States, residents of their states, and enrolled members of their Tribal Nations.[7] As a result, AI/AN peoples are eligible for health programs through the federal government such as Medicare (as US citizens), Medicaid (as state residents), and through the federally funded Indian Health Service (IHS; as Tribal citizens), Tribal health systems, and urban Indian health programs (I/T/U system). The complexity of providing comprehensive health services across diverse populations and multiple levels of government is challenging.[8]

Terminology

Each Tribe has a name in its language. The origin of the term *American Indian* has its roots in the misunderstandings of Christopher Columbus, who thought he had reached the Indian subcontinent. Understandably, many Indigenous peoples of North America

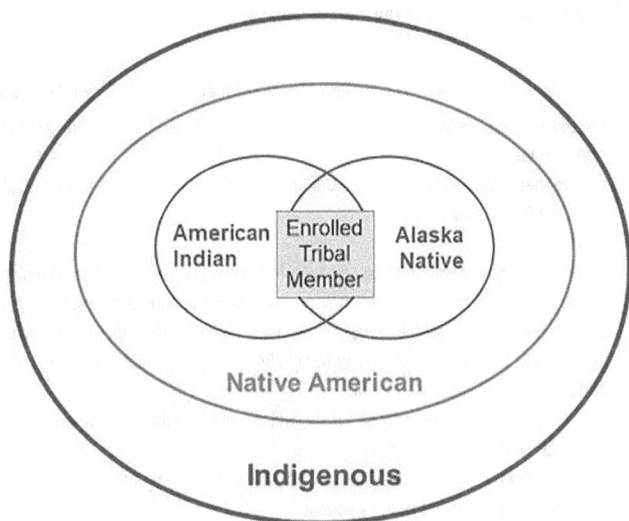

Figure 1-1. Terminology for Indigenous Peoples in the United States

do not value or connect with the term *Indian*. For example, the Indigenous peoples of Canada are commonly referred to as *First Nations*, *Metis*, or *Inuit*. The term *American* is derived from the first name of Amerigo Vespucci, another Italian explorer who recognized that the "New World" was not Asia. Ironically, the term *American Indian* pays homage to two Italians, Vespucci and Columbus. As the original inhabitants of various parts of the globe, the term *Indigenous* is more inclusive from an international perspective (see Figure 1-1).[9]

A LONG-STANDING HISTORY OF SYSTEMIC RACISM IN POLICY

Anti-Indigenous racism is insidious and deeply embedded within American society. As a result, the basic historical record that would presumably form a common understanding of the nation's past is tainted by myth and distortions of the truth. For this reason, a brief overview of the historical context is necessary to provide context to contemporary concerns, policies, and structures that stymie AI/AN populations and their health (see Box 1-1).[10,11]

AI/AN peoples have oral histories that describe eons of existence of multiple civilizations living in relationship with the ecosystems of North America. Each of these societies has unique and distinct languages, cultures, and beliefs. Corresponding genetic evidence suggests that human beings emerged from Africa between 1 and 2 million years ago.[12] Over the last 200,000 years, human beings began to migrate across the globe, and there

Box 1-1. Historic Timeline: Colonization of the United States

Pre-1400	Indigenous peoples lived in complex societies with autonomy and self-governance.
1400s	*Doctrine of Discovery*: Christian European nations believed they had the right to seize non-Christian lands.
1492	Christopher Columbus lands in the Caribbean under the direction of Spain (Columbus never set foot in what is now the US).
1492-1887	Removal Era
1609-1924	Indian Wars: starting with the First Anglo-Powhatan War (1609-1614) and spanning the continent and 3 centuries, the Indian Wars were a series of campaigns led by colonizing governments who intended to remove or eliminate AI/AN Nations. They include King Philip's War (1675-1676), the French and Indian War (1754-1763), the Great Sioux War (1876-1877), and the Apache Wars (1849-1924).
1800s	*Manifest Destiny*: the belief that it is the will of the (Christian) God to expand the US west ward across the North American continent.[11]
1819s-1969	Boarding School Era: forceful removal of AI/AN children from their families into placement in federal and religious boarding schools.
1924	Indian Citizenship Act: declares AI/AN peoples to be US citizens, granting them the right to vote in some states.
1819-1969	Assimilation Era
1932-1953	Reorganization Era
1953-1970	Termination Era
1970-present	Self-Determination Era

Source: Based on Dunbar-Ortiz.[10]
Note: AI/AN = American Indian or Alaska Native.

is evidence that the original inhabitants of what is now the United States migrated to this region between 14,000 and 40,000 years ago. It is these peoples who became what we now call AI/AN peoples.[13,14] However, we should also recognize and be respectful that cultures have their own belief systems regarding creation and the origins of their populations.[15]

Early Contact, Enslavement, and Colonization

There is evidence of transatlantic trade routes prior to 1492, including Leif Erikson, a Norse explorer who established settlements in Newfoundland, Canada in the 11th century.[16] The explorer who led the large-scale invasion and colonization of North America, however, was Christopher Columbus.[17] Upon his arrival in the Americas, Columbus noted in his journal that the peoples he encountered would make good servants. Columbus' policies toward these peoples included slavery and forced labor.[18] Columbus also sent thousands of Taino "Indians" from Hispaniola (now Haiti and the Dominican Republic) to Spain to be traded as slaves, losing untold numbers on the journey east. Those remaining faced tremendous hardships and were forced to mine for gold and work on plantations.[19] Within 60 years of Columbus' arrival, only a few hundred of what may have been a quarter million Taino peoples survived.[19] It is estimated that up to 5 million Indigenous Americans were forced into slavery during this early period of European contact.[18]

Shortly following Columbus' return to Europe, in May of 1493 Pope Alexander VI issued the papal bull *Inter Caetera*, commonly known as the *Doctrine of Discovery*.[20] Originally issued in support of Spain's holdings following Columbus' first journey, the Doctrine of Discovery ultimately became international law that supported claiming any lands not previously held or inhabited by Christians. Contained within the text of the document is both moral and legal justification for the colonization and ultimate genocide of Indigenous peoples This papal document provides the stipulation that forced conversion/education, also known as *cultural genocide*, was essential for European ownership of the land. In the 1830s, a subsequent US federal policy of western expansion was built upon the ideology of the Doctrine of Discovery. This movement, referred to as *Manifest Destiny*, suggested that a divine directive compelled white, Christian Americans to inhabit the entire North American continent, taking ownership of lands previously inhabited by Indigenous peoples.[21] Both the Doctrine of Discovery and Manifest Destiny are stark examples of white supremacy and racism, and they played significant roles in the displacement, oppression, and marginalization of Indigenous peoples, leaving lasting damage on their respective cultures, lands, rights, and health.

Settler colonization is defined as the inhabiting, controlling, and owning of a place that was not originally one's own, through the forceful removal of the original inhabitants.[22] A common element of settler colonization is to claim ownership of the land and to marginalize and subjugate its original inhabitants. Upon discovery of the "New World" by European explorers, most colonization of AI peoples in the lower 48 states was done by Western Europeans, specifically from Great Britain, Portugal, and Spain, although other European nations participated in colonization, including the Netherlands and France.[23] A multitude of Indigenous peoples in North America now speak French (largely in Canada), English, and Spanish (in the US Southwest and Mexico). Alaska was initially colonized by Russia in the 1800s.[24] Across the globe, there is a significant population of English-speaking Indigenous people, largely due to broad-based British colonization of North America, Australia, and the Pacific Islands, among other regions.[25]

Prior to establishment of the United States, relationships with original inhabitants were localized and influenced by the colonizing country of origin. Although the regions and colonizing nations vary, all have consistent themes of religious persecution and conversion, enslavement, assault, murder, illness, and brief periods of relative peace.[26] The US government used many of these tactics to annex land that was occupied by Indigenous peoples.

Unique Considerations for Alaska Native Peoples

In Alaska, our history is unique and distinct but related to other colonization experiences. Much of the initial colonization of Alaska Native peoples was done by Russians, and the intergenerational impact of Russian culture on Alaska Native peoples is

Box 1-2. Historic Timeline: Alaska

1784	First Russian colony established in Alaska.
1867	Treaty of Cession: Russia sells Alaska to the US for $7.2 million.
1880	Comity Agreement: Sheldon Jackson brings together all major denominations of the Western Church (1883 Roman Catholic inclusion) for first time in history to split up Alaska.
1884	Organic Act: establishes the civil and judicial District of Alaska.
1912	Alaska is made a US territory.
1913	Jules Jetté claims Alaska Natives are "probably doomed to disappear."[28(p407)]
1958	Alaska Statehood Act
1959	Alaska becomes the 49th US state.
1971	Alaska Native Claims Settlement Act

Source: Based on Blackhawk.[29]

significant, including among the Unangan peoples (known as Aleut by Russian fur traders) of the Aleutian Islands and other western coastal regions of Alaska.[24,27] As shown in Box 1-2, Russian colonization was followed by the cession of Alaska to the United States in 1867.[28,29] Though the nation claiming ownership of Alaska changed, colonial practices continued, and AN people were never conquered or involved in these early negotiations regarding their land. Disregard of the inherent human right to exist freely in traditional societies had a complex and detrimental impact on the population including loss of language, culture, and connection to family and Tribe, especially through boarding schools. Different religious factions divided Alaska for indoctrination into Christian religions, and Russian Orthodox (and later Jesuit) priests delegitimized AN religions.[28] In 1913, the US Department of War consulted Jules Jetté, a Catholic priest stationed in the interior AN village of Nulato, regarding the question of dispossessing AN peoples of their land and owing compensation to the original inhabitants. Jetté stated that AN peoples' "race is lower than ours ever was."[28(p407)] He also stated that the AN population was "probably doomed to disappear" and "the White man's intrusion can only hasten the result."[28(p407)]

Systematic displacement through dehumanization of its Indigenous peoples began early with the first ecumenical movement through the 1880 Comity Agreement, where future Secretary of Education of Alaska, Sheldon Jackson, met with major Protestant leaders and later with the Roman Catholic Church to split up Alaska based off the natural resources in the area.[30] With the rationale that AN peoples were nothing more than "heathen(s) of the frozen north,"[31(p100)] these various ecclesial institutions would commit cultural genocide through the creation of over 100 boarding schools to gain access to the natural resources in the area.[30] This "primitive," "heathen," "pagan," or "savage" designation first propagated by Jackson in Alaska became the motivation for dehumanization and systematic displacement of AN peoples through both religious and legal methods.

In 1912, Alaska became a US territory, and in 1958, Congress passed the Statehood Act, which made Alaska the 49th state. The law went into effect on January 3, 1959, and established a state government and described the types of public lands that the state could own and manage. However, this act did not address the land claims made by AN peoples, and the law declared that

> [t]he State must disclaim all right and title to lands and other property not granted or confirmed to the State including right or title which may be held by any Indians, Eskimos or Aleuts (natives) or is held by the United States in trust for said natives.[32]

The law further delineated that any land that belonged to Indigenous Alaskans would be under the jurisdiction and control of the US government. In 1971, the Alaska Native Claims Settlement Act (ANCSA) was a novel approach by Congress that established AN-owned, for-profit regional corporations which settled land and financial claims made by AN peoples and extinguished Indigenous title in Alaska.[33,34] To date, ANCSA is the largest land claims settlement in US history. It established 13 regional (of which 12 remain) and over 200 private, for-profit *Alaska Native village corporations*. These regional and village corporations are owned by enrolled AN shareholders. Each regional corporation engages with their stakeholders including shareholders, descendants, and communities to reflect their unique cultural values and financial priorities.[33] AN peoples have advocated for full control over their lands, rather than being subject to federal jurisdiction. AN peoples continue to engage in traditional and cultural practices and have policy history that is unique and different from AI peoples in the lower 48 states.

Federal Trust Responsibility

The *federal Indian trust responsibility* can be defined as fiduciary obligations on the part of the US government. It protects Tribes and their rights, lands, and assets with the power of the federal government. It was established by the Supreme Court decision *Seminole Nation v United States*[35] and has been reaffirmed numerous times since.[36] The federal government has historically adhered to this responsibility in an inconsistent manner.

Federal AI/AN Policy Eras

Federal AI/AN policy history can be broken into five major eras: Removal, Assimilation, Reorganization, Termination, and Self-Determination. Each era spans a period during which national leaders embraced policies that reflected the sentiment described. The first era, Removal, is best characterized through the systematic elimination and removal of AI/AN peoples from their traditional homelands through warfare, illness, or forced migration to a designated reservation.[37]

Removal Era (1492–1887)

The seizing of Indigenous lands was formal US policy through the Indian Removal Act of 1830, a law that removed original occupants from their homelands, primarily in the Southeastern United States, to what is now Oklahoma.[14,38] The act was designed to make lands available for white settlement and to facilitate national expansion. This proved to be devastating for AI/AN peoples. During relocation, entire Tribes were forced to walk to their new lands, causing tremendous suffering, hardship, and death.[14] The relocation and displacement subjugated AI/AN peoples to the church and crown under the papal bulls, creating a precedent for policies that eradicated traditional practices, healing knowledge, and other cultural assets. Within the context of the United States, the Doctrine of Discovery was recontextualized legally and socially through the 1823 Supreme Court case *Johnson v. McIntosh* alongside its Protestant interpretation, *Manifest Destiny*.[30,39] The act led to what is more commonly known as the *Trail of Tears*, which removed Cherokee, Choctaw, Creek, Chickasaw, and Seminole peoples from their homelands by military force. It is estimated that one-third of these people perished in the process.[40] The Homestead Act of 1862 allowed for predominantly white settlers to stake claim to 160 acres of land in the western United States for the purpose of developing the land for agricultural purposes.[41] As a result, millions of acres were claimed by settlers, and AI/AN peoples were excluded from their traditional homelands, denied the resources thereof, and many were forcibly relocated.

Between 1832 and 1871, hundreds of treaties were established between the US government and a multitude of Tribes.[10] These treaties were recognized as contracts between the Tribal and federal governments in which Tribes exchanged land and natural resources for several social services, including housing, education, and health care. Federal provision of these services today is largely based on language in the treaties as interpreted by the US Supreme Court and are considered the trust responsibility of the US government.[42] As stated in the Supremacy Clause of the US Constitution (Article VI, Clause 2), treaties are the supreme law of the land and take precedence over any other conflicting law.

Assimilation Era (1819–1969)

The Assimilation Era introduced a series of policies designed to eliminate AI/AN cultural and traditional practices, with the expectation that AI/AN culture could be eliminated through policy.[43] The policies were widespread and insidious, attempting to interrupt and eliminate AI/AN culture at all levels. They originated from the Code of Indian Offenses (1883), which restricted allowable religious practices and traditional medicine.[44] The Code of Indian Offenses criminalized participation in traditional ceremonies, punishable with incarceration. The Dawes Act (1887) broke up the large parcels of land contained within reservations and allocated those parcels to the individual members.[45,46] This undermined the collective ownership and historical land management systems and facilitated land sales to non-AI/AN peoples.

Boarding Schools

Education for Tribal children began with religious missionaries as early as the mid-1500s, and by 1611 missions were established across the northeastern United States and Canada.[47] Unknown numbers of AI/AN children were forcibly placed in boarding schools or residential schools between 1819 and the 1970s.[48] Government *boarding schools*, like the Hampton Institute in Virginia and Carlisle Indian Industrial School in Pennsylvania, were established to "civilize" Indians and assimilate them into mainstream American society. The motto of the Carlisle School was "kill the Indian, save the man."[49]

Boarding schools were used as tools for removal and assimilation, breaking up AI/AN families under the auspices of providing children with education and vocational training.[45] The primary aim of the boarding school system was to rid AI/AN children of their cultures, languages, traditions, and identities and replace them with Western values, beliefs, and behaviors.[45] The schools were operated by religious organizations or the federal government, including the Bureau of Indian Affairs (BIA). Congress created the Commission to the Five Civilized Tribes (also called the Dawes Commission) by the Act of 1893, authorizing BIA to "withhold rations, clothing and other annuities from Indian parents or guardians who refuse or neglect to send and keep their children of proper school age in some school a reasonable portion of each year."[50] Essentially, the choice was to give up their children or starve. As a result, well over 200,000 AI/AN and First Nations children attended boarding schools in the United States and residential schools in Canada.[51] The US Department of the Interior found that between 1819 and 1969 there were 408 federal schools across 37 states. There were also over 1,000 other federal or non-federal institutions that included Indian day schools, sanitariums, asylums, orphanages, and more.[45]

AI/AN children were forced to adopt Euro-American clothing, hairstyles, and names (see Figure 1-2), and were discouraged or punished for expressing their Indigenous identities.[45,52] Children at these schools were subjected to physical, emotional, and sexual abuse, neglect, and inadequate medical care.[45] The strict discipline, overcrowded conditions, and lack of cultural understanding left children traumatized. Additionally, many children died while at school, their bodies interred in unmarked or mass graves,[51] with little to no notification to the family regarding the last days of their loved one. The resultant intergenerational trauma has had profound and long-lasting effects, leading to ongoing health and social challenges in AI/AN communities.[53]

Indian Citizenship Act

Despite thousands of years of inhabiting the lands that are currently within the borders of the United States, AI people were not considered citizens until the Indian Citizenship Act (also known as the Snyder Act of 1924) which allowed AI peoples born in the United

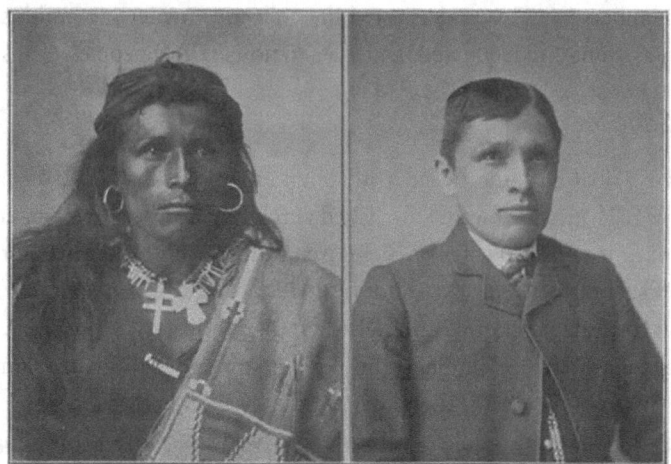

Source: Carlisle Indian School Digital Resource Center.[50] Reprinted under the terms of the CC BY license (https://creativecommons.org/licenses/by-nc-sa/4.0).

Figure 1-2. Carlisle Student Tom Torlino Upon Arrival at Carlisle (1882) and 3 Years Later

States to become full US citizens.[54] Although the Indian Citizenship Act granted citizenship to US-born AI/AN peoples, voting rights are determined by states, and some states did not allow AI/AN peoples to vote until the 1960s.[55]

Reorganization Era (1932–1953)

The Indian Reorganization Act (1934), commonly referred to as the Wheeler–Howard Act or the Indian New Deal, aimed to reverse some of the damaging effects of the Dawes Act of 1887 and provide a blueprint for the self-governance and preservation of Tribal Nations.[56] Under this act, Tribes were encouraged to form governments and write constitutions, building their political autonomy in the process. The act also sought to promote economic development on reservations by supporting agricultural initiatives and land consolidation.[56] The "one-size-fits-all" approach to establishing Tribal governance structures was in many cases culturally misaligned and ignored centuries of traditional Tribal governance practices.[57] Although there may have been good intentions, this act was met with mixed reactions among Tribes,[58] as it seemed to be "too little, too late" to reverse previous centuries of policies adversely affecting Tribal Nations.

Termination Era (1953–1968)

The Termination Era ushered in new policies intended to eliminate the federal trustee relationship guaranteed to AI/AN peoples through treaties. The Indian Relocation Act of 1952 was a policy aimed at relocating AI/AN peoples to cities in order to assimilate them into mainstream American society.[59]

From 1953 until 1970, Congress initiated 60 separate termination proceedings against American Indian Tribes, and over three million acres of Tribal lands were relinquished as a result. Although the Nixon administration repudiated termination in 1970 and shifted federal Indian policy toward self-determination, the effect of termination was nevertheless devastating for many tribes.[60]

Most AI/AN peoples who participated in relocation found themselves severed from their families, communities, and homelands. This created circumstances in which they experienced significant racism, discrimination, and substantial barriers in employment, education, and housing.[59]

Self-Determination Era (1968–Present)

The Self-Determination Era was established during the Civil Rights Movement. This complex time included the passage of the Voting Rights Act of 1965 and a series of laws that supported Tribal self-determination. These included the Indian Self-Determination and Education Assistance Act in 1975 and the Indian Health Care Improvement Act in 1976. The Indian Self-Determination and Education Assistance Act was instrumental in allowing Tribes to assume the management and operation of services provided by the federal government to Tribal control.[61] In 1978, the Indian Child Welfare Act was passed, protecting children from being fostered by and adopted into non-AI/AN families and prioritizing AI/AN communities when a child needed protective care.[62] The American Indian Religious Freedom Act of 1978 sought to end racist prohibitions on AI/AN ceremonial and spiritual practices at the federal level, reversing the Code of Indian Offenses of 1883.[63] The Affordable Care Act (ACA) of 2010 permanently reauthorized the Indian Health Care Improvement Act, and increased access to health resources through Medicaid expansion and other forms of health insurance.[64] A summary of the major court cases and legislation affecting AI/AN peoples in the United States can be found in Box 1-3.[56,65-67]

CULTURAL CONSIDERATIONS AND ORGANIZING FRAMEWORK

The intersectionality of social, historical, political, policy, and cultural forces have led to the significant health disparities we observe in AI/AN populations. The Indigenous-focused socioecological model illustrated Figure 1-3 demonstrates the broader ecological and systemic influences on community and individual health.[68] Within this framework, the individual comprises spiritual, mental, physical, and emotional forces. The systems we describe in this chapter, including health care, educational, and economic systems, directly impact the well-being of the community, organizations, and interpersonal relationships.

The Indigenous worldview and lived experience is vast and diverse and includes individual experience as well as temporal experience.[69] Due to the expansive nature of this subject, we have chosen three key areas to focus on in this chapter: medicine, education, and

Box 1-3. Timeline of Major Laws and Court Cases, United States

1830	Indian Removal Act: authorized the relocation of AI Tribes living east of the Mississippi River to lands west of the Mississippi River.
1832	*Worcester v Georgia* (state of Georgia vs. Cherokee Nation): supported the right of the Cherokee Nation to maintain sovereignty over and govern their Tribal lands.[65]
1871	Indian Appropriation Act: ended the practice of establishing treaties with AI Nations.[56]
1883	Code of Indian Offenses: restricted AI cultural and religious practices, resulting in the creation of the Courts of Indian Offenses.
1887	Dawes Act: broke up Native American reservations into individual allotments.
1893	Act of March 3, 1893: allowed BIA to penalize families who refused to send children to boarding school.
1934	Indian Reorganization Act (Wheeler-Howard Act/Indian New Deal): granted Tribes the ability to form Tribal governments and move toward self-determination.
1921	Snyder Act: allocated funds for health services for Tribes.[66]
1924	Indian Citizenship Act: granted AI/AN people US citizenship and granted the right to vote in many (not all) states.
1954	Transfer Act: IHS functions moved from the Dept of the Interior to the Dept of Health, Education, and Welfare (now HHS).[66]
1956	Indian Relocation Act: incentivized the relocation of AI people to urban areas in an attempt to assimilate them into mainstream culture.
1968	Indian Civil Rights Act: established regulations to guarantee AI/AN peoples received equal rights and treatment within Tribes.[67]
1975	Indian Self-Determination and Education Assistance Act: granted Tribes the ability to take over the management and operation of services from the federal government, including health services.[66]
1976	Indian Health Care Improvement Act: created infrastructure for IHS to function as a working health care system.[66]
1978	American Indian Religious Freedom Act: ended prohibitions on certain AI/AN ceremonial and spiritual practices.
1978	Indian Child Welfare Act: established minimum federal standards for the removal of AI/AN children and provided guidance regarding cases of child abuse and neglect of AI/AN children with the goal of preserving AI/AN families and communities.
2010	Affordable Care Act: permanently reauthorized the Indian Health Care Improvement Act and expanded Medicaid, including for AI/AN peoples.

Note: AI = American Indian; AI/AN = American Indian or Alaska Native; BIA = Bureau of Indian Affairs; HHS = US Department of Health and Human Services; IHS = Indian Health Service.

economics. These are illustrated in the Climate Change Model of Indigenous Resilience in Figure 1-4. AI/AN peoples are guaranteed health care through treaties according to the highest laws of the land. However, current health care paradigms omit essential aspects of wellness for AI/AN peoples. Within education, epistemicide has occurred and continues into the present as settler-colonial ideologies are prioritized.[70] Imposed economic systems fractionate populations even further, pitting extractive processes against maintaining intact ecosystems. The solution is weaving AI/AN epistemology and traditional

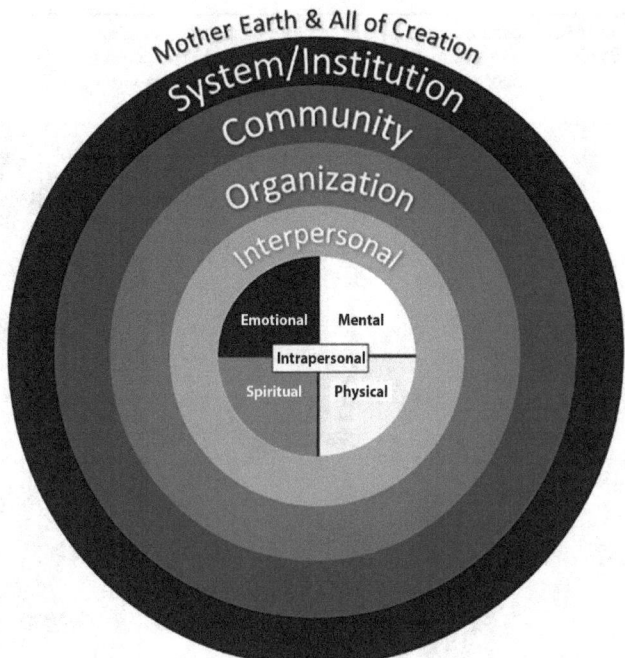

Source: Akbar et al.[68] Reprinted with permission of the authors.
Figure 1-3. The Integrated Indigenous-Ecological Model

and Indigenous approaches to wellness into medicine and collective and accessible economic and educational opportunities.

These systems are currently largely defined by the settler-colonial milieu. This includes what would be described in those terms as economics, medicine, and education. In the Indigenous worldview, they are interrelated and interwoven. The circles at the center of the diagram represent Indigenous lived experiences, providing for the needs of peoples across generations. As we face mounting environmental threats from climate change, we face similar threats to the health and wellness of our people, communities, and the integrity of our cultures. We represent these oppressive forces in the arenas below with tornadoes, forest fires, and droughts. Resistance is represented by the medicine wheel at the center of our diagram. It is characterized by actions to actively resist colonization, including promoting traditional practices and core values. The four directions of the medicine wheel are a meaningful framework that represent different stages of life, directions, plant medicines, and other aspects of well-being. These culturally specific traditional lifeways help AI/AN peoples to flourish despite oppressive forces and can protect not only our own peoples but the earth's ecosystem itself.

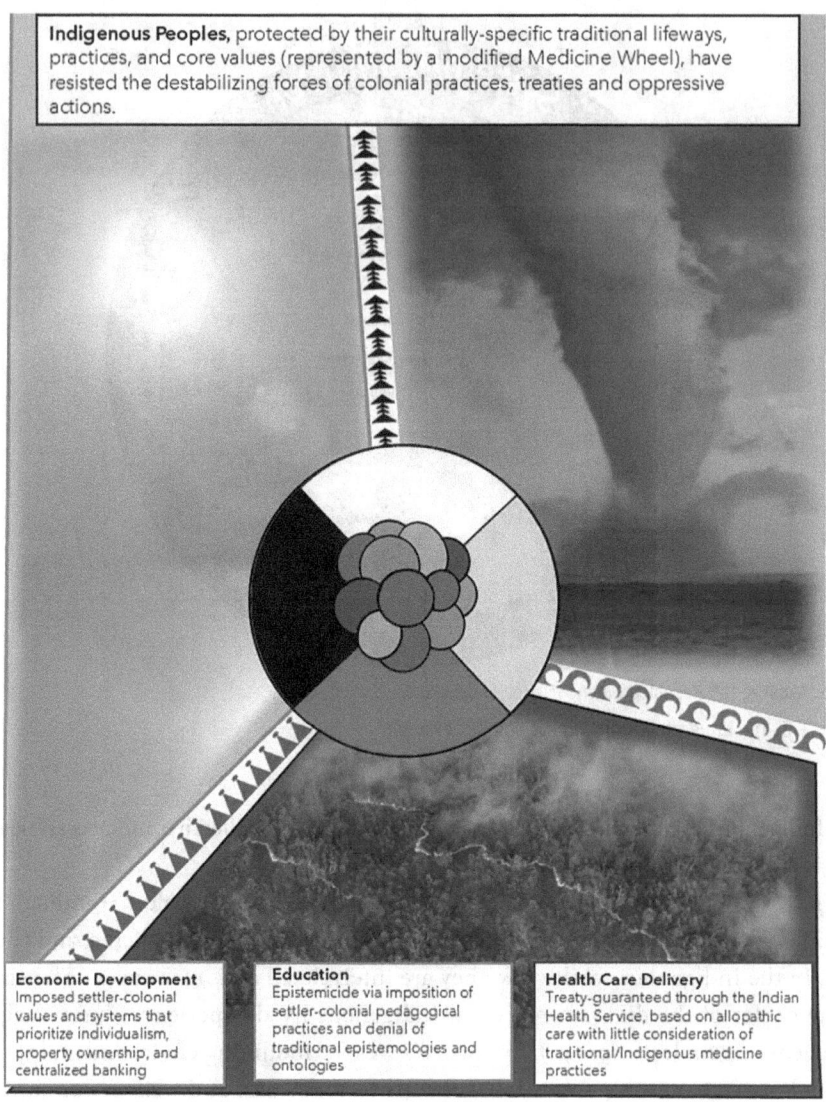

Figure 1-4. Climate Change Model of Indigenous Resistance

Reawakening and resurgence of AI/AN cultures, languages, knowledges, and practices are occurring despite the long history of harmful policies. Ceremonies and cultural practices are essential for maintaining health and wellness.[71] Despite repressive government policies, AI/AN peoples continue to gather, share, and express their cultures and celebrate ceremonies that were once illegal. Federal policies, including boarding schools, forced assimilation, relocation, and criminalization of traditional religious practices were intended to eliminate AI/AN peoples and have eroded trust. Traditional foods, medicines, languages, and practices have survived despite colonization. Traditional AI/AN cultures celebrate our connection to the natural world, including the environment, the health of our people, and the knowledge of who we are as Indigenous peoples.[70]

The Environment

The following section highlights AI/AN perspectives on the environment, followed by sections on sacred sites and traditional medicine and data sovereignty. Our environment and well-being have been interconnected in Indigenous worldviews for thousands of years. It is not surprising that colonizers systematically targeted land and disrupted traditional and intergenerational connections to the environment. The interconnectedness of land, identity, and health is a central principle in AI/AN communities.[72-74] However, intergenerational colonial barriers to land access and systemic discrimination regarding land well-being continue to plague Tribal health programs and communities, as we will discuss in the case of the Black Hills later.[53,75]

Environmental degradation, contamination, and climate change have disproportionately had negative impacts on Indigenous peoples.[76] Nearly a quarter of the 1,300 abandoned hazardous waste sites known as *Superfund sites* in the United States are located on Tribal lands, exposing AI/AN communities to increasingly toxic environments.[77] The degradation and contamination of land due to industrial activities, resource extraction, and failure to remediate can impede hunting, fishing, harvesting, and other land-based practices, limiting access to clean and safe environments necessary for healing ceremonies, gathering of medicinal plants, or engagement in cultural activities. Many AI/AN cultures that rely on subsistence foods including whale, bison, moose, caribou, salmon, birds, non–genetically-modified beans, native corn, wild rice, nuts, seeds, berries, wild greens, and roots are facing significant changes to cultures, lifestyles, and health status. Understanding and addressing these systemic barriers is crucial for promoting equity, cultural revitalization, and well-being. When coupled with historical and present-day trauma, loss of access to land and resources contributes to health disparities manifesting specifically with increased risks for addiction, chronic disease, mental illness, infectious disease, and physical distress.[78]

Sacred Sites and Traditional Medicine

Access to sacred sites and traditional medicine are essential to AI/AN well-being.[79] Before settler-colonialist contact in North America, traditional medicines were predominant, including land-based and place-based healing. Theft of land and diminished access to sacred and ceremonial sites has led to disruption of ceremonial practices and traditional healing. Many herbal remedies used by previous generations are no longer accessible, or, in some cases, the knowledge has been eradicated through colonization. The removal of AI/AN peoples from their traditional homelands has led to restricted use of these lands.

A stark example of this is in the Black Hills of South Dakota. According to the Fort Laramie Treaty of 1868,[80] the Black Hills region, which includes what is now known as Mount Rushmore, rightfully belongs to the Lakota Nation.[81] Unfortunately, many sacred and ceremonial sites in the Black Hills are held by the federal and state governments or are privately owned.[82] As a result, these sites are being desecrated, and Indigenous Peoples have limited access or are required to pay admission fees to sacred sites. This conflicts with Indigenous worldviews in which one is a natural part of the land, without ownership or governance over the earth.

Data Sovereignty

Accurate reporting of health conditions is vital to addressing inequities. AI/AN peoples are frequently omitted from datasets, either due to small sample sizes, misclassification, or because the data were not collected. When omitted or suppressed, AI/AN peoples are erased from the record, making our health outcomes impossible to know, investigate, or respond to.[83] *Indigenous data sovereignty* is defined as "the right of a [N]ation to govern the collection, ownership, and application of its data."[84] AI/AN data sovereignty addresses the sovereign rights of AI/AN Tribes to control what information is collected, where information is stored, and what is reported about their communities. Data sovereignty includes Tribal consultation, partnership with community advisory boards, data use agreements, and relevant informed consent.[85] Ongoing Tribal partnership and consultation ensures Tribal sovereignty is respected in addition to ensuring the interpretation of data accurately represents the Tribal communities being reported.[86,87] Tribal sovereignty allows Tribes to govern their data and ensure the welfare of Tribes.[88] Typically, the white population is used as a comparative population in assessing disparities in the United States. To promote AI/AN wellness, we must include diverse perspectives on data management and research. The Native BioData Consortium, led by Indigenous scientists and members, is one example of a project that aims to address underrepresentation in these matters. Tribes are now able to self-select if and how they want to participate in the use of their data. The Native BioData Consortium aims to address needs such as providing a biorepository to the benefit of all people by building Tribal capacity, building STEM capacity, fostering trust in research, and performing research that benefits Tribes.[89] Tribes have also taken the initiative to create their own institutional review boards (Tribal IRBs).[90]

STRUCTURAL AND SYSTEMIC BARRIERS THAT IMPACT AMERICAN INDIAN/ALASKA NATIVE HEALTH

The impact of colonization on AI/AN populations is profound. For over 500 years, Euro-American culture has been imposed on AI/AN populations through societal structures and systems. For AI/AN populations, the intersection of structural barriers, cultural misalignment of services and programs, and social determinants of health have resulted in some of the worst health disparities in the nation. Structural barriers include racism, marginalization, poverty, unemployment, and unequal access to health care, healthy and traditional foods, and adequate housing. Although structural racism permeates all aspects of AI/AN life, this section describes mechanisms within health care, education, and socioeconomic systems that contribute to substantial health inequities.

Access to Quality Health Care

Colonization and persistent underfunding of the treaty-guaranteed AI/AN health care have adversely impacted health. AI/AN peoples receive health care through a complex system that interlinks Tribal, state, and federal governments, the private sector, and both public and private health insurance programs.[66] IHS is the federal agency responsible for carrying out the trust responsibility to provide health services to the AI/AN population. A positive outcome of the Self-Determination Era is that over 60% of the IHS budget is now managed by Tribes under self-determination contracts and compacts.[66] In addition to underfunding as a structural barrier to health care, other access barriers include approachability, acceptability, availability, accommodation, affordability, and appropriateness.[91]

IHS is poorly integrated with the broader health system and suffers from longstanding underfunding because the treaties establishing funding and care are rooted in racism starting in the colonial era,[92] further complicating the challenges in providing high-quality health services. Although recent efforts have been made to improve integration, including interagency agreements between IHS and the Veterans Health Administration, much work needs to be done to create a comprehensive system of care, including funding medical residencies to serve AI/AN populations. As shown in Table 1-1, per capita expenditures for IHS are less than half of those for Medicare, Medicaid, or the Veterans Health Administration.[93-98] In 2024, the per capita spending for IHS was $3,043, compared with $12,889 for the Veterans Health Administration, $8,075 for Medicaid, and $12,778 for Medicare.

IHS requires a 10-fold increase in funding to meet its obligations. In financial year (FY) 2023, the appropriation for IHS was $4.9 billion. According to the IHS Budget Formulation Committee and the National Indian Health Board, full funding for IHS in FY 2023 would require $49.8 billion, a 10-fold increase in funding.[98] Addressing this issue requires a commitment to significant and long-term funding that will propel IHS's mission of ensuring the delivery of high-quality health services to AI/AN populations. The AI/AN population is unique nationally in that there are treaty-defined rights to health services. IHS underfunding contributes to significant health disparities and challenges in delivering adequate public health and medical services. Underfunding of IHS constitutes a treaty violation and breach of contract on the part of the United States in terms of providing all proper care and protection of Tribal members.

Table 1-1. Comparing 4 Federal Health Programs: IHS, VHA, Medicare, and Medicaid, 2024

Program	Service Population	Funding	Services/Coverage	Per Capita Spending
Non-Entitlement Programs (Health Care Providers)				
IHS	2.8 million (AI/AN)	Annual appropriations	Variable, primary care, water and sanitation, infection control	$3,043
VHA	>9 million (former/current US military)	Annual and advance appropriations	Inpatient, outpatient, mental health, disability, residential treatment, kidney dialysis	$12,889
Entitlement Programs (Health Care Payers)				
Medicare	68.4 million (aged >65 years)	Mandatory spending	Inpatient, outpatient, kidney dialysis, and more	$12,778
Medicaid & CHIP	79 million (low-income)	Annual appropriations	State-level coverage of inpatient/outpatient, long-term care	$8,075

Source: Based on data from Centers for Medicare and Medicaid Services,[85,86] IHS,[87] USAFacts,[88] and US Dept of Veterans' Affairs.[89]

Note: AI/AN = American Indian or Alaska Native; CHIP = Children's Health Insurance Program; IHS = Indian Health Service, VHA = Veterans' Health Administration.

In addition to funding challenges, the US health system is poorly equipped to address the needs of AI/AN communities from a cultural perspective. IHS and related programs were developed through the colonizer's lens, and as a result, there is frequently a mismatch between health services provided to AI/AN peoples and the cultural health needs of the population. AI/AN health and well-being require a holistic, intergenerational, and collective perspective that incorporates cultural knowledge. These concepts and other unique cultural components of Indigenous health are typically outside mainstream values, beliefs, and priorities. For example, a holistic understanding that health represents a balance among spiritual, mental, physical, and emotional forces[99] is a framework that is rarely implemented in modern health care.

Potential solutions in policy and funding exist. For example, through ACA, Medicaid expansion has substantially increased access to health services in expansion states, increasing rates of insured AI/AN peoples in those states and providing a needed infusion of funds to IHS and Tribal health centers.[95] Through ACA, AI/AN peoples can enroll in marketplace insurance programs outside the typical enrollment periods. However, inadequate integration with the broader health system and a lack of knowledge of IHS and the AI/AN population contributes to further marginalization in health care. Additionally, the inaccurate belief that IHS is a health insurance provider combined with nonpayment for health services provided through the IHS Purchased and Referred Care system due to underfunding of IHS overall can lead to discrimination toward AI/AN patients by the private sector.[64,100]

The intersectional experiences of structural racism and historical trauma compound the effects of marginalization and distrust, further separating AI/AN peoples from access to quality care.[92] A paucity of AI/AN physicians not only influences the ability of AI/AN peoples to access culturally safe care but also contributes to the health profession vacancy rate in IHS, which can be up to 60%.[101,102] Recent programs through the Association of American Indian Physicians and other national organizations are attempting to increase the numbers of AI/AN physicians and health professionals.[103]

Education and Workforce Development

A significant challenge that contributes to cultural erasure, discrimination, and pervasive misunderstanding of the AI/AN population is the lack of primary education in the United States regarding an accurate history of Indigenous peoples. AI/AN history is rarely taught as a stand-alone course, and many history books provide inaccurate or incomplete information.[104] As a result, intergenerational stereotypes and inaccurate perceptions of AI/AN peoples are commonplace.[105] In several of the authors' experiences, these stereotypes and assumptions exist among health care providers, educators, medical school administrators, and politicians. The pervasive misunderstanding of truth regarding the AI/AN population and history is a systemic threat to Indigenous peoples and leads to discrimination, marginalization, and racism. The US education system has failed to provide accurate and honest historical context.[106] In the authors' experience, in the few settings in which historical trauma is discussed, it is typically embedded within elective courses and primarily focused on mental health. This approach fails to create a broader understanding of AI/AN health disparities that are multifaceted, holistic, and also have an impact on chronic disease.[53]

A link exists between the educational system and barriers to effective health care that is rooted in systemic racism. The nature and extent of implicit and explicit biases in health care likely reflects systemic forces, including those biases that providers hold. By not including accurate AI/AN history, the education and workforce development systems are contributing to the challenges created by distrust and lack of cultural humility. Distrust of the health care system is a common issue in the AI/AN population[107] and contributes to decreased patient satisfaction of medical care among AI/AN peoples.[108] Improved provider–patient relationships can improve outcomes and compliance with medical recommendations.[109] Therefore, promoting trust in health care is deeply rooted in ensuring that health care providers are educated regarding the historical and cultural issues that contribute to the health disparities they are addressing in their patients.

American Indian/Alaska Native Educational System

In addition to the challenges posed by lack of truthful history of the AI/AN population, the educational system for AI/AN peoples is fraught with a history of discrimination, abuse, and lack of adequate resources.[45] The unique history of the AI/AN educational system is rarely understood by the non-Indigenous population and infrequently discussed in mainstream educational settings. Culturally competent education should be reflected in both curricula and personnel.

The consequences of the boarding school era described earlier in this chapter are long-lasting. Survivors of boarding schools have been found to have extensive personal health effects, including depression and suicidality.[110] Forced boarding school attendance has resulted in the extinction of over half of Indigenous North American languages and most Tribal people speaking English as their first and only language.[111] Boarding schools also damaged the Tribal family structure, introduced violence as a means of discipline,[45] and disrupted intergenerational knowledge, including parenting skills and processes that were originally rooted in community, kinship, and relationship. In addition, boarding school survivors would suffer from greater physical health disparities as adults.[112] Several authors of this chapter have parents who are survivors of attending boarding schools.

Present day reservation school systems are diverse with private, public, and Tribal governance, but most are rooted in the colonized model of American values, perspectives, and structure. Many school systems located in Tribal communities are in rural areas where there are challenges in recruiting and retaining teachers and staff. Despite challenges, Tribes have tailored programming including culture and language-based programs.[70,113] As the Bureau of Indian Education (BIE) website states, its mission is "to provide high-quality educational opportunities from early childhood through life in accordance with local needs for cultural and economic well-being, while respecting the diversity of AI/AN communities."[114] BIE takes into consideration the spiritual, mental, physical, and cultural aspects of students within their family and Tribal context. The BIE system employs thousands of teachers, administrators, and other personnel, while many more work in Tribal school systems.

BIE funds or operates off-reservation boarding schools and dormitories near reservations for students attending public schools. Over 180 BIE-funded elementary and secondary schools are located on numerous reservations in 23 states, with an enrollment of over 45,000 students. BIE also serves AI/AN postsecondary students through higher education scholarships and support funding for Tribal colleges and universities. A systemic challenge is that most teachers and staff are trained in systems that lack AI/AN cultural humility and culturally relevant pedagogies. This can create barriers to connecting with students who come from Tribal cultures in which there are different social norms and communication styles. There are examples of isolated efforts at multiple levels of education, including language nests and immersion schools, throughout North America that are Tribally driven and show promise. These programs need more resources to be scaled up to meet the equity needs of the AI/AN population. Other promising initiatives exist that incorporate AI/AN and Indigenous perspectives in education as mentioned in the United Nations Permanent Forum on Indigenous Issues.[115] For example, the University of New Mexico Public Health and General Preventive Medicine Residency Program has implemented a culturally based traditional healing curriculum that has been successful and well received.[116]

Unfortunately, the AI/AN population has the highest dropout rate in the nation. The overall dropout rate for those aged 16 to 24 years in 2022 was 5.3% compared with 9.9% for the AI/AN population.[117] Dropout rates vary extensively for on-reservation and off-reservation schools and by state. For example, between 2021 and 2022 the AI/AN dropout rate was 51% in Wyoming and 36% in Arizona.[118] Low graduation rates from high school lead to fewer AI/AN people with college degrees. For the AI/AN population aged 25 years or older, only 16.8% had earned a bachelor's degree or higher compared with the national rate of 36.2%.[119] In fall 2022, AI/AN students made up 0.7% of all postsecondary enrollment, and only 25.8% of the AI/AN population aged 18 to 24 years was enrolled in college, compared with 39% of the overall US population.[119] Tribal members are often required to leave their home communities to pursue advanced degrees, creating additional systemic challenges. Educational attainment is a well-established social determinant of health and is a systemic issue that needs to be improved to promote AI/AN health equity. This requires a multipronged approach through initiatives such as the Indigenous Healers and Educators Regional Taskforce, which encourages higher education and professional training for nurses, physician assistants, and other health care professions and collaborates with the American Indian Higher Education Consortium. Educational systems such as Tribal colleges and universities are working to provide culturally safe, appropriate, and needed programming to their populace.[120] The authors note that AI/AN peoples should not have to conform to the standards of the Western paradigm if they do not desire to. Current educational systems are implemented by Western dogma, though there is a movement toward Indigenous-led and Indigenous-influenced programming as illustrated through the American Indian Higher Education Consortium.

Health Care Workforce Development

In the United States, there are limited training programs that are delivered through an Indigenous lens and limited access to schools focused on AI/AN concepts, beliefs, and traditional cultures. In the health professions, the lack of relevant context regarding orientation to cultures, histories, and lived experiences grounded in Indigenous concepts has a negative impact on the delivery of culturally competent health services. Educational standards and accreditation requirements are generally determined from the priorities and perspectives of the settler-colonial experience, and these standards often exclude AI/AN histories and cultures.

Adding to the challenge of AI/AN workforce development in the health professions is the lack of Indigenous professors of medicine and academic leaders who could serve as role models and provide the lived experience to diversify curricula. According to the American Association of Medical Colleges, of over 176,000 full professors of medicine in the United States, only 274 are AI/AN, and there are zero AI/AN medical school deans.[102] The lack of role models in health profession higher education further limits AI/AN workforce development.

Economic System

Prior to colonization, most Indigenous cultures in North America did not have a system of currency, and the economic systems were based on trade, equality, relationships with the natural elements,[121] and communitarianism.[122] A common element of a communitarian societal structure is valuing the role that everyone has in society, and for many communitarian systems the goal is to treat everyone in an equitable manner. In these systems, the deep-rooted connection between individuals and the broader community creates a social identity and character that are largely shaped by these relationships. With the communal nature of many traditional societies, much less emphasis is placed on individualism. As a result, the "greater good" of relationships and priorities are focused on community benefit rather than personal gain.

Financial Systems, Cultural Differences, and Measures of Poverty

In addition to differences in governance and leadership principles, the economies of traditional Indigenous societies were multifaceted. Traditionally, many Indigenous Peoples lived in complex economies based on trade, production in harmony with the natural world, and real value. For many Tribal communities historically, there was no system of cash, which can be seen as an artificial proxy for value. According to David Graber, the difference "is between currencies that are used primarily to further the exchange of material goods, and those primarily used to transform social relationships."[123(p412)] Complex and intricate trade partnerships and relationships networked precontact North America, known to many Tribes as *Turtle Island*. Many of these relationships and practices continue today. For example, grease trails existed for over 6,000 years, allowing hooligan fish oil to be traded to areas that lacked this type of food and fuel.[124] Coastal peoples gathered a sufficient supply of oil and shells such as dentalium to use as trade items for inland goods such as tanned hides and crop seeds.[124] Traditional generative communal economic systems are overshadowed by extractive capitalist systems, which are harmful to the health of AI/AN peoples and the planetary ecosystems themselves. The capitalist system is based on human supremacy, whereas many Indigenous value systems recognized that humans are one component of the broader ecosystem. It was understood that the earth has been here for billions of years, and that we are merely outcroppings of earth. All our carbon, water, and minerals that make up the human body are of the earth, and when we die, we return to the earth. In essence, we belong to the earth, the earth does not belong to us. Hence, we call the earth *Mother Earth*.

Measures of poverty include concepts such as financial income and home/land ownership. Regarding financial income, for many AI/AN populations that did not have a historic concept of currency, the financial system imposed on the Americas from Europe was not only a foreign concept but also culturally inappropriate. Other contemporary measures of poverty and wealth include ownership of land and homes. Historically, Indigenous peoples of the United States generally did not have a concept of owning the earth. As a result, the AI/AN population experienced cultural misalignment between traditional Indigenous belief systems focused on living in harmony with nature and European-based concepts of ownership of land by individuals and states. AI/AN concepts of wealth include the value of traditional knowledges that allow us to live in close connection to nature, the ecosystem, and each other. We illustrate this later in this section with the example of Black Elk.

Another current issue in the economic system is a lack of financial institutions and business development located in Tribal communities. Geographic isolation, lack of infrastructure, and a complex policy history contribute to high prevalence of unbanked households in AI/AN populations.[92] Many AI/AN communities lack access to banks, Wi-Fi, and capital. According to the Federal Deposit Insurance Corporation (FDIC), AI/AN peoples have the highest rates for unbanked households of all races and ethnicities for which data are tracked.[125]

In our current political and economic climate, the need for our leaders to focus on community benefit is substantial. In positions of power and influence, a focus on personal financial and political gain over the collective benefit of society can lead to corruption and harm. Prior to colonization, these types of behaviors among traditional Indigenous leaders were not tolerated and could lead to banishment from the community.[126] A deep-rooted and spiritually based connection among people, the earth, and all living creatures provides a model for economics and leadership that would result in tremendous benefits to modern society.

Black Elk, a highly respected Lakota traditional healer and medicine man, was one of the American Indians who went to Europe as part of Buffalo Bill's Wild West Show. In the seminal book *Black Elk Speaks* by John Neihardt, he provides his observations of the economic conditions in Europe:

> I could see that the Wasichus (Europeans) did not care for each other the way our people did before the nation's hoop was broken. They would take everything from each other if they could, and so there were some who had more of everything than they could use, while crowds of people had nothing at all and maybe were starving. They had forgotten that the earth was their mother.[127(p135–136)]

Black Elk was saying that his traditional culture focused on equity and inclusion, while the colonizers' perspective focused on selfishness and greed. The imposed economic system of the United States is culturally misaligned with many traditional AI/AN cultures, values, and economies.

ACTIONABLE SOLUTIONS

Since systemic issues lead to health disparities that exist across a multitude of domains, the solutions need to be equally comprehensive and multidisciplinary. Although the needs are extensive, several steps can be taken to improve AI/AN peoples' health and well-being. These should focus on foundations in AI/AN lived experience, traditional knowledges, and practical applications of community-based action. Key organizational recommendations were reviewed in order to inform these solutions. This includes AI/AN expert opinions, including those of the National Indian Health Board (NIHB), American Heart Association, United Nations Permanent Forum on Indigenous Issues, and the National Center for American Indian Enterprise Development. We adapted recommendations from the national and international organizations listed below to create actionable solutions.

1. NIHB legislative and funding recommendations[128]
2. American Heart Association priorities to address the status of maternal cardiovascular health in AI/AN individuals[129]
3. The United Nations Permanent Forum on Indigenous Issues (UNPFII) recommendations on the Indigenous determinants of health, including intergenerational holistic healing, the health of Mother Earth, and decolonizing and re-Indigenizing culture as social determinants of health[130]
4. UNPFII and Indigenous Determinants of Health Working Group recommendations as recounted in *The Lancet Planetary Health*[71]
5. Recommendations from the National Center for American Indian Enterprise Development, the largest national Indian-specific business organization in the United States, which helps AI/AN businesses get the financing they need to reach their business goals. These describe providing access to capital and credit, addressing fairness and equity in federal economic regulation, promoting large- and small-scale business and sustainable economies such as food economies, ensuring tax fairness, and development of land, energy, infrastructure, and workforce. The authors note the importance of AI/AN representation and ownership of businesses, especially banking institutions.[131]

These organizations were selected based on their longstanding broad base of support among AI/AN stakeholders, leaders, and elected officials. These organizations and their publications are led by or inclusive of Indigenous peoples and reflect a broad base of input from AI/AN experts, community members, and leaders. Common aspects of the recommendations from these organizations include the need for adequate resources to promote health, promotion of cultural competence and awareness, linking educational and economic systems to public health, and implementation of culturally relevant services. Detailed recommendations and actionable solutions are provided in the following sections. In addition to health, education, and economic systems, *cross-cutting* and *foundational* issues include protecting and valuing intact ecosystems and preserving traditional knowledges by fostering intergenerational relationships with elders and knowledge bearers. The aim should be to include AI/AN peoples in all levels of health systems, including systems that protect and value intact ecosystems, intergenerational relationships, and include fully funding health systems, in addition to improving economic opportunities to include education and training, all from a relevant and safe cultural lens.

Overarching Priorities

Create a System to Protect and Value Intact Ecosystems

Supporting and valuing the efforts of Indigenous people to protect and maintain traditional lifeways, practices, and good stewardship for planetary health will foster wellness for Indigenous peoples. The health of Mother Earth and intact ecosystems with keystone species should be valued, including preserving salmon in Alaska and bison in the Plains and other appropriate initiatives as per local AI/AN peoples' self-identified priorities. Ensuring sustainable Indigenous food systems and land and water protections are essential for health. According to the United Nations, "Indigenous Peoples have deep traditional ecological knowledges that have sustained their communities for generations. They possess valuable insights into sustainable land management practices . . . recognizing and respecting these practices is crucial not only for the preservation of Indigenous cultures but also for global biodiversity and environmental sustainability."[130] For example, in Canada there has been progress in allowing for rivers to have legal personhood, entailing nine specific rights including biodiversity, freedom from pollution, and even the legal right to sue.[132] In the United States, a Tribal court moved to protect sacred plants and especially the Saguaro cactus.[133]

Foster Intergenerational Relationships With Elders and Knowledge Bearers

Intergenerational relationships include language and cultural practices that are protective of health. These relationships can address the multidisciplinary and intersectional experiences of social determinants of health. Promoting intergenerational holistic healing, the health of Mother Earth, and decolonizing and re-Indigenizing culture are AI/AN social determinants of health.

Health System Initiatives

Fully Fund the Indian Health Service

IHS has suffered from decades of significant underfunding even when compared with other federally funded health systems; as a result, the federal government has not complied with the hundreds of treaties with Tribal Nations. NIHB hosts the IHS Budget

Formulation Committee, and we recommend that Congress fully funds IHS at the level recommended by NIHB. In FY 2023, the appropriation for IHS was $4.9 billion. According to the IHS Budget Formulation Committee, full funding for IHS in FY 2023 would require $49.8 billion, a 10-fold increase in funding.[98] The US Department of Health and Human Services (HHS) budget in FY 2023 was $127.3 billion in discretionary and $1.7 trillion in mandatory budget authority for a total of $1.83 trillion.[134] An increase to the IHS budget of approximately $45 billion represents an increase of less than 2.5% of the HHS budget and would resolve the budget shortfall and underfunding issue.

Improve Coordination Across Indian Health Service, Tribal, and Urban Health Systems and Across Public and Private Sector Health Systems

The AI/AN health system, which comprises IHS, Tribal, and urban Indian health programs (I/T/U system), routinely engages public and private sectors to deliver health care services for AI/AN peoples. This is largely due to the underfunded AI/AN health system and the rural and remote nature of many Tribal communities. Due to underfunding, many health services are not directly provided or available in the I/T/U system, and AI/AN patients are frequently referred to non-I/T/U providers at federally qualified health centers, county hospitals, private sector, and other facilities. Outcomes of care coordination, discharge planning, and follow-up care are diverse in terms of quality and cultural competence. Optimizing AI/AN enrollment in Medicare and Medicaid will also improve access to resources and health services. Best practices in health services and resources coordination need to be established and promoted to improve AI/AN health outcomes.

Health Systems Actionable Solutions

- Develop an available, accessible, affordable, and competent workforce that integrates community voices and AI/AN traditions into culturally sensitive care.[129]
- Provide access to subspecialty care, particularly for the vulnerable, including prenatal, pediatric, and elder care. NIHB has actionable solutions regarding representation and sustainable funding to address infrastructure and training.[128]
- Ensure shared decision-making that includes AI/AN and Tribal representation.[129]
- Incorporate midwives, social workers, mental health counselors, doulas, AI/AN traditional healers, knowledge bearers, birth workers and peers, community health workers, and physician extenders into care.[129]
- Expand digital and telehealth in resource-limited areas as a supplement to existing care resources, but not as a substitute for care, and provide sufficient resources to these areas.[129]
- Provide appropriate screening for AI/AN people reflecting US Preventive Services Task Force standards and determine their effectiveness in the population in preventing

disease. Allow for modification when necessary and evidence based, as has become standard in Alaska, where screening begins at a younger age of 40 for colorectal cancer.[129]
- Improve health education and health promotion in Life's Essential 8 metrics from childhood throughout childbearing age, comprising physical activity, diet, smoking and other forms of nicotine exposure, sleep, body mass index, blood glucose, blood lipids, and blood pressure.[129]
- Build trust with respect, communication, and community knowledge, and understand the health needs of AI/AN peoples.[129]
- Deliver care tailored toward creating understanding of historical perspective, childhood trauma, and circumstances unique to AI/AN peoples.[129]
- Ensure Tribal sovereignty and ownership and control of data as discussed in the Data Sovereignty section.[135]

Economic System Initiatives

Invest in Economic Infrastructure in American Indian/Alaska Native Communities

Poverty is pervasive in tribal communities and is a key determinant of health disparities. As noted by the Board of Governors of the Federal Reserve System, "many tribal communities are underserved by financial institutions, a situation that limits their access to the credit and capital vital to their growth and development."[136(p88)] Geographic isolation, lack of infrastructure, and a complex policy history contribute to high numbers of unbanked households in AI/AN populations. Communities lack access to banks, Wi-Fi, and capital. According to FDIC, AI/AN peoples have the highest rates for unbanked households of all races and ethnicities. Promoting banking, business development, and economic sovereignty on reservations is necessary to promote wellness in Tribal communities. Tribal leaders, AI/AN entrepreneurs, and economic stakeholders should increase investment in on-reservation economic infrastructure.

Approach Economic Development as a Public Health Intervention

Scholars who study public health and equity in AI/AN populations should expand the focus to include the role of economics in promoting health equity. The intersectionality of public health research and academics needs to be linked to economics to better define challenges and to develop equitable solutions.

Economic System Actionable Solutions

- Increase the number of AI/AN-owned businesses.[131]
- Pass laws to ensure business funding for AI/AN peoples.[131]
- Launch financial institutions that can provide business funding for AI/AN peoples.[131]

- Reward and support Indigenous communities and land stewardship in ways that are meaningful to these communities and through funding, which is recognized by current economic systems.[137]

Educational System Initiatives

Incorporate Accurate American Indian/Alaska Native Peoples' History Into Educational Curricula

The lack of awareness of US history as it pertains to AI/AN policy, culture, and disparities contributes to ongoing stereotypes, assumptions, and marginalization. Educational curricula in the United States should include accurate AI/AN history and contemporary context beginning in elementary school. Curricula should be co-designed with AI/AN community leaders and educational stakeholders. This will also create opportunities for cultural exchange and promote tolerance, inclusion, and understanding of AI/AN cultures and histories among the broader US population.

Invest in American Indian/Alaska Native Schools and Tribal Colleges

Similar to IHS, BIE is underfunded. Educational attainment and quality of education are well-established social determinants of health. Many school systems located in Tribal communities are in rural areas, where the challenges in retaining teachers are substantial. The mission of BIE is to provide high-quality educational opportunities in accordance with local needs for cultural and economic well-being. We recommend full funding of BIE to achieve this mission. Schools, educational programs, policies, and research rooted in Indigenous culture and strengths can provide solutions to systemic educational issues.

Educational System Actionable Solutions

- Build capacity in the community.[135]
- Report in ways that are meaningful to tribal audiences as well as to funders.[135]
- Include AI/AN peoples in every step of the evaluation process, including, but not limited to, the following:[135]
  - Engage the community, not only the program, when planning and implementing an evaluation.
  - Determine milestones to accomplish funding and measure benefits to health outcomes related to increased funding.
  - Consider the context when constructing frameworks and involve AI/AN peoples in their creation.

- Allow for frameworks to be flexible and to be modified by local populations considering the unique needs of AI/AN peoples.
- Use participatory practices that engage stakeholders.
- Make evaluation processes transparent.
- Understand that programs may focus not only on individual achievement but also on restoring community health and well-being.
- Consider people not only as individuals but within the context of their culture, family and community.
- Include Tribal IRBs when applicable and follow Tribal IRB processes.

CONCLUSION

AI/AN populations are impacted by systemic and structural racism that contributes to health status and overall well-being. This dynamic creates an opportunity to address those structural elements to realize improved health by including relevant programming that addresses these underpinnings in a relevant way and allows AI/AN peoples access to health care and health care information in a way that is meaningful to our populations. We postulate that as climate change forces converge to influence our experience, the health care, education, workforce, and economics arenas can be prioritized to operationalize some antiracism countermeasures. In order to address the ongoing challenges of the current systems, we must integrate modern systems with traditional cultures. We should encourage and support healthy lifestyles that are consistent with our value systems and cultural traditions. The time between birth and death should include family, community, safe places to learn, and meaningful work. For AI/AN people, connection to the land and knowing our history and kinship allows us to live in balance with local ecosystems.

As we move forward toward equity, we must do so with genuine and inclusive involvement of AI/AN peoples. It is important to include AI/AN populations with unique considerations such as data sovereignty and differing and dynamic cultures and practices. For AI/AN peoples, inclusivity means involving Indigenous peoples longitudinally and respecting the value of our cultural knowledges, perspectives, and solutions.

REFERENCES

1. Smith LT. *Decolonizing Methodologies: Research and Indigenous Peoples*. Zed Books; 1999.
2. Battiste M. *Decolonizing Education: Nourishing the Learning Spirit*. University of Regina Press; 2013.
3. Casola L; National Academies of Sciences, Engineering, and Medicine. *Structural Racism and Rigorous Models of Social Inequity: Proceedings from a Workshop. Structural Racism and Rigorous Models of Social Inequity*. National Academies Press; 2022. doi:10.17226/26690

4. US Census Bureau. 2020 Census question on race: Information for American Indians and Alaska Natives. 2020. Accessed April 2, 2025. https://www2.census.gov/programs-surveys/decennial/2020/partners/outreach-materials/handouts/question-on-race-for-american-indians-alaska-natives.pdf
5. US Bureau of Indian Affairs. Bureau of Indian Affairs: Tribal Leaders Directory. Accessed April 2, 2025. https://experience.arcgis.com/experience/20ad1b9c9f4a40a586f3a4c72abe30bf
6. Thomas ME. The Alaska Native Claims Settlement Act: Conflict and controversy. *Polar Rec.* 1986;23(142):27–36. doi:10.1017/S003224740000677X
7. Wilkins DE, Stark HK. *American Indian Politics and the American Political System.* 4th ed. Rowman & Littlefield Publishers; 2017.
8. Bhatt J, Bathija P. Ensuring access to quality health care in vulnerable communities. *Acad Med.* 2018;93(9):1271–1275. doi:10.1097/ACM.0000000000002254
9. United Nations Dept of Economic and Social Affairs. Indigenous Peoples at the United Nations. Accessed July 9, 2023. https://www.un.org/development/desa/indigenouspeoples/about-us.html
10. Dunbar-Ortiz R. *An Indigenous Peoples' History of the United States.* Beacon Press; 2014.
11. Greenberg AS. *Manifest Destiny and American Territorial Expansion: A Brief History with Documents.* Bedford/St. Martin's; 2012.
12. Garcia T, Féraud G, Falguères C, de Lumley H, Perrenoud C, Lordkipanidze D. Earliest human remains in Eurasia: New 40Ar/39Ar dating of the Dmanisi hominid-bearing levels, Georgia. *Quat Geochronol.* 2010;5(5):443–452. doi:10.1016/j.quageo.2009.09.012
13. Deloria V Jr., Lytle CM. *American Indians, American Justice.* University of Texas Press; 2012.
14. Thornton R. *American Indian Holocaust and Survival: A Population History Since 1492.* University of Oklahoma Press; 1997.
15. Wilson S. *Research Is Ceremony: Indigenous Research Methods.* Fernwood Publishing; 2008.
16. Langmoen IA. The Norse discovery of America. *Neurosurgery.* 2005;57(6):1076–1087. doi:10.1227/01.neu.0000144825.92264.c4
17. Weidensaul S. *The First Frontier: The Forgotten History of Struggle, Savagery, and Endurance in Early America.* Harper; 2012.
18. Reséndez A. *The Other Slavery: The Uncovered Story of Indian Enslavement in America.* Houghton Mifflin Harcourt; 2016.
19. History.com editors. 2019. Why Columbus Day courts controversy. A+E Global Media. October 7, 2019. Updated March 10, 2025. Accessed April 2, 2025. https://www.history.com/news/columbus-day-controversy
20. Gilder Lehrman Institute of American History. The doctrine of discovery, 1493: A spotlight on a primary source by Pope Alexander VI. Accessed April 2, 2025. https://www.gilderlehrman.org/history-resources/spotlight-primary-source/doctrine-discovery-1493
21. Newcomb ST. The evidence of Christian nationalism in federal Indian law: The doctrine of discovery, Johnson v. McIntosh, and plenary power. *Rev Law Soc Change.* 1993;20(2):303–341. Accessed April 2, 2025. https://socialchangenyu.com/review/evidence-of-christian-nationalism-in-federal-indian-law-the-doctrine-of-discovery-johnson-v-mcintosh-and-plenary-power-the

22. Tuck E, Yang KW. Decolonization is not a metaphor. *Decolonization Indig Educ Soc.* 2012;1(1):1–40. Accessed August 13, 2025. https://jps.library.utoronto.ca/index.php/des/article/view/18630
23. National Geographic Society. Motivations for colonization. Accessed October 27, 2023. https://education.nationalgeographic.org/resource/motivations-colonization
24. Library of Congress. Russian colonization. 2000. Accessed April 2, 2025. https://www.loc.gov/collections/meeting-of-frontiers/articles-and-essays/alaska/russian-colonization
25. Trigger BG. *A History of Archaeological Thought*. Cambridge University Press; 1990.
26. Wolfe P. Settler colonialism and the elimination of the native. *J Genocide Res.* 2006;8(4):387–409. doi:10.1080/14623520601056240
27. Haigh JG. Unangan/Aleut, Sugpiaq/Alutiiq and Russian conquest. History of Alaska Natives. University of Alaska. 2018. Accessed April 2, 2025. http://sites.kpc.alaska.edu/jhaighalaskahistory/files/2018/02/Chapter-4-Unangan-and-Sugpiaq-.pdf
28. Clark ES. Jesuit missionaries in early-twentieth-century Alaska, colonialism, and categories of 'superstition.' *West Hist Q.* 2022;53(4):405–428;407. doi:10.1093/WHQ/WHAC046
29. Blackhawk N. *The Rediscovery of America: Native Peoples and the Unmaking of US History*. Yale University Press; 2023.
30. Jacuk BA. A historical overview of the Alaskan 'Comity Plan' and its continued effects on Indigenous peoples. *Alsk J Anthropol.* 2024;22(1–2):11–33. Accessed August 10, 2025. https://www.alaskaanthropology.org/product/volume_22_1-2_2024
31. Jackson S. *Sheldon Jackson Papers, Series V: Scrapbooks, 1885–1896*. Presbyterian Historical Society; 1885–1896. Accessed July 13, 2024. https://archive.org/details/sheldonjacksonpa49jack
32. Alaska Statehood Act, Pub L No. 85-508, 72 Stat 339 (1958). Accessed April 2, 2025. https://www.akleg.gov/basis/get_documents.asp?session=29&docid=29890
33. ANCSA Regional Association. Economic impacts. Accessed August 12, 2025. https://ancsaregional.com/economic-impacts
34. ANCSA Regional Association. About the Alaska Native Claims Settlement Act. Accessed August 12, 2025. https://ancsaregional.com/about-ancsa
35. *Seminole Nation v United States*, 316 US 286 (1942).
36. Advisory Council on Historic Preservation. *Consultation with Indian Tribes in the Section 106 Review Process: A Handbook*. June 2021. Accessed April 1, 2025. https://www.achp.gov/sites/default/files/2021-06/ConsultationwithIndianTribesHandbook6-11-21Final.pdf
37. Bowes JP. American Indian removal beyond the Removal Act. *Native Am Indigenous Stud.* 2014;1(1):65–87. doi:10.1353/nai.2014.a843652
38. Library of Congress. Indian Removal Act: Primary documents in American history. Accessed August 14, 2025. https://guides.loc.gov/indian-removal-act
39. Miller RJ. The doctrine of discovery: The international law of colonialism. *Indig Peoples J Law Cult Resist.* 2019;5:35–42. Accessed August 11, 2025. https://www.jstor.org/stable/48671863
40. Thornton R. Cherokee population losses during the Trail of Tears: A new perspective and a new estimate. *Ethnohistory.* 1984;31(4):289–300. doi:10.2307/482714
41. Wilm J. 'The Indians must yield': Antebellum free land, the Homestead Act, and the displacement of native peoples. *Bull German Hist Inst.* 2020;67:17–39. Accessed April 2, 2025. https://www.ghi-dc.org/fileadmin/publications/Bulletin/bu67/17.pdf

42. US Dept of Health and Human Services. American Indians and Alaska Natives - The trust responsibility. Accessed April 2, 2025. https://web.archive.org/web/20250202030015/https://www.acf.hhs.gov/ana/fact-sheet/american-indians-and-alaska-natives-trust-responsibility
43. Lomawaima KT, Ostler J. Reconsidering Richard Henry Pratt: Cultural genocide and native liberation in an era of racial oppression. *J Am Indian Educ*. 2018;57(1):79–100. doi:10.1353/jaie.2018.a798597
44. Price H. Rules governing the Court of Indian Offenses. US Dept of the Interior, Office of Indian Affairs. March 30, 1883. Accessed April 2, 2025. https://commons.und.edu/indigenous-gov-docs/131
45. Newland B. *Federal Indian Boarding School Initiative: Investigative Report*. Vol 1. US Dept of the Interior; 2022. Accessed April 2, 2025. https://www.bia.gov/sites/default/files/dup/inline-files/bsi_investigative_report_may_2022_508.pdf
46. Shelton BL. Legal and historical roots of health care for American Indians and Alaska Natives in the United States. Kaiser Family Foundation. February 2004. Accessed August 13, 2025. https://www.kff.org/wp-content/uploads/2013/01/legal-and-historical-roots-of-health-care-for-american-indians-and-alaska-natives-in-the-united-states.pdf
47. Penobscot Indian Nation. Tribal timeline. Accessed August 13, 2025. https://www.penobscotnation.org/departments/cultural-historic-preservation/historic-preservation/tribal-timeline
48. Truth and Healing Commission on Indian Boarding School Policies Act. HR Rep No. 117-595, 117th Cong, (2022). Accessed August 13, 2025. https://www.congress.gov/congressional-report/117th-congress/house-report/595
49. Moore G. The Carlisle Indian Industrial School. *The Friday Footnote* blog. November 10, 2021. Accessed April 2, 2025. https://footnote.wordpress.ncsu.edu/2021/11/10/the-carlisle-indian-industrial-school-11-12-21
50. An act making appropriations for current and contingent expenses and fulfilling treaty stipulations with Indian tribes (Act of March 3, 1893), 25 USC §283 (1893).
51. Truth and Reconciliation Commission of Canada. *Honouring the Truth, Reconciling for the Future: Summary of the Final Report of the Truth and Reconciliation Commission of Canada*. 2015. Accessed April 2, 2025. https://publications.gc.ca/pub?id=9.800288&sl=0
52. Carlisle Indian School Digital Resource Center. Tom Torlino, 1882 and 1885. Accessed August 13, 2025. https://carlisleindian.dickinson.edu/images/tom-torlino-1882-and-1885
53. Warne D, Lajimodiere D. American Indian health disparities: Psychosocial influences. *Soc Personal Psychol Compass*. 2015;9(10):567–579. doi:10.1111/spc3.12198
54. Deloria PJ, Lomawaima KT, Brayboy BMJ, et al. Unfolding futures: Indigenous ways of knowing for the twenty-first century. *Daedalus*. 2018;147(2):6–16. Accessed August 14, 2025. https://www.jstor.org/stable/48563014
55. *Montoya v. Bolack*, 372 P2d 387 (NM 1962). Accessed April 2, 2025. https://law.justia.com/cases/new-mexico/supreme-court/1962/7103-0.html
56. Indian Reorganization Act (Act of June 18, 1934), 25 USC §5101–5129 (1934).
57. Kalt JP. Statement before the US Senate Committee on Indian Affairs. Harvard Project on American Indian Economic Development. December 8, 2021. Accessed August 11, 2025. https://hwpi.harvard.edu/files/hpaied/files/senatfnl.pdf

58. Otis MDS. *The Dawes Act and the Allotment of Indian Lands.* University of Oklahoma Press; 2014.
59. Bessel R, Haake CB. The federal Indian relocation programme of the 1950s and the urbanization of Indian identity. In: Bessel R, Haake CB, eds. *Removing Peoples: Forced Removal in the Modern World.* Oxford University Press; 2009:107–129.
60. National Archives. Bureau of Indian Affairs Records: Termination. Accessed April 1, 2025. https://www.archives.gov/research/native-americans/bia/termination
61. Warne D. Policy issues in American Indian health governance. *J Law Med Ethics.* 2011;39 (suppl 1):42–45. doi:10.1111/j.1748-720X.2011.00564.x
62. Bureau of Indian Affairs. Indian Child Welfare Act. Accessed August 12, 2025. https://www.bia.gov/bia/ois/dhs/icwa
63. Native American Rights Fund. "We Also Have A Religion": The American Indian Religious Freedom Act and the Religious Freedom Project of the Native American Rights Fund. 1979. Accessed August 13, 2025. https://narf.org/nill/documents/nlr/nlr5-1.pdf
64. Frerichs L, Bell R, Hassmiller Lich K, Reuland D, Warne DK. Health insurance coverage among American Indians and Alaska Natives in the context of the Affordable Care Act. *Ethn Health.* 2019;27(1)174–189. doi:10.1080/13557858.2019.1625873
65. Blackhawk M. Federal Indian law as paradigm within public law. *Harvard Law Rev.* 2019;132(7):1787–1877. Accessed August 13, 2025. https://harvardlawreview.org/print/vol-132/federal-indian-law-as-paradigm-within-public-law
66. Warne D, Frizzell LB. American Indian health policy: Historical trends and contemporary issues. *Am J Public Health.* 2014;104(suppl 3):S263–S267. doi:10.2105/AJPH.2013.301682
67. Indian Civil Rights Act, 25 USC §1301–1303 (1968).
68. Akbar L, Zuk AM, Tsuji LJS. Health and wellness impacts of traditional physical activity experiences on Indigenous youth: A systematic review. *Int J Environ Res Public Health.* 2020;17(21):8275. doi:10.3390/ijerph17218275
69. Cajete G. *Native Science: Natural Laws of Interdependence.* Clear Light Publishers; 2000.
70. Cajete G. *Look to the Mountain: An Ecology of Indigenous Education.* Kivaki Press; 1994.
71. Redvers N, Celidwen Y, Schultz C, et al. The determinants of planetary health: An Indigenous consensus perspective. *Lancet Planet Health.* 2022;6(2):e156-163. doi:10.1016/S2542-5196(21)00354-5
72. Jennings D, Lowe J. Photovoice: Giving voice to Indigenous youth. *Pimatisiwin.* 2013;11(3):521–536. Accessed April 2, 2025. https://journalindigenouswellbeing.co.nz/wp-content/uploads/2014/02/15Jennings.pdf
73. Johnson-Jennings M, Billiot S, Walters K. Returning to our roots: Tribal health and wellness through land-based healing. *Genealogy.* 2020;4(3):91. doi:10.3390/genealogy4030091
74. Johnson-Jennings M. (Re)connecting to the land and centering the land in order to conduct healing. Presented at: National Academy of Medicine Workshop on Indigenous Knowledge and Health; March 22, 2023; Washington, DC. Accessed August 11, 2025. https://nam.edu/wp-content/uploads/2023/03/Dr.-Michelle-Johnson-Jennings.pdf
75. Walters KL, Johnson-Jennings M, Stroud S, et al. Growing from our roots: Strategies for developing culturally grounded health promotion interventions in American Indian, Alaska Native,

and Native Hawaiian communities. *Prev Sci.* 2020;21(suppl 1):54–64. doi:10.1007/s11121-018-0952-z
76. United Nations. Climate change. Accessed October 27, 2023. https://www.un.org/development/desa/indigenouspeoples/climate-change.html
77. Hansen T. Kill the land, kill the people: There are 532 superfund sites in Indian Country! *Intercontinental Cry.* June 18, 2014. Accessed April 2, 2025. https://intercontinentalcry.org/kill-land-kill-people-532-superfund-sites-indian-country-24366
78. Evans-Campbell T. 2008. Historical trauma in American Indian/Native Alaska communities: A multilevel framework for exploring impacts on individuals, families, and communities. *J Interpers Violence.* 2008;23(3):316–338. doi:10.1177/0886260507312290
79. Ahmed F, Zuk AM, Tsuji LJS. The impact of land-based physical activity interventions on self-reported health and well-being of Indigenous adults: A systematic review. *Int J Environ Res Public Health.* 2021;18(13):7099. doi:10.3390/ijerph18137099
80. National Archives. Treaty of Fort Laramie. Accessed April 2, 2025. https://www.archives.gov/milestone-documents/fort-laramie-treaty
81. Jimenez S. Standing up for the Sacred Black Hills and native sovereignty. *Cultural Survival.* July 15, 2020. Accessed April 2, 2025. https://www.culturalsurvival.org/news/standing-sacred-black-hills-and-native-sovereignty
82. American Civil Liberties Union, Lakota Peoples' Law Project, Great Plains Tribal Chairman's Association, Black Hills Clean Water Alliance. Desecration and exploitation of the Black Hills, South Dakota Indigenous sacred site. 2023. Accessed April 2, 2025. https://www.aclu.org/wp-content/uploads/2023/10/9.12.23-ICCPR-Shadow-Report-Desecration-of-the-Black-Hills.pdf
83. Srinivasan S, Moser RP, Willis G, et al. Small is essential: Importance of subpopulation research in cancer control. *Am J Public Health.* 2015;105(suppl 3):S371–S373. doi:10.2105/AJPH.2014.302267
84. United States Indigenous Data Sovereignty Network. Promoting Indigenous data sovereignty through decolonizing data and Indigenous data governance. The Public History Project. 2021. Accessed April 2, 2025. https://www.publichistoryproject.org/2021/11/04/united-states-indigenous-data-sovereignty-network
85. Carroll SR, Rodriguez-Lonebear D, Martinez A. Indigenous data governance: Strategies from United States native nations. *Data Sci J.* 2019;18:31. doi:10.5334/dsj-2019-031
86. Haozous EA, Lee J, Soto C. Urban American Indian and Alaska Native data sovereignty: Ethical issues. *Am Indian Alsk Native Ment Health Res.* 2021;28(2):77–99. doi:10.5820/AIAN.2802.2021.77
87. Rainie SC, Schultz JL, Briggs E, Riggs P, Palmanteer-Holder NL. Data as a strategic resource: Self-determination, governance, and the data challenge for Indigenous Nations in the United States. *Int Indig Policy J.* 2017;8(2). doi:10.18584/iipj.2017.8.2.1
88. National Congress of American Indians. Tribal Nations & the United States: An introduction. Accessed July 18, 2024. https://archive.ncai.org/about-tribes
89. Native BioData Consortium. Accessed July 13, 2024. https://nativebio.org
90. Hull SC, Wilson DR. Beyond Belmont: Ensuring respect for AI/AN communities through Tribal IRBs, laws, and policies. *Am J Bioeth.* 2018;17(7):60–62. doi:10.1080/15265161.2017.1328531

91. Jindal M, Chaiyachati KH, Fung V, Manson SM, Mortensen K. Eliminating health care inequities through strengthening access to care. *Health Serv Res.* 2023;58(suppl 3):300–310. doi:10.1111/1475-6773.14202
92. Solomon TGA, Starks RRB, Attakai A, et al. The generational impact of racism on health: Voices from American Indian communities. *Health Aff.* 2022;41(2):281–288. doi:10.1377/hlthaff.2021.01419
93. Centers for Medicare and Medicaid. November 2024 Medicaid & CHIP enrollment data highlights. Accessed April 16, 2025. https://www.medicaid.gov/medicaid/program-information/medicaid-and-chip-enrollment-data/report-highlights
94. Centers for Medicare and Medicaid. Medicare enrollment dashboard. 2024. Accessed April 16, 2025. https://data.cms.gov/tools/medicare-enrollment-dashboard
95. Indian Health Service. 2024. Indian Health Service health equity report fact sheet. Accessed April 16, 2025. https://www.ihs.gov/sites/newsroom/themes/responsive2017/display_objects/documents/factsheets/IHS_Health_Equity_Report_FactSheet_2024.pdf
96. USA Facts. This chart tells you all you need to know about government spending. February 6, 2025. Accessed April 16, 2025. https://usafacts.org/articles/this-chart-tells-you-everything-you-want-to-know-about-government-spending
97. US Dept of Veterans' Affairs. Serving America's veterans. 2024. Accessed April 16, 2025. https://department.va.gov/veterans-experience/wp-content/uploads/sites/2/2024/08/VA-FY2024-Q3-Trust-Report_Final.pdf
98. National Tribal Budget Formulation Workgroup. *Building Health Equity With Tribal Nations: The National Budget Formulation Workgroup's Recommendations on the Indian Health Service Fiscal Year 2023 Budget.* 2021. Accessed April 2, 2025. https://www.nihb.org/wp-content/uploads/2025/01/FY-2023-Tribal-Budget-Formulation-Workgroup-Recommendations-Vol-1.pdf
99. Steele L. Holistic well-being: Mental, physical, and spiritual. In: Filho WL, Wall T, Marisa Azul A, Brandli L, Özuyar PG, eds. *Good Health and Well-Being.* Springer; 2019:373–382.
100. Frerichs L, Bell R, Hassmiller Lich K, Reuland D. Regional differences in coverage among American Indians and Alaska Natives before and after the ACA. *Health Aff.* 2019;38(9):1542–1549. doi:10.1377/hlthaff.2019.00076
101. US Government Accountability Office. Indian Health Service: Agency faces ongoing challenges filling provider vacancies. August 2018. Accessed April 2, 2025. https://www.gao.gov/assets/gao-18-580.pdf
102. Association of American Medical Colleges. Diversity in medicine: Facts and figures 2019. Association of American Medical Colleges. Accessed April 1, 2025. https://www.aamc.org/data-reports/workforce/report/diversity-medicine-facts-and-figures-2019
103. Association of American Medical Colleges, Association of American Indian Physicians. (2018). *Reshaping the Journey: American Indians and Alaska Natives in Medicine.* Association of American Medical Colleges; 2018. Accessed July 13, 2024. https://store.aamc.org/reshaping-the-journey-american-indians-and-alaska-natives-in-medicine.html
104. Journell W. An incomplete history: Representation of American Indians in state social studies standards. *J Am Indian Educ.* 2009;48(2):18–32. Accessed April 2, 2025. https://www.jstor.org/stable/24398743

105. Mihesuah DA. *American Indians: Stereotypes & Realities*. Clarity Press; 2009.
106. Haozous EA. Native America 101—Why are health researchers teaching high school history? *Res Nurs Health*. 2023;46(3):279–281. doi:10.1002/nur.22311
107. Jacob M, Poole M, Gonzales K, Jim H, Duncan G, Manson S. Exploring an American Indian participatory medical model. *J Particip Med*. 2015;7:e8. Accessed April 2, 2025. https://participatorymedicine.org/journal/evidence/research/2015/05/30/exploring-an-american-indian-participatory-medical-model
108. Guadagnolo BA, Cina K, Helbig P, et al. Medical mistrust and less satisfaction with health care among Native Americans presenting for cancer treatment. *J Health Care Poor Underserved*. 2009;20(1):210–226. doi:10.1353/hpu.0.0108
109. Gonzales KL, Garcia GE, Jacob MM, Muller C, Nelson L, Manson SM. Patient-provider relationship and perceived provider weight bias among American Indians and Alaska Natives. *Obes Sci Pract*. 2017;4(1):76–84. doi:10.1002/osp4.135
110. Running Bear U, Thayer ZM, Croy CD, et al. The impact of individual and parental American Indian boarding school attendance on chronic physical health of Northern Plains Tribes. *Fam Community Health*. 2019;42(1):1–7. doi:10.1097/FCH.0000000000000205
111. Lutz EL. Saving America's endangered languages. *Cult Surv Q*. 2007;31(2). Accessed April 2, 2025. https://www.culturalsurvival.org/publications/cultural-survival-quarterly/saving-americas-endangered-languages
112. Running Bear U, Croy CD, Kaufman CE, et al. The relationship of five boarding school experiences and physical health status among Northern Plains Tribes. *Qual Life Res*. 2018;27(1):153–157. doi:10.1007/S11136-017-1742-Y
113. Alaska Native Languages. Immersion schools. Accessed July 18, 2024. https://www.alaskanativelanguages.org/immersion-schools
114. Bureau of Indian Education. Our mission. Accessed April 16, 2025. https://www.bie.edu/topic-page/our-mission
115. Redvers N, Reid P, Carroll D, et al. Indigenous determinants of health: a unified call for progress. *Lancet*. 2023;402(10395)7–9. doi:10.1016/s0140-6736(23)01183-2
116. Kesler DO, Hopkins LO, Torres E, Prasad A. Assimilating traditional healing into preventive medicine residency curriculum. *Am J Prev Med*. 2015;49(5 suppl 3):S263–S269. doi:10.1016/j.amepre.2015.07.007
117. National Center for Education Statistics. Fast facts: Dropout rates. US Dept of Education. 2024. Accessed April 16, 2025. https://nces.ed.gov/fastfacts/display.asp?id=16#fr1
118. Annie E. Casey Foundation. 2025 KIDS COUNT data book interactive: Education. Accessed August 12, 2025. https://www.aecf.org/interactive/databook?c=race&d=ed
119. Postsecondary National Policy Institute. Native Americans in higher education. February 2025. Accessed April 16, 2025. https://pnpi.org/wp-content/uploads/2025/02/NativeAmerican_FactSheet_Feb25.pdf
120. American Indian Higher Education Consortium. Vision & mission. Accessed July 13, 2024. https://www.aihec.org/vision-mission-2
121. Dick A (Kwaxsistalla Wathl'thla), Sewid-Smith D (Mayanilth), Recalma-Clutesi K (Oqwilowgwa), Deur D (Moxmowisa), Turner NJ (Galitsimġa). 'From the beginning of time': The colonial

reconfiguration of native habitats and Indigenous resource practices on the British Columbia coast. *Facets*. 2022;7:543–570. doi:10.1139/facets-2021-0092
122. Kuokkanen R. Indigenous economies, theories of subsistence, and women. *Am Indian Q*. 2011;35(2):215–240. doi:10.5250/amerindiquar.35.2.0215
123. Graeber D. On social currencies and human economies: Some notes on the violence of equivalence. *Soc Anthropol*. 2012;20(4):411–428. doi:10.1111/j.1469-8676.2012.00228.x
124. Byram RS, Lewis DG. 2001. Ourigan: Wealth of the Northwest Coast. Oregon Historical Quarterly. 2001;102(2):126–147. Accessed April 1, 2025. https://www.jstor.org/stable/20615134
125. Federal Deposit Insurance Corporation. 2023 FDIC National Survey of Unbanked and Underbanked Households. Updated November 14, 2024. Accessed April 2, 2025. https://www.fdic.gov/analysis/household-survey/index.html
126. Fletcher MLM. *American Indian Tribal Law*. 2nd ed. Aspen Publishing; 2020.
127. Neihardt JG. *Black Elk Speaks: Being the Life Story of a Holy Man of the Oglala Sioux*. William Morrow & Company; 1932.
128. National Indian Health Board. 2023 legislative and policy agenda for Indian health. 2023. Accessed April 2, 2025. https://www.rmtlc.org/wp-content/uploads/2023/02/Draft-Explanatory-Version-2023-Legislative-Policy-Agenda-2.22.23.pdf
129. Sharma G, Kelliher A, Deen J, et al. Status of maternal cardiovascular health in American Indian and Alaska Native individuals: a scientific statement from the American Heart Association. *Circ Cardiovasc Qual Outcomes*. 2023;16:e000117. doi:10.1161/HCQ.0000000000000117
130. Secretariat of the Permanent Forum of Indigenous Issues, Economic and Social Council. Improving the health and wellness of Indigenous peoples globally: Operationalization of Indigenous determinants of health. February 2, 2024. Accessed April 2, 2025. https://digitallibrary.un.org/record/4039161?v=pdf
131. National Center for American Indian Enterprise Development. Indian Country policy priorities. Accessed July 13, 2024. https://www.ncaied.org/indian-country-policy-priorities
132. Berge C. This Canadian river is now legally a person. It's not the only one. *National Geographic*. April 15, 2022. Accessed July 13, 2024. https://www.nationalgeographic.com/travel/article/these-rivers-are-now-considered-people-what-does-that-mean-for-travelers
133. Tohono O'odham Legislative Council. Resolution of the Tohono O'odham Legislative Council: Recognition and Protection of the Sacred Ha:san. (Resolution No. 21-137). 2021. Accessed April 2, 2025. https://www.tolc-nsn.org/docs/Actions21/21137.pdf
134. US Dept of Health & Human Services. FY 2023 Budget in Brief. 2023. Accessed April 2, 2025. https://web.archive.org/web/20240821000358/https://www.hhs.gov/sites/default/files/fy-2023-budget-in-brief.pdf
135. LaFrance J, Nichols R. Reframing evaluation: Defining an Indigenous evaluation framework. *Can J Program Eval*. 2008;23(2):13–31. doi:10.3138/cjpe.23.003
136. Board of Governors of the Federal Reserve System. *Annual Report 2002*. 2002. Accessed April 1, 2025. https://www.federalreserve.gov/boarddocs/rptcongress/annual02/ar02.pdf
137. Campaign for Nature. 30x30 and Indigenous peoples and local communities. Accessed April 1, 2025. https://www.campaignfornature.org/30x30-and-indigenous-peoples-and-local-communities

2

Structural Racism, Asian American Communities, and Health Equity: A Historical, Transnational, and Intersectional Perspective

Mienah Zulfacar Sharif, PhD, MPH, Marshall H. Chin, MD, MPH, Ignatius Bau, JD, Melissa Borja, PhD, Nadia Islam, PhD, Nadia Kim, PhD, LeiLani Nishime, PhD, Paul M. Ong, PhD, MUP, and Gilbert C. Gee, PhD

INTRODUCTION

As noted in the introduction of this book, structural and systemic racism organizes the societal institutions, systems, rules, and practices in the United States to enshrine white supremacy, within the United States and globally.[1,2] Racism also shapes the conditions that foster health and illness, including systems that can either promote and/or undermine health (e.g., educational system, legal system, media). When polluted with racism, these systems exacerbate and sustain racialized inequities in health. Throughout history, Asian American communities have grappled with the impacts of how racism structures social systems, including, but not limited to, media representations that reinforce stereotypes of Asian Americans as perpetual foreigners, carriers of diseases, being over- and under-sexual, and as a model minority. Consequently, these images contribute to scapegoating of Asian-descent groups for social, legal, and health challenges, as seen recently with the surge of Anti-Asian violence during the COVID-19 pandemic. At the same time, the contradictory stereotype that Asian Americans are a universally "successful" and privileged model minority often leads policymakers and researchers to ignore the pressing needs of these communities, rendering them invisible and neglected. This concern is amplified when Asian ethnic communities—including Hmong, Bangladeshis, and Filipinos—are considered a single racial category, rather than diverse communities with distinct experiences, histories, and health and social issues and varying inequities across and within ethnic groups.

CHALLENGES OF DEFINING "ASIAN AMERICANS"

Defining who is Asian American is a two-pronged problem: (1) The continent of Asia is characterized as a monolithic construct with little conceptual basis; and (2) defining which countries are considered "Asian" is arbitrary. "Asia" is a European concept that artificially imposes uniformity on diverse groups east of the Western world.[3] Throughout history, the US Office of Management and Budget (OMB) has continuously redefined which groups are considered "Asian." The general idea is that people are *Asian Americans* if they or their ancestors hail from Asian countries. This seems straightforward, yet a recent study demonstrated the arbitrariness—and historic inconsistencies—of these definitions promulgated by the Census and OMB.[4] For example, Afghanistan shares a border with China and Pakistan, includes many residents with Pakistani and Indian heritage, and resides on the continent of Asia. This applies to other Middle Eastern countries described in Chapter 5. Yet, OMB classified people from Afghanistan as "white" until the most recent revisions to the categories in 2024 that now categorize Afghans as "Asian."[4]

These racial classifications are not simply neutral taxonomies, but social and political categories shaped by racism and by resistance to that racism. For example, in 1922, the US Supreme Court ruled in *Ozawa v United States* that citizenship privileges belonged to persons who were of the "Caucasian" race and therefore excluded a Japanese American.[5] A year later, Bhagat Singh Thind, an Indian Sikh immigrant, petitioned for citizenship on grounds that he was "Caucasian" based on scientific reports at the time. Yet, the court ruled that people of India would not be considered "white" in the eyes of the "common man."[6] Thus, the political process of (re)creating the "Asian" category—often in contradictory ways—undoubtedly influences who is and is not counted/included.

RACISM IN THE ASIAN AMERICAN CONTEXT: FOUR FUNDAMENTAL CHALLENGES

Racism impacts health for all groups, yet four distinct challenges are especially pertinent and harmful to Asian Americans: the perpetual foreigner stereotype, the model minority myth, the aggregation fallacy, and invisibility.

The Perpetual Foreigner Stereotype

First, Asian Americans are often viewed as *perpetual foreigners*, or outsiders who are inherently unassimilable, and by implication, a threat to American society.[7] The fate of Asians in America has been tightly interwoven with politically contentious US relations with Asian countries (e.g., colonial rule, war, political/military interventions, trade, economic competition). Such tensions have fostered the idea that Asians and Asian Americans are a "yellow peril" or "brown peril" that threaten the safety and prosperity of the United States. *Yellow peril* fears led to policies targeting East Asian communities and those who resemble them, which manifested as immigration exclusion laws, "English only" ordinances, the mass incarceration of Japanese Americans, and heightened scrutiny of researchers with suspected ties to China.[8,9] *Brown peril*, similarly, represents the oppression faced by South Asian Americans who in the 1800s were referred to as the "Hindoo Invasion" (although most South Asian immigrants at the time were Sikh or Muslim), thereby signaling their association with the perpetual foreigner stereotype.[10]

These racist characterizations have persisted, leading to heightened surveillance, stigmatization, and criminalization of South Asian and South West Asian and North African (SWANA; also called Middle Eastern and North African [MENA]) Americans, particularly in the post-9/11 context (e.g., the "Muslim Ban").[11] Grounded in white supremacist ideologies, the consequences of such characterization have resulted in widespread violence against South Asian and SWANA/MENA people (see Chapter 5). *Brown peril* (a racist term referring to Asians with perceived darker phenotype) has also referred to the US perception of Filipino farmworkers as "stealing" white women at taxi dance halls (which culminated in the 1930 Watsonville, California race riots) and to Vietnam (and Cambodia and Laos) and the waves of refugees from those countries as threats to US global economic dominance and domestic resources and culture.

Model Minority Myth

The *model minority myth* portrays Asian Americans as universally "successful," socioeconomically privileged, hyper-studious, passive, meek, and apolitical.[12] This myth contributes to harmful, racist assumptions with implications for health, including the systematic exclusion of Asian Americans from mainstream dialogue on racism and health inequities.[13,14] This image also conflates the heterogeneity of Asian American communities into a single, homogeneous group, focusing on the "highest achievers" or more socioeconomically advantaged in ways that hide and dismiss the lifelong burdens of poverty and racism among many Asian Americans who are not so well-off or privileged.[15]

Moreover, proponents of the model minority myth, which emerged in the middle of the 20th century, framed Asian Americans as disciplined, family-oriented, upwardly mobile, and politically docile, with these characteristics seen as a product of an essentialized Asian "culture"; this myth was often used to oppress other groups. Opponents of the Civil Rights Movement and Black Power activism used these arguments about Asian American success to undermine Black Americans in their struggles for political, economic, and social equality in the 1960s.[16]

In subsequent decades, the model minority myth has continued to be deployed as a strategy to justify anti-Black racism and create intergroup conflict across racially minoritized groups.[17] The perpetual foreigner and model minority racialization have a dynamic, bidirectional relationship. Being a passive, "good" minority can assuage animosity towards the "yellow/brown peril," but being high achieving has also prompted anti-foreigner racism,[18] as many children of Indian descent have experienced in national spelling bee competitions.[19] Indeed, as a form of internalized racism, Asian Americans themselves can perpetuate the model minority myth to counter the perpetual foreigner myth. This myth has sometimes been adopted by Asian Americans as a form of internalized racism, which then plays out in current debates on affirmative action.[20,21]

Aggregation Fallacy

When multiple Asian ethnic groups are lumped together, it results in the *aggregation fallacy*, referring to erroneous inferences about subgroups based upon the group mean.[4] Table 2-1 displays the heterogeneity across Asian American ethnic groups.[22] For example, on average, about 55.7% of Asian Americans have a bachelor's degree or higher. Yet, this ranges from 16.4% for Laotian Americans to 75.7% for Indians. This illustrates how poorly the average for all Asian ethnic groups represents the actual educational level for each subgroup. Further, aggregation across nationality groups does not account for the tremendous variation in migration trajectories, employment types, and socioeconomic backgrounds of Asian immigrants from large countries such as India and China. Equally important, it obscures intragroup heterogeneity and inequities, such as those among Punjabi and Sikh members of the Indian community and Fujianese individuals from China who are overrepresented in lower-wage occupations. In addition, health status and access to health services vary across subgroups. For example, relative to non-Hispanic white persons, a study conducted in California showed that Vietnamese Americans reported high rates of their health being fair or poor, Filipinos and Japanese Americans had high rates of obesity or overweight and hypertension, and Korean Americans reported high rates of serious distress and lacking a usual source of care.[23]

Moreover, it is important to recognize within-group heterogeneity. For example, Vietnamese Americans are very diverse themselves: some are refugees, some are immigrants, and some are US born.[24] With this diversity comes variation in access to privileges (e.g., citizenship) as well as multiple forms of social disadvantages (e.g., restrictive immigration policies). Their histories, politics, and health profiles vary along these dimensions, as well as several others, such as (but not limited to) gender identity and education level.[25] Accordingly, it is imperative to thoughtfully and critically disaggregate Asian subgroups through an intersectional lens in policy discourse, research, and interventions.

Invisibility

Invisibility results from the model minority image and the perception that the Asian American population is "too small to matter" at the national or federal level.[26,27] Despite the fact that Asian Americans are the fastest growing racial or ethnic group,[28] they often

Table 2-1. Recalculation of Asian American Ethnic Groups Only

Ethnic Group	Population	% of total Asian population	Population Aged ≥25 with ≥Bachelor's Degree (%)	Unemployed Civilian Labor Force (%)	Households With Food Stamps/SNAP Benefits (%)	Uninsured (%)	Poverty Rate	% Foreign Born	Median Household Income ($)
Indian	4,240,466	23.75	75.7	2.4	3.5	5.2	5.9	70.9	126,705
Chinese (except Taiwanese)	4,216,922	23.62	56.7	2.1	6.7	6.1	13.1	69	85,424
Filipino	2,983,596	16.71	49.8	2.6	5.7	5.5	5.8	64.5	100,273
Vietnamese	1,873,707	10.5	32	2.4	9.9	8.3	10.9	67.1	72,161
Korean	1,461,843	8.19	58.9	1.9	6.3	10	11.2	69.3	76,674
Japanese	755,672	4.23	53.7	1.6	2	2.8	7.3	41.4	85,007
Pakistani	506,193	2.84	59.8	2.4	9.3	8.4	12.6	63.7	87,509
Hmong	308,803	1.73	24.4	3.3	16.6	7.3	14	35.2	73,373
Cambodian	258,052	1.45	22.3	2.7	15.3	8.9	10.3	56.4	72,038
Thai	224,463	1.26	45.9	2.5	7.3	9.6	11.9	75.5	66,763
Bangladeshi	198,628	1.11	49.1	2.7	16	8.4	18.1	73.2	67,944
Laotian	192,689	1.08	16.4	2.7	16.3	9.5	14	56.1	66,117
Nepalese	189,399	1.06	44.3	3	17	12.6	13.8	81.5	63,619
Taiwanese	187,756	1.05	78.8	1.4	1.4	4.9	8.8	67.1	102,405
Burmese	173,586	0.97	26.2	1.6	29.8	12.1	24.3	78	45,903
Indonesian	81,269	0.46	55.8	3.8	4.2	9.9	8.9	72.8	93,501
Weighted means			55.7	2.3	6.7	6.6	9.6	66.7	94,204
Reweighted means			46.5	2.5	13.2	9.5	14.1	71.2	75,432

Source: Based on data from US Census Bureau.[22] Population weighted estimates are calculated from the 2019 American Community Survey.

Note: SNAP = Supplemental Nutrition Assistance Program.

are still excluded or are lumped into a racial and ethnic "other" category in almost all national polls, surveys, and data. This institutionalized form of erasure makes it easy for policymakers to overlook the needs of Asian Americans when they are seen erroneously as a monolithic model minority who do not face multiple forms of inequity, all of which have implications for health.

RACISM ACROSS FOUR SYSTEMS AND HEALTH INEQUITIES

This chapter explains how structural racism undermines health across Asian American communities by discussing four systems that vary across historical periods within the United States as well as internationally and by recognizing that racism intersects with other forms of oppression, such as sexism. The conceptual framework for this chapter is illustrated in Figure 2-1. We discuss how structural racism drives health and social inequities that impact Asian American communities via fewer resources, less privilege, lower social status, and diminished power within these systems. Although each system is discussed separately, structural racism sustains health inequities through the interconnectedness of systems.[29] Given page constraints, we could not focus on other equally important systems in detail (e.g., transportation, education), but instead focused on four systems that we thought were relevant for (re)producing racial inequity, particularly in Asian American experiences.

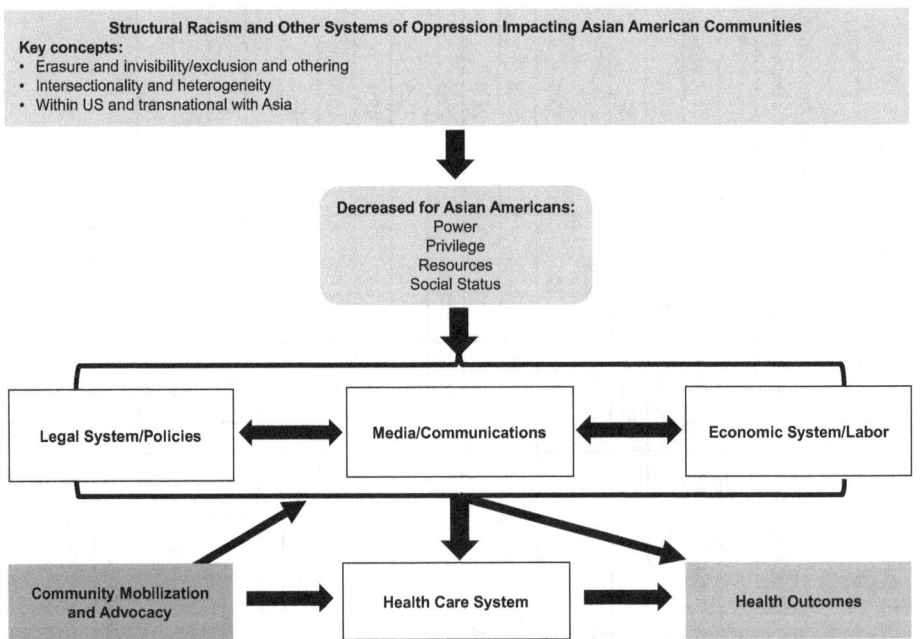

Figure 2-1. Conceptual Framework

The legal and policy system shapes which Asians are allowed entry, defines citizenship rights, and sets the foundation for other systems; the economic system is relevant for determining basic social drivers of health, and is connected both domestically and globally (as seen when Asians in America are used as scapegoats during conflicts with Asian countries); the media/communications system has played a pivotal role in shaping the ever-changing image of Asians as a yellow peril or model minority; and the health care system is relevant to individual health and well-being. Although we do not focus on other systems explicitly, our conceptualization of structural racism[29] underscores the many ways in which systems (and how racism permeates within/across them) are interconnected and influence one another.

We caution that the research on structural racism and the health of Asian Americans is still nascent, but strong evidence for such connections exists and is growing. Certainly, there is a long history of research on racism and Asian Americans, including some of the early works by LaPiere, who studied the basic connections between prejudicial attitudes and discriminatory behavior faced by Chinese people in the United States in the 1930s.[30] This research grew primarily in the social sciences and in ethnic studies but started to enter into the health sciences in the 1980s and 1990s. For example, in 1981 Streltzer and Wade found that Asian American patients received less postoperative analgesia than white patients because nurses stereotyped Asians as being more stoic.[31] A report by Lee in 1993 described a connection between Asian Americans and living in communities with uncontrolled toxic waste sites.[32] In 1999, Noh et al. found that self-reported discrimination was related to poor mental health among Southeast Asians.[33] Since that time, much more research has been conducted, primarily focused at the individual level.[3,34-39] Nonetheless, the connections we lay out between structural racism and health inequities serve as a template for future research.

Legal System

The legal system shapes the general policies that affect well-being for all (e.g., Medicare, Clean Air Act) and those specific to Asian Americans (e.g., Chinese Exclusion Act, "Muslim Ban"). These actions have direct socioeconomic consequences on communities. For example, immigration policy, which historically suppressed the number of Asians permitted to enter the United States and currently selects for high-skilled workers, contributes to the model minority myth that *all* Asian Americans are successful. We describe a long history of white supremacist anti-Asian laws that have limited immigration and civil rights, impacted family formation, and compromised access to education, land, housing, employment, political power, and health care.[40,41]

These laws and policies have negative implications for socioeconomic opportunities which limit resources, social status, privilege, and power, ultimately impacting individual- and family-level health and well-being via multiple social drivers of health.

In addition to federal laws and policies, some state and local laws governing employment, property rights, and judicial processes also present unequivocal examples of the structural racism experienced by Asian Americans.[42]

There was early immigration of Filipinos to Louisiana and Chinese, Japanese, Filipino, Okinawan, and Korean workers to the Kingdom of Hawaiʻi, but the largest cohorts began migrating from China in 1849 to "Gold Mountain" (California) during the California Gold Rush. Many Chinese immigrants worked throughout the western states and territories, including constructing the transcontinental railroad.[43,44] The resentment of white workers of the competition from Chinese workers resulted in exclusion from the country (i.e., the Chinese Exclusion Act), denial of citizenship, the exclusion of women and families,[45] and widespread discrimination and violence, including lynching.[46,47] The prevalence of Chinese laundries and restaurants today dates back to racial discrimination in the labor market, reinforced by laws and policies, which limited Chinese male immigrants to such service-oriented small ethnic enterprises[48] and spawned racialized gender stereotypes of Chinese men as effeminate and homosexual for doing "women's work" and living in male-only communities.[45] The early history of Chinese immigrants reflects how immigration law has always been linked both to the need for cheap labor and white supremacy, that is, needing cheap, exploitable labor domestically and abroad for white nation-building and empire.

In 1854, the California Supreme Court applied an existing state law, already in place to prevent Black Americans and American Indians from testifying against white Americans, to Chinese immigrants living in California, leaving all three racialized, minoritized groups legally defenseless against the crimes of violence and economic exploitation.[49] The court ruled that the Chinese were "a race of people whom nature has marked as inferior, and who are incapable of progress or intellectual development beyond a certain point, as their history has shown; differing in language, opinions, color, and physical conformation; between whom and ourselves nature has placed an impassable difference."[49]

In 1888, however, two Chinese laundry owners, Yick Wo and Wo Lee, successfully challenged a San Francisco, California policy that denied operating permits to all Chinese-owned laundries under the pretense that they were fire hazards. The US Supreme Court ruled that although the ordinance as written was neutral, its implementation violated the 14th Amendment of the US Constitution ensuring equal protection of the law and therefore prohibited discrimination based on race.[50] This repudiation of racial discrimination was an important application of the protections of the post-Civil War constitutional amendments to all racial and ethnic groups.

The scapegoating of Chinese immigrants by white laborers and political leaders in the western United States resulted in the 1882 Chinese Exclusion Act. This was one of the first federal laws to discriminate by race/ethnicity, based on a false rationale that Chinese persons and Chinatowns were the source of diseases.[51] The Chinese Exclusion Act and its subsequent recodifications resulted in near-total exclusion of additional Chinese immigrants and separated hundreds of thousands of Chinese men from their families. Thereafter, Japan agreed to limit the migration of laborers to the United States under the Gentlemen's Agreement of 1907, while the Immigration Act of 1917 established the Asiatic Barred Zone, which banned immigration from much of Asia and the Pacific Islands. Although the Chinese Exclusion Act was repealed in 1943, it was not until the Immigration Act of 1965 that significant immigration from Asia was allowed.[52]

Racially based laws targeting Asian Americans were not isolated to Chinese Americans. President Franklin D. Roosevelt's Executive Order 9066 in 1942 authorizing the incarceration of Japanese Americans, one of the only executive orders to discriminate by ethnicity/country of origin, was rationalized by false assumptions about the disloyalty of Japanese Americans after Japan's attack on Pearl Harbor, based on the narrative of Asian Americans as perpetual foreigners.[53] In the 1940s, 120,000 Japanese Americans—two-thirds of whom were US citizens—were taken from their homes, schools, and jobs and incarcerated for three years without due process by presidential and US military actions. Gordon Hirabayashi, Minoru Yasui, and Fred Korematsu challenged the curfew, relocation, and incarceration under the executive order, but the policies were upheld by the Supreme Court.[54-56] In his dissent in *Korematsu v United States*, Justice Robert Jackson called the executive order "the legalization of racism." The three cases were reopened in the 1980s when evidence was discovered of false and intentionally misleading US military and intelligence assessments rooted in racism, and the three convictions were vacated.[56] After Japanese Americans waged a powerful movement for redress and reparations, Congress enacted the 1988 Civil Liberties Act, issuing an apology and authorizing monetary reparations of $20,000 for each surviving Japanese American who had been incarcerated.[57]

Laws targeting specific Asian American communities persist. Since 9/11, the surge of anti-Muslim racism resulted in extraordinary government policies and practices including widespread surveillance, searches, arrests, and indefinite detention, often with secretive processes and without due process or judicial review,[58] and even reports of torture (see Chapter 5). There is evidence of the adverse mental health impacts on immigrants who are detained.[59,60] The conflation of race, ethnicity, national origin, language, and religion in the eyes of much of the public and law enforcement agencies only compounded the applications of these policies with disproportionate impacts on populations that include South Asian Americans.[61] Congress authorized additional actions through the USA PATRIOT Act that targeted Middle Eastern people, and those who are, or "perceived to be," Muslim, including many South Asian Americans. Congress also created the Department of Homeland Security, which began to use national security ("homeland" security) as the framework and justification for all immigration policy[62,63] and facilitated ongoing, excessive surveillance. These policies continue to contribute to scapegoating that can result in violence against these targeted communities, such as the massacre of Sikh congregants at an Oak Creek, Wisconsin gurudwara (temple) in 2012.[64]

Similarly, race-based restrictions on economic security were not limited to the 19th century. In 2023, Florida enacted a state law prohibiting Chinese individuals from owning land or homes in that state, with similar laws pending in Texas, Louisiana, and Alabama. This is the modern manifestation of the 1913 California Alien Land Laws that prohibited Asians from owning property.

More recently, certain national origin limits continue race-based restrictions on immigration, disproportionately preventing immigrants from the Philippines, India, China, and other Asian countries from joining their families or pursuing employment opportunities. Currently, backlogs in both family-based[65] and employment-based[66] visas are both overrepresented by applicants from Asian countries. More recently, the number of Chinese nationals crossing the United States' southern border has dramatically increased (they are the largest group from outside the Americas entering via this path),[67] thereby making US border control and immigrant detention policies more relevant to Asian populations.[68] These exclusionary race-based immigration laws and policies continue to suppress the Asian American population.

Yet, as immigration from Asia continues, support for civic participation among Asian Americans is vital, including access to US citizenship and voting rights. These are undermined by the aforementioned backlogs in applications for citizenship[69] as well as growing restrictions on voting rights.[70] For example, limits on mail-in ballots, including translated ballots, make it more difficult for Asian Americans who need language assistance to vote. Moreover, there is some evidence that Asian Americans, like other minoritized voters, face active suppression of their voting rights.[71] Several states have begun requiring individuals who are assisting US citizens registering to vote to be US citizens themselves,[72] which decreases naturalization rates for Asian Americans as well as other racially minoritized communities.

Such laws and policies are connected to health outcomes. For example, one study showed that the "Muslim ban" was related to increased risk of missing primary care appointments and increased risk of emergency department visits among Muslim-origin people in Minneapolis.[73] These findings may be driven by increased stress among Muslim-origin people following the ban. Similarly, another study found that women with Arab names had a higher risk of poor birth outcomes in the six months following the 9/11 attacks, presumably due to higher experiences of discrimination and stress. Other studies have found that the type of visa held by Filipino immigrants was related to health outcomes, possibly because the type of visa issued reflects social stratification arising from immigration policy.[74] Moreover, a systematic review showed that Hmong refugees were at elevated risk for psychiatric disorders and symptoms (and reported the highest rates of depression among Southeast Asian communities).[75] The authors of the study suggested that early separation from their country of origin and other Hmong communities in the United States may have exacerbated the trauma experienced by refugees, leading to these outcomes. Thus, the policy and legal systems can contribute to health inequities among Asian Americans through various pathways that include stress as well as inequitable access to care and other health-promoting resources.

Economic System and Labor

The economic system is complex, involving local, national, and international laws, policies, and practices that govern everything from relations among nation-states to individual worker experiences. While it is not possible to cover all this ground, we focus on a subset of ideas that are particularly relevant to Asian Americans in the context of structural racism.

The characterization of Asian Americans as a model minority has obscured the underlying internal economic disparities and inequalities within the population.[76] Asian Americans have the largest intragroup income inequality of any other racial group,[77] yet the misguided model minority narrative is reinforced by rudimentary statistical averages (*aggregation fallacy*, described earlier) that situate the relative position of Asians within the economic hierarchy in the US. This simplistic metric, however, hides a complex reality and history, one anchored in selective migration patterns and resulting economic diversity, with systematic disparities along ethnic lines. The economic reality and dynamics undeniably contribute to health inequities, especially considering that socioeconomic position is one of the most consistent predictors of health outcomes.[23,78]

The current internal economic inequality of Asian Americans is the product of multiple manifestations of racism, including colonialism and imperialism during the latter half of the 20th century. The first of two pivotal events was the 1965 Immigration Act, which ended nearly a century of racist anti-Asian restrictions and facilitated large-scale Asian immigration. One outcome has been the arrival of highly educated immigrants, initially through preferential quotas for skilled workers and subsequently through family-based migration.[79] This selective migration created a much-needed labor pool for America's growing technology and health sectors, and this socioeconomic class would serve as a cultural and institutional foundation for the reproduction of a highly educated second and third generation of Asian Americans.[80] The second major event was part of the US government's effort to dominate the global economic order in the second half of the 20th century, particularly against forces of communism and socialism; this included the Vietnam War. Following the US loss in the Vietnam War in 1975, hundreds of thousands of Southeast Asian refugees who had either directly assisted the US military or were now on the losing side of the conflict resettled in the United States and elsewhere from Vietnam, Laos, and Cambodia.[81] A disproportionate number of these political refugees had limited education and fewer marketable skills, which marginalized them to the bottom segments of the labor market.[82] Many of the refugees' economic disadvantages have been reproduced among their children, leaving them trapped at the lower economic rungs.[83] Five years later, the United States finally codified post–World War II international law by enacting the Refugee Act of 1980, adopting the United Nations definition of a refugee and resulting in the one million Asian refugees in the United States today. From 2012 to 2022, of the over 500,000 refugees admitted to the United States, about 19% were from Myanmar and 10% were from Bhutan.[84]

Extending from the legacy of historical imperialism and colonialism, current dual migration patterns to the United States are anchored in racialized neocolonialism, revealing the complexity and reach of structural racism.[85] *Neocolonialism* is the effort by "first world" nations to use economic, political, and cultural power to reestablish control of former "third world" colonies. These unequal global relationships are also defined along racial lines, with people racialized as white having power over people racialized as non-white. An integral part of this system is the international flow of people due to both economic needs and political dynamics. The nexus between the global and domestic phenomena can be seen in the migration of political refugees, which is tied to displacement resulting from the struggle of previously colonized nations against world powers. Such events that induced refugee migration include the Vietnam War,[86] the overthrow of the CIA-sponsored dictatorship in Iran,[87] and anti-communist interventions in Latin American countries and their civil wars.[88] The global movement is also shaped by first world demand for both high-skill labor discussed earlier, a phenomenon known as *brain drain*,[79] and low-skill labor. These global structures and dynamics in turn have shaped the economic disparities among highly heterogeneous Asian American groups.

The economic effects of the systematic bias towards highly educated immigrants and the intergenerational reproduction of high educational levels among some US-born Asian Americans are evident in the labor market, where the "typical" fully employed Asian American, prior to the COVID-19 pandemic, was economically well-off.[23] However, this does not take into account the fact that Asian Americans are concentrated in US regions with a high cost of living.[89] While Asian Americans are above parity with non-Hispanic whites nationally, they are below parity when accounting for regional differences.[90] The 2022 American Community Survey shows that per capita income for Asians was 8% higher than non-Hispanic whites nationally but 20% lower in the three largest metropolises where a third of Asians reside (the high-cost regions of Greater Los Angeles and the San Francisco Bay Area in California and the New York City, New York metro area).

The duality of Asian immigration has created considerable internal disparities among workers along ethnic lines. The inequality is evident when looking at the distribution of earnings in California. Approximately 1 in 10 (10.5%) Asian American workers earned less than $25,000 per year while 16% earned $150,000 or more. The degree of inequality between Asians in the top category and those in the bottom category is staggering, nearly 15 times as much in earnings. There are dramatic ethnic disparities in the relative concentration at the two ends of the spectrum. Among refugees composed of Cambodians, Hmong, and Laotians, 18% were low earners and only 3% were high earners. On the other hand, among Indians, many of whom benefited directly or indirectly from high-skilled migration, 33% were high earners and only 6% were low earners.

Earnings inequality creates disparities among households. For example, the median income for Cambodians, Hmong, and Laotians was $59,000, with 21.3% falling below the federal poverty line. In comparison, the median for Indians was $150,000, with only 5.4% in poverty.[91] The socioeconomic position of Indian Americans, on the other hand, does not represent all South Asian communities, as one-quarter (25%) of the Bangladeshi and Nepali American population is considered low income (i.e., living in households in the lowest Asian American and Pacific Islander income quintile).[28] Other researchers using more recent data have also found similarly large disparities in economic status across ethnic lines.[92]

Wealth is a different dimension of economic status; it is related to income (money earned and received from labor or capital over a given period) but also measures the value of assets such as savings, stocks, investments, real estate, and other physical property, as well as debt. Pre-pandemic empirical evidence revealed that the median net worth for Asian Americans at the national level was lower than for non-Hispanic whites despite higher household income[92-94]; however, more recent data indicate that Asian Americans now have greater wealth.[95,96] Indirect evidence and one local survey show that there are considerable disparities across ethnic subgroups and that wealth disparities by ethnicity are far greater than inequalities in earnings and household income.[97,98]

Thus, overall, the model minority depiction of Asian Americans is erroneous. After adjusting for regional cost of living, Asians are not "out whiting whites," although Asians fare better than other people of color. The economic achievement of the average Asian American is largely due to immigration laws and policies favoring the highly educated, rather than a simplistic narrative of a group "bootstrapping" themselves up. There are other structural factors that have contributed to the changing economic position of Asian Americans during the latter half of the 20th century, including the enactment and implementation of civil rights legislation in the 1960s.[92] This removed some of the discriminatory barriers in employment and housing, which benefited some Asian Americans, particularly the highly educated. The model minority mythology is also problematic because it obscures the enormous inequalities along ethnic lines. The disproportionate number of economically disadvantaged Asian Americans is the result of US political and economic interference in Southeast Asia (i.e., US foreign policy) and failure to assist refugees to succeed in the labor market (i.e., US domestic policy). Unfortunately, governmental policies and programs often fail to recognize this heterogeneity, and the needs of structurally disadvantaged Asian Americans are ignored under the belief that the population as a whole is economically successful—or "should be."

We can see how these disparities manifest by looking at relationships between socioeconomic class and health. Certainly, there is a robust literature that shows that persons of higher class enjoy lowered mortality and morbidity. For example, among Vietnamese

Americans, employment in nail salons was related to lower cognitive functioning relative to those who did not work in these salons[99] demonstrating how health outcomes are patterned across socioeconomic lines. Similarly, among Asian Americans, increased education is related to lower dementia incidence. Further, Filipino Americans suffered disproportionately higher COVID-19 mortality relative to non-Hispanic whites and other Asian ethnic groups, plausibly due to their higher representation in nursing and other health care occupations.[100,101] Yet, there is some indication that these relationships are not so straightforward among Asian Americans. For example, Walton has shown that despite the expected gradient in education and health among Asians educated in the United States, there is no such gradient among Asians educated abroad,[102] thereby posing significant implications to health outcomes—specifically indicators of health equity—given the large proportion of immigrants in the Asian American population. Although future work focusing on these factors can provide more evidence to delineate specifics, what this suggests is an important interaction between both person-level factors (i.e., educational attainment) and global connections. This aligns with our framework that suggests that structural racism plays a role in shaping the economic system that has implications for personal level well-being.

Media and Communications

The landmark *New York Times* article in 1966 by William Pettersen helped popularize the model minority mythology and underscores how the media shapes harmful stereotypes.[103] The media plays a key role in perpetuating *cultural racism*, which refers to the structures, practices, norms, and values that reinforce the ideology of white supremacy (see the Introduction).[29,104] Media and communications profoundly shape how people perceive Asian Americans. Words and images convey messages, stories, narratives, and ultimately the value-driven, "baked in," deep narratives that all too often harm Asian Americans.[105] For example, one study found that media stereotypes of the "nerdy" and "antisocial" Asian American lowered social acceptance of the young adult populace, a key predictor of social functioning across the life course.[106-109] Racist, anti-Asian representations in the media not only perpetuate harmful images but create a sociopolitical climate conducive to anti-Asian policies, regulations, and rhetoric. Furthermore, negative images and cultural climate impact health vis-a-vis several pathways, including marginalization from employment, housing and educational opportunities, lower quality of care in the health care system, and acts of violence, harassment, and discrimination that bring both physical and mental injury.[110-112]

Nonetheless, the US has witnessed a recent increase in media representations of Asians and Asian Americans. Films like the Oscar-winning *Everything Everywhere All at Once* as well as *Beef*, the most streamed television series in April 2023, demonstrate the growing visibility of Asian-descended people in American media. In addition, Americans are increasingly exposed to images of Asian people due to the global spread of media from places like India and South Korea. The popularity of Bollywood films and the enormous success of Korean pop groups like BTS indicate a long-awaited shift toward a greater diversity of images of Asians and Asian Americans for US audiences. Yet, these optimistic signs should not be mistaken for fair or equitable representation, nor does this progress remediate the long-lasting historical effects of minimal or stereotypical representation. A recent study of the top 1,300 grossing films from 2007 to 2019 include only six movies that featured an Asian-descent woman in a leading role, and more than 40% did not include even one Asian-descent character.[113] Moreover, after the period of *yellow face* in which white Americans played East Asian–descended characters (with pulled-back eyes and prosthetics),[114] more Asian Americans have appeared in mainstream media, but they are often stereotyped, relegated to tokenized roles and/or treated as a source of humor. Most Americans are familiar with the three dominant images of Asian-descent groups, as the yellow peril, the perpetual foreigner,[115] and the "terrorist."[116]

One of the few places where we do see Asian Americans represented in media is as health professionals, yet even these representations tend to perpetuate the model minority myth and usually reinforce stereotypes, including a narcissistic focus on professional success and poor bedside manner. Asian Americans have responded with creative use of user-generated content on platforms such as TikTok and Instagram. Their grassroots media combats stereotyping and creates new communities. Digital media scholars have noted the importance of online spaces for Asian Americans to develop a sense of group identity, to create alternative public spaces, and to view themselves as participants in activist movements.[117–119] They produce this alternative media despite the fact that Asian Americans, and Asian American women in particular, are frequently targeted by racist and sexist users who use harassment and intimidation to limit Asian American participation online.[118]

While the portrayal of Asian Americans in fictional media is caricatured, their representation in news media is even worse. Scholars have found a consistent pattern of underrepresentation and stereotyping of Asians and Asian Americans in news stories.[120] Asian American journalists have also reported a pressure to maintain white hegemonic norms in the newsroom.[121,122] We can see the results of this absence or underrepresentation following 9/11 as media-fueled brown peril has grown in significance for South Asian and Muslim Asian Americans, who disproportionately contend with accusations of terrorism and treason both in society and through media portrayals (see Chapter 5). In recent years, the coverage of the impact of COVID-19 on the Asian American population betrays a similar bias.[123,124]

Asian Americans were (and still are) impacted by anti-Asian rhetoric and misinformation related to the pandemic in the media, particularly about the origins of the virus, even before geographic origins of background of the first confirmed case was known.[125] Such media stories awakened long-standing associations of Asian bodies with invasive illness and disease.[126] This continues the history of racist rhetoric of Chinatowns being referred to as sources of moral corruption and spreadable disease, merging discourse around invasive agricultural pests with that of Asian immigration at the turn of the 20th century and beyond.[127,128] Believed to be carriers of syphilis, smallpox, and bubonic plague, public officials passed laws and policy such as the 1882 Chinese Exclusion Act partly out of fear of such contagion, containing Chinese American communities and reducing or reversing the flow of immigration from China.[127,128] Madhavi Mallapragada traces these earlier histories into the current COVID-19 context and argues that the convergence of these narratives with nativist tropes demonstrates the insecurity of Asian American citizenship.[129]

Health Care

Structural racism impacts Asian Americans' health directly and via pathways that involve the health care system. Specifically for health care, structural racism limits access to care and upholds a system of health care that often does not meet the needs of Asian Americans and can increase the cost of care for this populace.

Access to Care

Multiple factors, including jobs, language barriers, and citizenship status, undergirded by structural racism, contribute to many Asian Americans not having health insurance or being underinsured. Explained previously, structural racism contributes to many Asian Americans having low-wage jobs without employer-sponsored health insurance. According to the American Community Survey, in 2021 25% of Asians were noncitizens.[130] Currently, Asian Americans are the fastest-growing undocumented group (currently 13%–16% of the Asian American population) as one in seven Asian immigrants are undocumented.[131] Eligibility varies across states, but in general, undocumented immigrants and refugees are restricted to care from emergency departments and free or low-cost clinics.[131] Noncitizens have limited access to public insurance including Medicaid, the Children's Health Insurance Program (CHIP), and health insurance offered on the Affordable Care Act (ACA) Marketplace.[132] Some lawfully present immigrants can qualify for Medicaid and CHIP within specific eligibility requirements. To be eligible for Medicaid or CHIP, immigrants must have a qualified immigration status and usually must wait five years after getting this status. Addressing the health care needs (physical and mental) of people of Asian descent with precarious immigration status is a timely and pressing concern, especially considering the increasing rates of undocumented Chinese immigrants entering the United States through the Mexican border since 2023.[67]

Noncitizens have a higher rate of uninsurance than citizens[130,132]; this has important consequences, especially considering the physical and emotional toll the immigration process takes.[133] Undocumented immigrant adults are more likely to report barriers to health care than immigrant adults with less precarious immigration status and naturalized citizen adults as measured by no usual source of care other than emergency room (38%, 18%, 12%, respectively); no doctor visit in the past 12 months (37%, 26%, 18%); and skipped or postponed care in the past 12 months (31%, 22%, 19%).[132] Ultimately, health insurance is associated with better health outcomes.[134] Thus, the ACA, which was supported by a majority of Asian Americans, reduced health inequities in part by increasing health insurance coverage.

Other politically-motivated barriers, however, have further diminished access to and enrollment in health insurance.[132] For example, the Trump administration cut funding for navigators who would help people enroll in the ACA Marketplace health plans and Medicaid insurance; these navigators are especially important for those with limited English proficiency or literacy issues.[135,136] The Trump administration also implemented a public charge rule, which considers a noncitizen's probability of depending on the government for subsistence when determining whether to grant a green card or visa.[137] The public charge rule created a culture of mistrust which made it less likely that noncitizens would explore and understand their health insurance options, or even seek care from health care institutions. After Trump, the Biden Administration reversed the public charge rule and increased funding for navigators. However, mistrust takes a long time to overcome.

While undocumented immigrants are not eligible for federal health insurance through Medicaid, CHIP, or the ACA insurance exchanges, as of September 2023, five states and the District of Columbia provide state-funded health insurance or subsidies to them.[130]

Quality of Care

Patients with limited English proficiency require interpreter services and patient information materials in their native language.[130] In 2019, 31% of Asian American adults across diverse native languages had limited English proficiency.[139] Unfortunately, the health care system inadequately supports culturally tailored approaches to meet the physical and mental health needs of Asian American and other ethnic subpopulations.[140–143] These services are often not available, leading to reduced access to care.[3,144] For example, in 2018 Asians were 60% less likely than non-Hispanic whites to receive mental health treatment.[145] The health care workforce is not well trained in either antiracism or cultural humility, health care institutions are not set up to be culturally tailored, and payment systems lack strong incentives to address these inequity issues. Moreover, the health care workforce lacks diversity of some Asian American ethnic subpopulations, and there are limited Asian American voices in senior health care leadership positions.[146,147] The recent and increasing political pushback against diversity, equity, and inclusion in some states and institutions poses an increasing threat to addressing these forms of structural racism and health inequity.

Cost of Care

The health care payment system is not structured to advance health equity[148] and is not designed to support and incentivize those care transformations that can successfully address the medical and social needs of Asian Americans and other socially marginalized groups to improve health.[149] To reverse this, major national efforts are attempting to align payment reform and care transformation to advance health equity, including the Centers for Medicare and Medicaid Services Health Care Payment Learning and Action Network Health Equity Advisory Team and the Robert Wood Johnson Foundation's Advancing Health Equity: Leading Care, Payment, and Systems Transformation Program, which explicitly incorporates an antiracist approach.[150-154] Such state and national payment and care delivery reform efforts are necessary for the long-term sustainability of interventions to improve health equity for Asian American communities.

Not only is the health care payment system not designed to advance health equity but also a sizable body of research suggests that immigrants, especially undocumented immigrants, are subsidizing the health care of citizens because of the combination of lower health care utilization and medical expenditures by immigrants, greater difficulty for undocumented immigrants in accessing government health insurance, and payment of taxes and health insurance premiums by immigrants.[155,156] For example, a 2022 study found that immigrants paid the same amount of premiums and taxes that fund health care as citizens but had lower third-party expenditures for health care.[155] Thus, not only do many Asian Americans have difficulty accessing health insurance and the health care system in part from structural racism, immigrants are likely subsidizing the care of citizens.

SYNTHESIS ACROSS SYSTEMS

Structural racism is viewed as the interaction and interconnections among institutions that perpetuate racial inequities. For the purposes of this chapter, we lay out four systems in separate sections. However, in actuality they work in a mutually reinforcing manner by decreasing access to opportunity and increasing risk to harmful exposures, leading to cumulative disadvantage within and across Asian American communities. For example, media portrayals of Asian Americans are inextricably tied to the labor and economic systems, which are connected to immigration policies that simultaneously select for immigrants who are highly skilled workers and penalize other immigrants for being "public charges." The media frequently stereotypes and dehumanizes Asians as perpetual foreigners who are different from "real" Americans. Even the model minority myth, superficially about the overall economic success of Asians in America, makes invisible Asians encountering social inequities such as low-income Hmong Americans. The result is that Asians are generically deemed unworthy of additional support in social policies, meaning that low-income laborers and service workers within the population suffer.

These immigration and economic policies also intersect with health care, given that access to health insurance and quality health care in the United States is tied to employment. Importantly, immigration policy is neither neutral nor uniform across and within communities; rather, immigration policy restricted entry of persons from Asian countries who were undesirable to politicians and their working-class supporters due to their exploitation as low-cost laborers. Immigrants from Asia were also accused of spreading "pestilential diseases" from Asia. Eugenics beliefs rooted in an ideology of the superiority of white genetics and culture underlay many of these racist views and policies[157–159] and these ideas have persisted across time in policies that screen immigrants for health problems. Indeed, they prominently resurfaced in the wake of COVID-19, as terms like "Kung Flu" and "China virus" spread across both traditional media and newer social media,[160–162] concomitant with a rise in anti-Asian hate crimes. Policy and research initiatives should employ methodologies that explicitly model the complexities within and across Asian American communities. Research ranging from case studies to system sciences approaches should span multiple levels of analysis and incorporate these complex interactions. Just as importantly, such research cannot be ahistorical. Time and intergenerational interactions are key dimensions of the effects of structural racism.

CASE STUDIES

Two case studies, environmental justice and COVID-19, discuss how structural racism leads to health inequities across communities via direct effects (e.g., exposure to environmental toxicants, anti-Asian violence) and indirectly through socioeconomic disadvantage, decreased political power, diminished access to high-quality health care, and from living in ethnic concentrations (ethnoburbs) that are near polluting sources.[117]

Environmental Justice

Environmental racism is the denial of a safe and healthy environment on the basis of white supremacy and systemic racism, much of which is promulgated by social institutions such as governmental agencies and corporations. Placing themselves disproportionately in communities of color as enabled by the US history of racist residential segregation, industries such as fossil fuel are backed by banks and enabled by government bodies that barely regulate them.[163] Further, the government—in cooperation with corporations and banks—oversees military operations that contribute to pollution concentrated in minoritized and low-income communities, such as in Hawai'i, and in the Global South.[117,164] Although understudied, some Asian American groups suffer disproportionate rates of environmental contamination and health hazards such as asthma.[165] Filipino Americans suffer the highest lifetime asthma prevalence rate at 21.5% to 23%, compared with 12.2% among white children, according to the 2023 California Health Interview Survey.[166]

Asian Americans who tend to be more impoverished and live in inner cities also have higher asthma prevalence rates than those in wealthier, suburban areas, although smoking and tobacco use are also risk factors for these health outcomes. Southeast Asian Americans, for example, have a rate of lung cancer 18% higher than white Americans.[167] California's Chinese Americans, likely those in inner-city Chinatown and other urban Chinese ethnic concentrations, also have a higher incidence of asthma than white Americans by two percentage points—not what we tend to expect of a "model minority" population.[168]

A case study of environmental racism appears in the city of Carson, California (Los Angeles County), which boasts a large Filipino/a community. Amidst the goods movement apparatus to shift China-made goods from dock to store, Carson is located close to the ports of Los Angeles and Long Beach and the nation's most cancerous freeway (Interstate 710) and houses a diesel-spewing rail yard and Marathon and Phillips 66 oil refineries. The exposures there include pollutants (e.g., particulate matter 2.5) that are related to high rates of asthma and other health issues.[168,169]

In addition, an interview-based and ethnographic study of Carson in line with residents' own community surveys revealed that Filipina/o and other Asian American activists suffered regular headaches, bloody noses, fainting spells, and fibromyalgia, which is often not captured by academic studies focused on asthma.[117] The concentrated pollution in this area arose due to multiple factors, including corporations seeking convenient and inexpensive areas, as well as governmental incentives to entice industry (e.g., providing tax breaks to corporations for locating in their city). Thus, these findings evidence structural racism, as they involve the collaboration of multiple systems that perpetuate health inequities. In these racially segregated neighborhoods, local governments and their policies prioritize corporations and industry over the health of residents of color. Those who work in these systems know that they are sickening and prematurely killing people of color, yet laws and cultural frames paint the corporations as caring and looking out for the best interests of the residents and children by providing jobs and funding local schools, hospitals, and police departments.[117,170] However, this "philanthropic" funding is a conflict of interest, as school administrations and the police are those who quell and punish the youth and community mobilizations against the goods movement industry (that chooses diesel as its main fuel source and does not work for more domestic manufacturing) and against oil refinery pollution that is slowly killing them all.[117] Taken together, disproportionate contamination propagated by the state, corporations, the capitalist market, racist residential segregation, and racist and anti-immigrant ideologies are all designed to prop up neoliberal racial capitalism, that is, capitalism based and founded on racial hierarchies and injustices.[117,171]

Importantly and as noted, community members in Carson have been actively fighting back. Immigrant women, in particular, have been instrumental in leading these efforts and creating organizations such as the Filipino/American Coalition for Environmental Solutions (FACES) and the Asian Pacific Environmental Network (APEN), a Northern

California organization.[172] APEN, for instance, led a campaign against toxic industrial and oil pollution in the heavily contaminated Richmond, California area where Southeast Asian Americans have been disproportionately falling ill and dying prematurely.

COVID-19 Pandemic

Anti-Asian racism in the media, including circulating the term "Kung Flu virus" in relation to COVID-19, cannot be disentangled from other pandemic-related adverse outcomes across Asian American communities.[173] Specifically, almost half of Asian businesses reported "catastrophic losses." The scapegoating, particularly towards Chinese Americans, was especially deleterious to economic revenue and employment since many Chinese American restaurants and small businesses, particularly those in Chinatowns, were vandalized, lost customers, and had to shut down owing to the view that Chinatowns spread the virus.[174] As early as February 2020, small businesses, especially those in Chinatowns and other Asian American enclaves, reported substantial loss in revenue.[175] Compared with other non-Asian owned restaurants, Asian American restaurants experienced an 18.4% larger decrease in traffic (estimated $7.42 billion lost revenue in 2020), with greater decreases in areas where more people supported Donald Trump.[176]

Blamed for the pandemic, Asian Americans experienced a greater increase in unemployment rates than any other racialized group.[177] Moreover, impacts on employment levels varied across ethnic populations such that Asian Americans with lower levels of education were particularly vulnerable (1 in 10 workers were impacted), with Vietnamese Americans experiencing the largest impact earlier on in the pandemic.[178] Having a lower educational level was also associated with significantly slower employment regrowth, particularly among lower wage workers.[179] Employment status is a critical driver of health, considering the strong role it plays in insurance coverage and therefore health care access and as a source of income and social connections.

These economic impacts have implications for other drivers of health including housing. A study in California discussed how Asian American households disproportionately fell behind on their rent and mortgage payments because of enormous economic disruptions created by pandemic.[180] Individuals with lower educational levels, a subgroup that was already financially vulnerable as they pay more than half of their income to cover housing costs, were most affected, with over 1 in 4 less-educated Asian Americans more likely to be behind on their housing payments.[180] This segment of Asian American households is predominantly composed of renters, impoverished families, immigrants with limited English-language proficiency, and makes up one-fifth of all Asian households. The study also found disparities across ethnic groups, with Korean, Vietnamese, Cambodians, Hmong, and Laotians more likely to be at risk because of extremely high housing burdens.[180]

Disease-Related Violence

Throughout history, Asian Americans have been particularly vulnerable to violence during moments of crisis and tension, including war and geopolitical conflict and heightened economic competition.[128] For example, in the early 20th century, Asian Americans were scapegoated and targeted during an outbreak of the bubonic plague in San Francisco and Los Angeles.[123] During the 1980s, Asian Americans were targeted in attacks, which federal civil rights officials attributed to international economic tensions with Japan as well as local economic tensions related to the arrival of refugees displaced by war in Southeast Asia.[129] Also, following 9/11, South Asians were targeted in incidents of street violence as well as federal policy and media reports.[181] Not surprisingly, Asian Americans faced racist rhetoric, scapegoating and a surge of targeted attacks and violence related to the COVID-19 pandemic.

In 2020, hate crimes against Asian Americans increased by almost 150% from the year prior.[182] By 2021, 1 in 5 Asian Americans had reported experiencing a hate incident (interpersonal verbal and written harassment, inappropriate gestures, physical violence, shunning or deliberate avoidance, and civil rights violations, such as experiencing workplace or business-based discrimination).[183] Chinese Americans, women, and older adults were most likely to report a hate incident.[184,185] The racist rhetoric regarding the pandemic is also associated with an increase in verbal harassment of youth at school, in public, and online, all of which can have lifelong implications for mental health and well-being.[186,187] In an effort to address these surges in anti-Asian attacks, the COVID-19 Hate Crimes Act was passed by President Biden in May of 2021. Yet, crimes targeting Asian Americans increased by almost 339% in 2021 compared with 2020.[188]

Asian American communities experience indirect, racially motivated COVID-related violence in the form of news reports, online hate, or through social media.[162] At the start of the pandemic in 2020, the online usage of inflammatory words substantially increased. After the televised usage of racially charged and offensive phrases, such as the "China virus," the "Wuhan virus," and the "Kung Flu virus" by popular news outlets and political figures, there was a 650% increase of such terms on Twitter and 800% increase in news articles online.[173] Another study found that the number of anti-Asian hashtags increased by a staggering 17,400% in relation to #Chinesevirus after a tweet by (then President) Donald Trump.[160] Since the beginning of the pandemic, the number of cyberbullying incidents among youth has increased, with Asian American youth experiencing higher rates of online victimization. Asian American and Pacific Islander youth also reported an increase in verbal and physical assaults in other settings.[186]

The hostile sociopolitical climate and targeted violence towards Asian Americans during the pandemic has adversely affected health across age ranges. Some studies specifically focused on the adverse effects on social–emotional indicators of health among Asian American and Pacific Islander youth during the pandemic.[187,189] As of 2022, a study reported that 25% of their Asian American adolescent (aged 13–17) and young adult (aged 18–29) study participants had experienced an increase in the frequency and/or severity of anti-Asian harassment in addition to two-thirds of individuals noting that their depression had worsened since the start of the pandemic.[190] In 2021, a national survey among Asian American adults found almost half (49%) reported experiencing anxiety and depression, with 72% identifying COVID-related discrimination as their main source of stress.[183] Older Asian American adults also reported increased fear, stress, and anxiety as a result of the pandemic. Social isolation was a major contributor to worsened mental health (e.g., depression, anxiety) and some physical health outcomes. Older adults also described limited access to mental health services due to barriers such as language and mental health stigma.[184]

COVID-19 impacted Asian Americans' sense of belonging, well-being, and safety, all of which can influence behavior including seeking health care. A 2023 study reported that half of Asian Americans felt unsafe due to their race, and 80% felt they did not belong or were not accepted in the United States because of their race.[191] They also reported feeling unsafe across multiple settings including on public transportation, in school, in their neighborhood, at markets, and at work.[191] Immigrants have reported fear of deportation or being detained during COVID-19 due to policies passed during President Trump's administration.[192] Among Asian Americans, younger respondents (aged 16–24) and females exhibited the lowest likelihood of feeling like they belong or were accepted.[191] Importantly, anti-Asian racism is coupled with another public health crisis of increased gun violence. Purchases of firearms among Asian Americans have surged in recent years due to elevated concerns about personal safety in an era of anti-Asian racism and violence.[193]

Community Mobilizing and Advocacy

Contrary to the model minority myth that depicts Asian Americans as docile and apolitical, Asian Americans have actively resisted racism and other forms of social, political, and economic injustice. Mobilizing for change in a variety of settings, they have endeavored to change both the state and its policies as well as the hearts and minds of the broader public, including members of their own communities. Some of the most visible forms of mobilization have focused on the United States at the local, state, and national levels. However, Asian American activism has also been transnational. Because many are immigrants with social, economic, and political ties to their home countries, Asian Americans have organized events, demonstrations, and advocacy campaigns responding to developments overseas, such as the democracy movement in Hong Kong.[194]

Asian American communities have a rich history of community mobilizing, advocacy, and solidarity with other groups to resist racism and other injustices (see Table 2A-1 in Appendix 2A), and such efforts persisted in response to the surge of COVID-19 violence and discrimination targeting Asian Americans (see Table 2-2). The activists involved

Table 2-2: Selected Examples of Community Mobilization During COVID-19 Among Asian American Communities

Type of Community Mobilization	Examples
Health data and resources	• AAs advocated for disaggregated data about COVID-19 in New York and other places and supported efforts by NH/PIs to report COVID-19 data separately from AAs. • AA-serving community health centers organized COVID-19 testing sites and ensured language access for COVID-19 testing. • AA health providers led efforts to educate and provide access to COVID-19 vaccines. • AA health providers and community organizations helped AAs gain access to telehealth and other virtual services while paying special attention to the impact of the digital divide. • AA mental health providers offered culturally and linguistically appropriate health resources for AAs. Pandemic-era racism contributed to worsening mental health among AAs, who historically have been the least likely group to seek mental health support.
Advocacy	• AAs called for an end to stigmatizing rhetoric and for improved resources to support victims of racism, violence, and discrimination. Their efforts resulted in the 2021 Presidential Memorandum Condemning and Combating Racism, Xenophobia, and Intolerance Against Asian Americans and Pacific Islanders in the United States. • AA organizations lobbied for robust government responses to the rise in anti-Asian hate crimes. Their efforts resulted in the COVID-19 Hate Crimes Act (2021), a law that some AA groups opposed because of its focus on using law enforcement to address acts of anti-Asian violence and racism.
Community organizing	• Stop AAPI Hate and other AA community organizations tracked anti-Asian attacks, raised public awareness, sought to hold elected officials accountable, and created new systems for reporting hate incidents. • AA activists, attentive to the mass mobilization and protests after the murder of George Floyd, called for solidarity and unity in addressing racism.
Education	• AA educators planned teach-ins and shared resources to put recent anti-Asian attacks in broader historical context • AA activists called for improved AA studies in both K–12 education and higher education.
Mutual aid and community care	• AA organizers provided resources for victims of attacks and support for vulnerable groups (e.g., children and elders) who felt unsafe. • AA organizations such as Asian Americans Advancing Justice Chicago worked with the organization Hollaback! to provide the public with bystander intervention training. • AA religious leaders worked within and across faith communities to provide support for victims of anti-Asian attacks. • AA joined others in advocating for relief to small businesses as part of the American Recovery and Reinvestment Act.
Arts and media	• AA filmmakers, podcasters, and artists created projects that called for solidarity and pushed back against "China virus" language. • AA journalists created guidelines for respectful and responsible reporting on the pandemic. • The Asian American Feminist Collective produced the *Asian American Feminist Antibodies: Care in the time of Coronavirus* online zine (see: https://perma.cc/2MSJ-SE63).

Note: AA = Asian American; NH/PI = Native Hawaiian or Pacific Islander.

in the Asian American Movement in the 1960s and 1970s identified solidarity with other systematically marginalized "third world peoples," including the Black Panthers and United Farm Workers, as a guiding principle of their work.[195] Today many Asian American activists continue to work in solidarity with Black, Latinx, Middle Eastern, Pacific Islander, Native Hawaiian, and Indigenous communities, contending with resurgent white supremacist movements, environmental racism, police violence, anti-labor policies and the degradation of working conditions for non-standardized workforces, and severe restrictions or bans on refugees and asylum seekers. Japanese Americans, for example, have drawn on their experience with being racially profiled and incarcerated during the World War II to express their solidarity for migrant families separated at the United States–Mexico border and Muslim Americans facing anti-Muslim racism during the War on Terror.[196,197]

At times, different political ideologies, including different approaches to understanding and addressing racism, have contributed to tensions and fissures within Asian American groups. Differences among Asian Americans about how to address the rise in anti-Asian racism and violence during the pandemic offers an instructive example. Some Asian American politicians and community organizations supported solutions focused on law enforcement, such as the COVID-19 Hate Crimes Act, which was signed into law in 2021. However, that bill found only muted support and sometimes even explicit opposition from other Asian American organizations and activists who believed that investing more resources in policing could harm Black and Brown communities affected by long-standing police violence and mass incarceration.[198,199] The opposition to the COVID-19 Hate Crimes Act reflects a long and rich history of Asian Americans striving to work in solidarity with Black and Brown communities in the effort to combat racism, along with efforts by Asian Americans to confront the problem of anti-Black racism within their own ethnic and racial communities.[16,200-202]

Asian American community mobilization and advocacy has often reflected a sensitivity to the diversity of the Asian American community. This sensitivity includes a commitment to viewing social inequities through an intersectional lens and attending to diverse identities and experiences of oppression; recognizing the needs of particular times, people, and places; and tailoring grassroots advocacy to reflect specific local histories, demographics, issues, transnational ties, and political contexts.[203] For example, community activists responding to Islamophobia and anti-Muslim racism during the War on Terror have embraced an intersectional approach and highlighted the overlap of white supremacy and Christian privilege in the United States.[204] In addition, increased public attention to the problem of anti-Asian racism and violence during the COVID-19 pandemic created a favorable political context for community organizers to advocate for changes to K–12 social studies curriculum so that it includes more content about Asian Americans. For example, in 2021, activists in Illinois successfully pushed for the passage of a state law mandating the teaching of Asian American history in K–12 public schools.[205]

Activists in other states have pursued similar education measures, though their goals and strategies have varied, reflecting local demographics and political coalitions. In 2023, for example, activists in Ohio championed legislation that would expand multicultural social studies education in K–12 schools and ensure that children learn not just about Asian Americans, but also Black, Latino, Jewish, Arab, and Native Americans.[206]

PROPOSED SOLUTIONS FOR CHANGE

Addressing the impact of structural racism on health in the Asian American context requires a transnational, intersectional, and historical perspective. Considering Asian American experiences through a transnational lens illuminates the ongoing impact of US imperialism and international military intervention on the health of Asian American communities. Over the past 150 years, US-backed wars throughout Asia displaced populations, contaminated and sickened their countries, and spurred the migration of Asian people, many of whom arrived with injuries and traumas associated with war. Moreover, an intersectional perspective recognizes that racism is just one of many interlocking systems of oppression, including, *but not limited to*, those based on gender, sexual orientation, social class, religion, and nativity. Lastly, it is imperative that contemporary experiences are placed in historical context to better understand that ongoing forms of structural racism are undergirded by long-standing systems and institutions that have sustained such practices and norms and are highly pervasive in present day political and social narratives.

Next, we outline six domains that encapsulate the many determinants of health (e.g., employment, immigration policies) discussed earlier, as well as some additional factors to consider (e.g., hiring and curricula within educational contexts) that, without critical interrogation, uphold the many ways racism operates across systems, including the specific systems discussed earlier. Our approach to the proposed solutions aligns with our overall conceptualization of structural racism, such that racism in any one system is influenced by and influences other interrelated systems. Effectively and appropriately challenging structural racism requires a transdisciplinary, systems-level approach that disrupts both the overt and covert manifestations of racism across systems. We are guided by extant empirical evidence that has demonstrated health linkages with the strategies we present below.

Data Infrastructure and Research Agenda

- Increase active engagement of diverse Asian Americans in research and policy advocacy by systematically including Asian American ethnic subgroups in all data collection, analyses and dissemination efforts.

- Incentivize institutions of higher education and research entities to recruit and retain scholars specializing in Asian American studies and Asian American health.
- Invest in innovative methodologies to disaggregate data (e.g., use data from smaller populations through oversampling, pooling multiple years of data) for research and programmatic and policy approaches.
- Partner with Asian American–led organizations to facilitate the creation of a data infrastructure that allows for iterative and ongoing input from community advocates.[207,208]
- Synergize the unique assets of quantitative data, qualitative data, evidence from lived experiences, and other forms of evidence that community advocates prioritize.

Legal System

- Reform immigration laws and policies to reestablish fair border policies consistent with international law and prohibit indefinite detention of immigrants for violations of civil immigration law; provide pathways to citizenship for all immigrants already in the United States (including Deferred Action for Childhood Arrivals youth); relieve immigrant visa backlogs; preserve family reunification; and expand employment-based opportunities.
- Remove barriers to citizenship (high fees and long backlogs) and voting (additional documentation requirements for voter registration and voting, limits on mail-in ballots and on times and places for early and same-day voting); promote citizenship (naturalization), proactive and automatic voter registration, and language access in voting and in all public services (e.g., climate warning systems).
- Increase representation of Asian Americans from a diverse range of ethnicities in leadership across sectors (e.g., government, academia, health care).
- Enforce civil rights laws to eliminate English-only laws and barriers to equal access because of primary language or immigration status.
- Mandate the teaching of Asian American history and issues in K–12 curriculum.
- Discourage xenophobic foreign relations rhetoric and policies that spur anti-Asian animosity.
- Increase and expand policies promoting Asian American communities who are underrepresented in the labor market, housing, contracting, and higher education.

Economic System and Labor

- Provide economic assistance to Asian American businesses, particularly those that were impacted by the COVID-19 pandemic, with low-interest loans and grants.
- Increase the federal minimum wage with automatic cost-of-living increases.

- Expand paid family leave.
- Support subsidies for childcare.
- Reduce student loan debt.
- Eliminate the penalties related to assistance programs that discourage savings and economic advancement.
- Increase economic assistance programs addressing the extreme economic heterogeneity among Asians along ethnic and socioeconomic lines (e.g., focus on subgroups who have been historically marginalized and systematically overlooked, such as refugees and their children) and along age lines, given higher levels of poverty among the elderly. Such policies would also address the issue of unemployment/precarious employment, including people with H-1B visas being laid off.

Media and Communications Systems

- Work with news media and entertainment industry to promote accurate narratives of heterogeneous Asian American communities and to discontinue portrayals of Asians as perpetual foreigners, yellow peril, the "other," and the model minority.
- Recognize and represent the diversity of Asian American cultures and languages when disseminating health information.
- Implement policies to protect Asian Americans and other targeted groups from online harassment.
- Prioritize research to identify and address media/communications systems' impact on the health inequities of Asian American communities.

Health Care System

- Increase access to, and affordability of, health insurance:
    - Expand support for health insurance navigators and assisters; increase enrollment of small businesses in public insurance options.
    - Eliminate barriers to insurance based on immigration status.
    - Repeal the public charge law.
- Provide culturally safe and appropriate care:
    - Support health care services that are covered by insurance plans and are patient-, family-, and community-centered and include proactive engagement of patients, families, and caregivers during care. Examples include integrating non-Western conceptions of health and well-being (e.g., practices that are aligned with health-promoting behaviors and norms within/across Asian American communities).

- Clarify requirements and increase enforcement of language access in all health care programs and services, including ensuring access to qualified health care interpreters and translations of written materials in multiple Asian languages.
- Expand the role of community health workers and patient advisors to mitigate access, cultural, and structural barriers to health care systems.
- Increase health care workforce diversity and ensure federally funded training and diversity programs create sustainable employment opportunities for underrepresented groups (e.g., Southeast Asians).
• Reform payment systems.
• Support and incentivize care systems tailored to meet the medical and social needs of Asian subgroups.

Community Mobilization and Advocacy

• Partner with communities with the goal of redistributing and/or sharing power, and attend to local needs, the diversity of experiences, and potential solutions specific to the opportunities and constraints of each diverse community.
• Create and sustain infrastructure for Asian American, Native Hawaiian, and Pacific Islander community advocacy and government accountability.
• Make the White House Initiative on Asian Americans, Native Hawaiians, and Pacific Islanders and the President's Advisory Commission permanent, with increased staffing, resources, and community engagement.
  - Hold every governmental department and agency accountable for measurably increasing disaggregated data collection.[209]
  - Expand state-level institutions/entities such as the Michigan Asian Pacific American Affairs Commission and the California Commission on Asian Pacific Islander Affairs to all 50 states and provide them with sustainable funding for staffing and programmatic costs.

CONCLUSION

Racism is an unequivocal core driver of health inequities and a long-standing barrier towards achieving health equity. Throughout history, structural racism has sustained social and health inequities across Asian American communities. This chapter highlights insidious structural racism within four systems: (1) legal/policy, (2) media/communications, (3) economy/labor, and (4) health care. It also presents concrete antiracist strategies and emphasizes the need to end the invisibility of Asian American voices and experiences in discussions on racism and health. Multisector approaches should center equitable partnerships with community advocates and recognize the vast heterogeneity within and across communities, so programs and policies do not exacerbate inequities and instead advance equity. Asian Americans represent the fastest-growing ethnic group in the United States and addressing the social and health inequities this community experiences is an increasingly pressing policy concern. Public health and health care professionals, social service professionals, industry leaders, media and entertainment leaders, and policymakers have a professional and ethical responsibility to directly combat the myriad ways racism undermines health.

REFERENCES

1. Bailey ZD, Krieger N, Agénor M, Graves J, Linos N, Bassett MT. Structural racism and health inequities in the USA: Evidence and interventions. *Lancet*. 2017;389(10077):1453–1463. doi:10.1016/S0140-6736(17)30569-X
2. Gee GC, Ford CL. Structural racism and health inequities: Old issues, new directions. *Du Bois Rev*. 2011;8(1):115–132. doi:10.1017/S1742058X11000130
3. Muramatsu N, Chin MH. Battling structural racism against Asians in the United States: Call for public health to make the "invisible" visible. *J Public Health Manag Pract*. 2022;28(suppl 1):S3–S8. doi:10.1097/PHH.0000000000001411
4. Gee GC, Chien J, Sharif MZ, Penaia C, Tran E. East is east … or is it? Racialization of Asian, Middle Eastern, and Pacific Islander persons. *Epidemiol Rev*. 2023;45(1):93–104. doi:10.1093/epirev/mxad007
5. *Ozawa v United States*, 260 US 178 (1922).
6. *United States v Bhagat Singh Thind*, 261 US 204 (1923).
7. Lee SJ, Wong NWA, Alvarez AN. The model minority and the perpetual foreigner: Stereotypes of Asian Americans. In: Tewari N, Alvarez AN, eds. *Asian American Psychology: Current Perspectives*. Psychology Press; 2009:69–84.
8. Tran AG, Lee RM. You speak English well! Asian Americans' reactions to an exceptionalizing stereotype. *J Couns Psychol*. 2014;61(3):484–490. doi:10.1037/cou0000034
9. Lee E. *America for Americans: A History of Xenophobia in the United States*. Basic Books; 2019.
10. Chalana M. 2021. Whither the "Hindoo Invasion"? South Asians in the Pacific Northwest of the United States, 1907–1930. *Int J Reg Local Hist*. 2021;16(1):14–38. doi:10.1080/20514530.2021.1908719
11. Siu L, Chun C. Yellow Peril and techno-Orientalism in the time of COVID-19: Racialized contagion, scientific espionage, and techno-economic warfare. *J Asian Am Stud*. 2020;23(3):421–440. doi:10.1353/jaas.2020.0033
12. Chou R, Feagin J. *Myth of the Model Minority: Asian Americans Facing Racism*. 2nd ed. Routledge; 2010.
13. Yip T, Cheah CSL, Kiang L, Hall GCN. Rendered invisible: Are Asian Americans a model or a marginalized minority? *Am Psychol*. 2021;76(4):575–581. doi:10.1037/amp0000857
14. Đoàn LN, Takata Y, Sakuma KK, Irvin VL. Trends in clinical research including Asian American, Native Hawaiian, and Pacific Islander Participants funded by the US National Institutes of Health, 1992 to 2018. *JAMA Netw Open*. 2019;2(7):e197432. doi:10.1001/jamanetworkopen.2019.7432

15. Ko M, Ngo V, Zhang AY, Mabeza RM, Hahn M. Asian Americans and Racial Justice in Medicine. *N Engl J Med*. 2024;390(4):372–378. doi:10.1056/NEJMms2307748
16. Wu ED. *The Color of Success: Asian Americans and the Origins of the Model Minority*. Princeton University Press; 2015.
17. Shams T. Successful yet precarious: South Asian Muslim Americans, Islamophobia, and the model minority myth. *Sociol Perspect*. 2020;63(4):653–669. doi:10.1177/0731121419895006
18. Yi SS, Kwon SC, Suss R, et al. The mutually reinforcing cycle of poor data quality and racialized stereotypes that shapes Asian American health. *Health Aff (Millwood)*. 2022;41(2):296–303. doi:10.1377/hlthaff.2021.01417
19. Bever L. Scripps National Spelling Bee draws racially charged comments after Indian Americans win again. *Washington Post*. May 30, 2014. Accessed April 7, 2025. https://www.washingtonpost.com/news/morning-mix/wp/2014/05/30/scripps-national-spelling-bee-draws-racially-charged-comments-after-indian-americans-win-again
20. Hwang WC. Demystifying and addressing internalized racism and oppression among Asian Americans. *Am Psychol*. 2021;76(4):596–610. doi:10.1037/amp0000798
21. Yi J, Todd NR. Internalized model minority myth among Asian Americans: Links to anti-Black attitudes and opposition to affirmative action. *Cultur Divers Ethnic Minor Psychol*. 2021;27(4):569–578. doi:10.1037/cdp0000448
22. US Census Bureau. 2019 American Community Survey single-year estimates. September 17, 2020. Accessed August 11, 2025. https://www.census.gov/newsroom/press-kits/2020/acs-1year.html
23. Adia AC, Nazareno J, Operario D, Ponce N. Health conditions, outcomes, and service access among Filipino, Vietnamese, Chinese, Japanese, and Korean adults in California, 2011–2017. *Am J Public Health*. 2020;110(4):520–526. doi:10.2105/AJPH.2019.305523
24. Kula SM, Tran VQ, Garcia I, Saito E, Paik SJ. Vietnamese Americans: History, education, and societal context. *J Southeast Asian Am Educ Adv*. 2021;16(1):14. doi:10.7771/2153-8999.1201
25. Meyer OL, Park VT, Kanaya AM, et al. Inclusion of Vietnamese Americans: Opportunities to understand dementia disparities. *Alzheimers Dement (NY)*. 2023;9(2):e12392. doi:10.1002/trc2.12392
26. Muramatsu N, Chin MH. Asian, Native Hawaiian, and Pacific Islander Populations in the US—Moving from invisibility to health equity. *JAMA Netw Open*. 2024;7(5):e2411617. doi:10.1001/jamanetworkopen.2024.11617
27. Datar S. Asian Americans are often invisible in polling. That's changing. *The New York Times*. February 24, 2024. Accessed April 7, 2025. https://www.nytimes.com/2024/02/24/us/asian-americans-polling.html
28. Budiman A. Asian Americans are the fastest-growing racial or ethnic group in the US electorate. Pew Research Center blog. May 7, 2020. Accessed April 7, 2025. https://www.pewresearch.org/short-reads/2020/05/07/asian-americans-are-the-fastest-growing-racial-or-ethnic-group-in-the-u-s-electorate
29. Gee GC, Hicken MT. Structural racism: The rules and relations of inequity. *Ethn Dis*. 2021;31(suppl 1):293–300. doi:10.18865/ed.31.S1.293
30. LaPiere RT. Attitudes versus actions. *Soc Forces*. 1934;13(2):230–237. doi:10.2307/2570339

31. Streltzer J, Wade TC. The influence of cultural group on the undertreatment of postoperative pain. *Psychosom Med.* 1981;43(5):397–403. doi:10.1097/00006842-198110000-00002
32. Lee C. Beyond toxic wastes and race. In: Bullard RD, ed. *Confronting Environmental Racism: Voices from the Grassroots*. South End Press; 1993:41–52.
33. Noh S, Beiser M, Kaspar V, Hou F, Rummens J. Perceived racial discrimination, depression, and coping: A study of Southeast Asian refugees in Canada. *J Health Soc Behav.* 1999;40(3):193–207. doi:10.2307/2676348
34. Gee GC, Ro A, Shariff-Marco S, Chae D. Racial discrimination and health among Asian Americans: evidence, assessment, and directions for future research. *Epidemiol Rev.* 2009;31:130–151. doi:10.1093/epirev/mxp009
35. Nadimpalli SB, Hutchinson MK. An integrative review of relationships between discrimination and Asian American health. *J Nurs Scholarsh.* 2012;44(2):127–135. doi:10.1111/j.1547-5069.2012.01448.x
36. Forbes N, Yang LC, Lim S. Intersectional discrimination and its impact on Asian American women's mental health: A mixed-methods scoping review. *Front Public Health.* 2023;11:993396. doi:10.3389/fpubh.2023.993396
37. Kim HJ, Park E, Storr CL, Tran K, Juon HS. Depression among Asian-American adults in the community: Systematic review and meta-analysis. *PLoS One.* 2015;10(6):e0127760. doi:10.1371/journal.pone.0127760
38. Raman P, Chu CT, Chong SK, Mukherjea A, Kue J. Assessing structural racism measures on health outcomes of Asian Americans, Native Hawaiians, and Pacific Islanders: A scoping review. *J Racial Ethn Health Disparities.* doi:10.1007/s40615-024-01987-1
39. Wang J, Vela MB, Chin MH. Addressing bias and racism against Asian American, Native Hawaiian, and Pacific Islander individuals: A call to action to advance health equity and leadership. *JAMA Netw Open.* 2023;6(7):e2325872. doi:10.1001/jamanetworkopen.2023.25872
40. Lee JP, Lee RM, Hu AW, Kim OM. Ethnic identity as a moderator against discrimination for transracially and transnationally adopted Korean American adolescents. *Asian Am J Psychol.* 2015;6(2):154–163. doi:10.1037/a0038360
41. Sudhinaraset M, To TM, Ling I, Melo J, Chavarin J. The influence of Deferred Action for Childhood Arrivals on undocumented Asian and Pacific Islander young adults: Through a social determinants of health lens. *J Adolesc Health.* 2017;60(6):741–746. doi:10.1016/j.jadohealth.2017.01.008
42. Jenkins A. Racial equity and US law. *Health Equity.* 2023;7(1):61–69. doi:10.1089/heq.2022.29022.aje
43. Chang GH. *Ghosts of Gold Mountain: The Epic Story of the Chinese Who Built the Transcontinental Railroad*. Mariner Books; 2019.
44. National Park Service. A Legacy from the Far East. US Dept of the Interior. Accessed April 30, 2025. https://web.archive.org/web/20220803033022/https://www.nps.gov/gosp/learn/historyculture/a-legacy-from-the-far-east.htm
45. Espiritu YL. *Asian American Women and Men: Labor, Laws, and Love*. Sage Publications; 1997.
46. Pfaelzer J. *Driven Out: The Forgotten War Against Chinese*. University of California Press; 2008.
47. Lew-Williams B. *The Chinese Must Go: Violence, Exclusion, and the Making of the Alien in America*. Havard University Press; 2021.

48. Jung J. *Chinese Laundries: Tickets to Survival on Gold Mountain*. Yin and Yang Press; 2007.
49. *People v Hall*, 4 Cal 399 (1854).
50. *Yick Wo v Hopkins*, 118 US 356 (1888).
51. Yiu M. COVID-19 is a "yellow peril" redux: Immigration and health policy and the construction of the Chinese as disease. *Asian Am Res J*. 2022;2. doi:10.5070/RJ42057359
52. Hing BO. *Making and Remaking Asian America Through Immigration Policy, 1850-1990*. Stanford University Press; 1993.
53. National Archives. Japanese-American incarceration during World War II. August 15, 2016. Accessed April 7, 2025. https://www.archives.gov/education/lessons/japanese-relocation
54. *Hirabayashi v United States*, 320 US 81 (1943).
55. *Yasui v United States*, 320 US 115 (1943).
56. *Korematsu v United States*, 323 US 214 (1944).
57. Office of Art and Archives, US House of Representatives. Long road to redress. Accessed May 27, 2023. https://history.house.gov/Exhibitions-and-Publications/APA/Historical-Essays/Exclusion-to-Inclusion/Redress
58. South Asian Americans Leading Together. Profiling and immigration in a post-9/11 world. March 2010. Accessed April 8, 2025. https://saalt.org/wp-content/uploads/2012/09/SAALT-Issue-Briefs-Immigration-March-2010.pdf
59. von Werthern M, Robjant K, Chui Z, et al. The impact of immigration detention on mental health: A systematic review. *BMC Psychiatry*. 2018;18(1):382. doi:10.1186/s12888-018-1945-y
60. Hampton K, Mishori R, Griffin M, Hillier C, Pirrotta E, Wang NE. Clinicians' perceptions of the health status of formerly detained immigrants. *BMC Public Health*. 2022;22(1):575. doi:10.1186/s12889-022-12967-7
61. Iyer D. *We Too Sing America: South Asian, Arab, Muslim, and Sikh Immigrants Shape Our Multiracial Future*. The New Press; 2017.
62. Sekhon V. The civil rights of "others": Antiterrorism, the Patriot Act, and Arab and South Asian American rights in post-9/11 American society. *Texas Forum Civ Lib Civ Rights*. 2003;8(1):117–148. Accessed April 8, 2025. https://sites.utexas.edu/tjclcr/files/2022/11/Sekhon_The-Civil-Rights-of-Others.pdf
63. New York City Profiling Collaborative, Desis Rising Up and Moving (DRUM), The Sikh Coalition, United Sikhs, South Asian Youth Action (SAYA!), Coney Island Avenue Project, Council of Peoples Organization, South Asian Americans Leading Together. *In Our Own Words: Narratives of South Asian New Yorkers Affected by Racial and Religious Profiling*. March 2012. Accessed April 7, 2025. https://saalt.org/wp-content/uploads/2012/09/In-Our-Own-Words-Narratives-of-South-Asian-New-Yorkers-Affected-by-Racial-and-Religious-Profiling.pdf
64. Goode E, Kovaleski SF. Wisconsin killer fed and was fueled by hate-driven music. *The New York Times*. August 6, 2012. Accessed April 7, 2025. https://www.nytimes.com/2012/08/07/us/army-veteran-identified-as-suspect-in-wisconsin-shooting.html
65. US Dept of State. Annual report of immigrant visa applicants in the family-sponsored and employment-based preferences registered at the National Visa Center as of November 1, 2023. 2023. Accessed April 2, 2025. https://travel.state.gov/content/dam/visas/Statistics/Immigrant-Statistics/WaitingList/WaitingListItem_2023_vF.pdf

66. Bureau of Consular Affairs. Visa bulletin: Immigrant numbers for June 2024. US Dept of State. June 2024. Accessed April 8, 2025. https://travel.state.gov/content/dam/visas/Bulletins/visabulletin_June2024.pdf
67. Yeung P. "Disillusioned about China," more Chinese aim for US via risky Darien Gap. *Al Jazeera*. February 22, 2024. Accessed April 8, 2025. https://www.aljazeera.com/economy/2024/2/22/disillusioned-about-china-more-chinese-aim-for-us-via-risky-darien-gap
68. Palmer J. Why are more Chinese migrants arriving at the US southern border? *Foreign Policy*. June 28, 2024. Accessed April 8, 2025. https://foreignpolicy.com/2024/05/07/china-us-southern-border-migration-darien-gap
69. National Immigration Forum. Eliminating the naturalization backlog. May 11, 2023. Accessed April 7, 2025. https://immigrationforum.org/article/eliminating-the-naturalization-backlog
70. Wong JS, Ramakrishnan K. Asian Americans and the politics of the twenty-first century. *Annu Rev Polit Sci*. 2023;26(1):305–323. doi:10.1146/annurev-polisci-070621-032538
71. Enjeti A. Reckoning with Georgia's increasing suppression of Asian American voters. *Longreads*. December 19, 2018. Accessed April 7, 2025. http://longreads.com/2018/12/19/reckoning-with-georgias-increasing-suppression-of-asian-american-voters
72. Alexander A. Voter outreach groups targeted by new laws in several GOP-led states are struggling to do their work. *AP News*. May 28, 2024. Accessed April 2, 2025. https://apnews.com/article/voting-rights-outreach-republican-states-new-laws-70e034dd46baf474998259a2b737c096
73. Samuels EA, Orr L, White EB, et al. Health care utilization before and after the "Muslim ban" executive order among people born in Muslim-majority countries and living in the US. *JAMA Netw Open*. 2021;4(7):e2118216. doi:10.1001/jamanetworkopen.2021.18216
74. Morey BN, Bacong AM, Hing AK, de Castro AB, Gee GC. Heterogeneity in migrant health selection: The role of immigrant visas. *J Health Soc Behav*. 2020;61(3):359–376. doi:10.1177/0022146520942896
75. Vang C, Sun F, Sangalang CC. Mental health among the Hmong population in the US: A systematic review of the influence of cultural and social factors. *J Soc Work*. 2021;21(4):811–830. doi:10.1177/1468017320940644.
76. Muhammad DA, Kurani M. Racial wealth snapshot: Asian Americans and the racial wealth divide. National Community Reinvestment Commission. August 23, 2023. Accessed April 8, 2025. https://www.ncrc.org/racial-wealth-snapshot-asian-americans-and-the-racial-wealth-divide-2023
77. Kochhar R, Moslimani M. 3. How wealth and wealth gaps vary by income. Pew Research Center. December 4, 2023. Accessed April 8, 2025. https://www.pewresearch.org/2023/12/04/how-wealth-and-wealth-gaps-vary-by-income
78. Park H, Choi E, Wenzel JA. Racial/ethnic differences in correlates of psychological distress among five Asian-American subgroups and non-Hispanic Whites. *Ethn Health*. 2020;25(8):1072–1088. doi:10.1080/13557858.2018.1481495
79. Ong PM, Lucie C, Evans L. Migration of highly educated Asians and global dynamics. *Asian Pac Migration J*. 1992;1(3–4):543–567. doi:10.1177/011719689200100307.
80. Lee J, Zhou M. *The Asian American Achievement Paradox*. Russel Sage Foundation; 2015.
81. Rumbaut RG. The structure of refuge: Southeast Asian refugees in the United States, 1975–1985. *Int Rev Comp Public Policy*. 1989;1:97–129. Accessed April 8, 2025. https://papers.ssrn.com/abstract=1886685

82. Bach R, Bach JB. Employment patterns of Southeast Asian refugees. *Mon Labor Rev.* 1980;103(10):31–38. Accessed April 30, 2025. https://fraser.stlouisfed.org/title/monthly-labor-review-6130/october-1980-611406?page=33
83. Portes A, Zhou M. The new second generation: Segmented assimilation and its variants. *Ann Am Acad Pol Soc Sci.* 1993;530:74–96. doi:10.1177/0002716293530001006
84. Ward N, Batalova J. Refugees and asylees in the United States. Migration Policy Institute. June 15, 2023. Accessed April 8, 2025. https://www.migrationpolicy.org/article/refugees-and-asylees-united-states
85. Jackson M. 2022. Neo-colonialism, same old racism: A critical analysis of the United States' shift toward colorblindness as a tool for the protection of the American colonial empire and white supremacy. *Berkeley J Af Am Law Policy.* 2022;11(1):156–192. Accessed April 7, 2025. https://ssrn.com/abstract=3699715
86. Ngô FIB, Nguyen MT, Lam MB. Southeast Asian American Studies special issue: Guest editors' introduction. *Positions.* 2012;20(3):671–684. doi:10.1215/10679847-1593492
87. Bozorgmehr M. From Iranian studies to studies of Iranians in the United States. *Iran Stud.* 1998;31(1):5–30. Accessed April 7, 2025. https://www.jstor.org/stable/4311116
88. Stanley WD. Economic migrants or refugees from violence?: A time-series analysis of Salvadoran migration to the United States. *Latin Am Res Rev.* 1987;22(1):132–154. doi:10.1017/S0023879100016459
89. Greenwood MJ, Hunt GL, Rickman DS, Treyz GI. Migration, regional equilibrium, and the estimation of compensating differentials. *Am Econ Rev.* 1991;81(5):1382–1390. Accessed April 7, 2025. https://www.jstor.org/stable/2006927
90. Ong P, Ong E, Ong J. The future of Pacific Islander America in 2040. *AAPI Nexus J.* 2016;14(1):1–13. doi:10.17953/nx.014.01.1
91. Beine M, Docquier F, Rapoport H. Brain drain and human capital formation in developing countries: Winners and losers. *Econ J.* 2008;118(528):631–652. doi:10.1111/j.1468-0297.2008.02135.x
92. Tian Z, Ruiz NG. Key facts about Asian Americans living in poverty. Pew Research Center. March 27, 2024. Accessed April 8, 2025. https://www.pewresearch.org/short-reads/2024/03/27/key-facts-about-asian-americans-living-in-poverty
93. Patraporn, RV, Ong PM, Houston D. Closing the Asian-White wealth gap? *Asian Am Policy Rev.* 2009;18(January):35–49. Accessed August 10, 2025. https://www.academia.edu/10327739/Closing_the_Asian_White_Wealth_Gap
94. Patraporn RV, Ong PM, Pech C. Wealth inequality among Asian Americans: The continuing significance of ethnicity and immigration. *Asian Am Policy Rev.* 2021;31(1):43–56. Accessed April 8, 2025. https://studentreview.hks.harvard.edu/wealth-inequality-among-asian-americans-the-continuing-significance-of-ethnicity-and-immigration
95. Kochhar R, Moslimani M. 2. Wealth gaps across racial and ethnic groups. Pew Research Center. December 4, 2023. Accessed April 8, 2025. https://www.pewresearch.org/2023/12/04/wealth-gaps-across-racial-and-ethnic-groups
96. Aladangady A, Chang AC, Krimmel J, Ma E. Greater wealth, greater uncertainty: Changes in racial inequality in the survey of consumer finance. FEDS Notes. Board of Governors of the Federal Reserve System. October 18, 2023. Accessed April 2, 2025. https://www.federalreserve.gov/econres/notes/feds-notes/greater-wealth-greater-uncertainty-changes-in-racial-inequality-in-the-survey-of-consumer-finances-20231018.html

97. Cheng A, Ong PM, de La Cruz-Viesca M. Revisiting works on Asian American wealth and inequality through graphics. *AAPI Nexus J*. 2016;14(2):129–134. doi:10.36650/nexus14.2_129-134_ChengEtAl
98. de La Cruz-Viesca M, Chen Z, Ong P, Hamilton D, Darity W. *The Color of Wealth in Los Angeles*. Duke University Research Network on Racial and Ethnic Inequality; The Milano School of International Affairs, Management and Urban Policy at The New School; UCLA Asian American Studies Center; 2016. Accessed April 7, 2025. https://www.aasc.ucla.edu/besol/Color_of_Wealth_Report.pdf
99. Nguyen TN, Chen S, Chan K, Nguyen MT, Hinton L. Cognitive functioning and nail salon occupational exposure among Vietnamese immigrant women in northern California. *Int J Environ Res Public Health*. 2022;19(8):4634. doi:10.3390/ijerph19084634
100. Bacong AM, Chu R, Le A, Bui V, Wang NE, Palaniappan LP. Increased COVID-19 mortality among immigrants compared with US-born individuals: A cross-sectional analysis of 2020 mortality data. *Public Health*. 2024;231:173–178. doi:10.1016/j.puhe.2024.03.016
101. Escobedo LA, Morey BN, Sabado-Liwag MD, Ponce NA. 2022. Lost on the frontline, and lost in the data: COVID-19 deaths among Filipinx healthcare workers in the United States. *Front Public Health*. 2022;10:958530. doi:10.3389/fpubh.2022.958530.
102. Walton E, Takeuchi DT, Herting JR, Alegría M. Does place of education matter? Contextualizing the education and health status association among Asian Americans. *Biodemography Soc Biol*. 2009;55(1):30–51. doi:10.1080/19485560903054648
103. Pettersen W. Success story, Japanese-American Style. *The New York Times*. January 9, 1966. Accessed April 8, 2025. https://www.nytimes.com/1966/01/09/archives/success-story-japaneseamerican-style-success-story-japaneseamerican.html
104. Michaels EK, Lam-Hine T, Nguyen TT, Gee GC, Allen AM. The water surrounding the iceberg: Cultural racism and health inequities. *Milbank Q*. 2023;101(3):768–814. doi:10.1111/1468-0009.12662
105. American Medical Association, Association of American Medical Colleges. Advancing health equity: A guide to language, narrative and concepts. Accessed April 2, 2025. https://www.ama-assn.org/about/ama-center-health-equity/advancing-health-equity-guide-language-narrative-and-concepts-0
106. McElhaney KB, Antonishak J, Allen JP. "They like me, they like me not": Popularity and adolescents' perceptions of acceptance predicting social functioning over time. *Child Dev*. 2008;79(3):720–731. doi:10.1111/j.1467-8624.2008.01153.x
107. Zhang Q. Asian Americans beyond the model minority stereotype: The nerdy and the left out. *J Int Intercult Commun*. 2010;3(1):20–37. doi:10.1080/17513050903428109
108. Siy JO, Cheryan S. Prejudice masquerading as praise: The negative echo of positive stereotypes. *Pers Soc Psychol Bull*. 2016;42(7):941–954. doi:10.1177/0146167216649605
109. Xie M, Fowle J, Ip PS, Haskin M, Yip T. Profiles of ethnic-racial identity, socialization, and model minority experiences: Associations with well-being among Asian American adolescents. *J Youth Adolesc*. 2021;50(6):1173–1188. doi:10.1007/s10964-021-01436-w
110. Santos PMG, Dee EC, Deville C Jr. Confronting Anti-Asian racism and health disparities in the era of COVID-19. *JAMA Health Forum*. 2021;2(9):e212579. doi:10.1001/jamahealthforum.2021.2579

111. Misra S, Kwon SC, Abraído-Lanza AF, Chebli P, Trinh-Shevrin C, Yi SS. Structural racism and immigrant health in the United States. *Health Educ Behav*. 2021;48(3):332–341. doi:10.1177/10901981211010676
112. Sharif MZ, García JJ, Mitchell U, Dellor ED, Bradford NJ, Truong M. Racism and structural violence: Interconnected threats to health equity. *Front Public Health*. 2022;9:676783. doi:10.3389/fpubh.2021.676783
113. Yuen NW, Smith SL, Pieper K, Choueiti M, Yao K, Dinh D. The prevalence and portrayal of Asian and Pacific Islanders across 1,300 popular films. USC Annenberg Inclusion Initiative. 2021. Accessed April 8, 2025. https://assets.uscannenberg.org/docs/aii_aapi-representation-across-films-2021-05-18.pdf
114. Yuen NW. *Reel Inequality: Hollywood Actors and Racism*. Rutgers University Press; 2017.
115. Ono K, Pham V. *Asian Americans and the Media*. Polity Press; 2009.
116. Alsultany E. *Arabs and Muslims in the Media: Race and Representation After 9/11*. New York University Press; 2012.
117. Kim NY. *Refusing Death: Immigrant Women and the Fight for Environmental Justice in LA*. Stanford University Press; 2021.
118. Saraswati LA. *Pain Generation: Social Media, Feminist Activism, and the Neoliberal Selfie*. New York University Press; 2021.
119. Lee JJ, Lee J. #StopAsianHate on TikTok: Asian/American women's space-making for spearheading counter-narratives and forming an ad hoc Asian community. *Soc Media Soc*. 2023;9(1). doi:10.1177/20563051231157598
120. Josey C, Riles JM, Cen X. Making the model: How news media perpetuate harmful model minority stereotypes of Asian Americans. In: Dixon TL, Mastro D, eds. *US Media and Diversity: Representation, Dissemination, and Effects*. Routledge; 2024;21–41.
121. Walker D, Anders AD. "China Virus" and "Kung-Flu": A critical race case study of Asian American journalists' experiences during COVID-19. *Cult Stud Crit Methodol*. 2022;22(1):76–88. doi:10.1177/15327086211055157
122. Oh DC, Min SJ. *Navigating White News: Asian American Journalists at Work*. Rutgers University Press; 2023.
123. Long H, van Dam A, Fowers A, Shapiro L. The covid-19 recession is the most unequal in modern US history." *Washington Post*. September 30, 2020. Accessed April 8, 2025. https://www.washingtonpost.com/graphics/2020/business/coronavirus-recession-equality
124. Li Y, Nicholson HL Jr. When "model minorities" become "yellow peril"—Othering and the racialization of Asian Americans in the COVID-19 pandemic. *Sociol Compass*. 2021;15(2):e12849. doi:10.1111/soc4.12849
125. Campanile C, Hogan B. First case of coronavirus confirmed in New York City. *New York Post*. March 1, 2020. Accessed April 7, 2025. https://nypost.com/2020/03/01/first-case-of-coronavirus-confirmed-in-manhattan
126. Gee GC, Ro MJ, Rimoin AW. Seven reasons to care about racism and COVID-19 and seven things to do to stop it. *Am J Public Health*. 2020;110(7):954–955. doi:10.2105/AJPH.2020.305712
127. Eng D. *Racial Castration: Managing Masculinity in Asian America*. Duke University Press; 2001.
128. Shah N. *Contagious Divides: Epidemics and Race in San Francisco's Chinatown*. University of California Press; 2021.

129. Mallapragada M. Asian Americans as racial contagion. *Cult Stud*. 2021;35(2–3):279–290. doi:10.1080/09502386.2021.1905678.
130. Pillai D, Ndugga N, Artiga S. Health care disparities among Asian, Native Hawaiian, and other Pacific Islander (NHOPI) people. KFF. May 24, 2023. Accessed April 8, 2025. https://www.kff.org/racial-equity-and-health-policy/issue-brief/health-care-disparities-among-asian-native-hawaiian-and-other-pacific-islander-nhopi-people
131. Ramakrishnan K, Shah S. One out of every 7 Asian immigrants is undocumented. *AAPI Data* blog. September 8, 2017. Accessed April 8, 2025. https://aapidata.com/blog/asian-undoc-1in7
132. Kaiser Family Foundation. Key facts on health coverage of immigrants. January 15, 2025. Updated June 2, 2025. Accessed August 10, 2025. https://www.kff.org/racial-equity-and-health-policy/fact-sheet/key-facts-on-health-coverage-of-immigrants
133. Shastri D. Migrants in cities across the US may need medical care. It's not that easy to find. *AP News*. November 2, 2023. Accessed April 8, 2025. https://apnews.com/article/immigration-migrants-border-health-care-us-mexico-79353b08f07933f66961a7f07cf3e397
134. Institute of Medicine Committee on Health Insurance Status and Its Consequences. *America's Uninsured Crisis: Consequences for Health and Health Care*. National Academies Press; 2009.
135. Pear R. Trump officials slash grants that help consumers get Obamacare. *The New York Times*. July 10, 2018. Accessed April 8, 2025. https://www.nytimes.com/2018/07/10/us/politics/trump-affordable-care-act.html
136. Myerson R, Li H. Information gaps and health insurance enrollment: Evidence from the Affordable Care Act navigator programs. *Am J Health Econ*. 2022;8(4):477–505. doi:10.1086/721569
137. Huynh N. Public charge: An injustice and its chilling effects on AAPI and low-income communities. *Asian American Policy Review* blog. Harvard University. October 4, 2020. Accessed April 7, 2025. https://studentreview.hks.harvard.edu/public-charge-an-injustice-and-its-chilling-effects-on-aapi-and-low-income-communities
138. Green AR, Ngo-Metzger Q, Legedza AT, Massagli MP, Phillips RS, Iezzoni LI. Interpreter services, language concordance, and health care quality. Experiences of Asian Americans with limited English proficiency. *J Gen Intern Med*. 2005;20(11):1050–1056. doi:10.1111/j.1525-1497.2005.0223.x
139. Haley JM, Zuckerman S, Rao N, Karpman M, Stern A. Many Asian American and Native Hawaiian/Pacific Islander adults may face health care access challenges related to limited English proficiency. Urban Institute. December 2022. Accessed April 7, 2025. https://www.urban.org/research/publication/many-asian-american-and-native-hawaiianpacific-islander-adults-may-face-health
140. Kim SB, Lee YJ. Factors associated with mental health help-seeking among Asian Americans: A systematic review. *J Racial Ethn Health Disparities*. 2022;9(4):1276–1297. doi:10.1007/s40615-021-01068-7
141. Than V, Doroud N, O'Brien L. Mental health service utilization and help seeking behaviours of adult Cambodians living in Western countries: A systematic scoping review. *Int J Soc Psychiatry*. 2024;70(4):778–791. doi:10.1177/00207640241230848
142. Weng SS, Spaulding-Givens J. Strategies for working with Asian Americans in mental health: Community members' policy perspectives and recommendations. *Adm Policy Ment Health*. 2017;44(5):771–781. doi:10.1007/s10488-016-0784-8
143. Fadiman A. *The Spirit Catches You and You Fall Down: A Hmong Child, Her American Doctors, and the Collision of Two Cultures*. Farrar, Straus and Giroux; 1997.

144. Jang Y, Kim MT. Limited English proficiency and health service use in Asian Americans. *J Immigr Minor Health.* 2019;21(2):264–270. doi:10.1007/s10903-018-0763-0
145. Office of Minority Health. Mental and behavioral health—Asian Americans. US Dept of Health and Human Services. 2021. Accessed April 30, 2025. https://minorityhealth.hhs.gov/mental-and-behavioral-health-asian-americans
146. Lee TH, Volpp KG, Cheung VG, Dzau VJ. Diversity and inclusiveness in health care leadership: Three key steps. *NEJM Catalyst.* 2021;2(3). doi:10.1056/CAT.21.0166
147. Dzau VJ, Lee TH. Conversation: Confronting racial disparities in C-suite health care leadership. *NEJM Catalyst.* December 17, 2021. doi:10.1056/CAT.21.0449
148. Berwick DM. Salve lucrum: The existential threat of greed in US health care. *JAMA* 2023;329(8):629–630. doi:10.1001/jama.2023.0846.
149. Chin MH. Uncomfortable truths—What Covid-19 has revealed about chronic-disease care in America. *N Engl J Med.* 2021;385(18):1633–1636. doi:10.1056/NEJMp2112063
150. Health Care Payment Learning & Action Network Health Equity Advisory Team. Advancing health equity through APMs: Guidance for equity-centered design and implementation. 2021. Accessed August 5, 2025. https://hcp-lan.org/workproducts/APM-Guidance/Advancing-Health-Equity-Through-APMs.pdf
151. Health Care Payment Learning & Action Network Health Equity Advisory Team. Guidance for health care entities partnering with community-based organizations: Addressing health-related social needs in alternative payment models. 2023. Accessed August 5, 2025. https://hcp-lan.org/workproducts/APM-Guidance/HEAT-CBO-Partnership-Guidance.pdf
152. Health Care Payment Learning & Action Network Health Equity Advisory Team. Value of health care redefined: Social return on investment. 2024. Accessed August 5, 2025. https://hcp-lan.org/wp-content/uploads/2024/11/HCPLAN-Social-ROI-Publication_vFinal.pdf
153. Cook SC, Todić J, Spitzer S, et al. Opportunities for psychologists to advance health equity: Using liberation psychology to identify key lessons from 17 years of praxis. *Am Psychol.* 2023;78(2):211–226. doi:10.1037/amp0001126
154. Singletary KA, Chin MH. What should antiracist payment reform look like?. *AMA J Ethics.* 2023;25(1):E55–E65. doi:10.1001/amajethics.2023.55
155. Ommerborn MJ, Ranker LR, Touw S, Himmelstein DU, Himmelstein J, Woolhandler S. Assessment of immigrants' premium and tax payments for health care and the costs of their care. *JAMA Netw Open.* 2022;5(11):e2241166. doi:10.1001/jamanetworkopen.2022.41166
156. Ku L. Who pays for immigrants' health care in the US?. *JAMA Netw Open.* 2022;5(11):e2241171. doi:10.1001/jamanetworkopen.2022.41171
157. Kilty KM. Race, immigration, and public policy: The case of Asian Americans. *J Poverty.* 2002;6(4):23–41. doi:10.1300/J134v06n04_03
158. Abel EK. 'Only the best class of immigration': Public health policy toward Mexicans and Filipinos in Los Angeles, 1910–1940. *Am J Public Health.* 2004;94(6):932–939. doi:10.2105/ajph.94.6.932
159. Takaki RT. *Strangers from a Different Shore: A History of Asian Americans.* Rev ed. eBookIt.com; 2012.
160. Hswen Y, Xu X, Hing A, Hawkins JB, Brownstein JS, Gee GC. Association of "#covid19" versus "#chinesevirus" with Anti-Asian sentiments on Twitter: March 9–23, 2020. *Am J Public Health.* 2021;111(5):956–964. doi:10.2105/AJPH.2021.306154

161. Darling-Hammond S, Michaels EK, Allen AM, et al. After "The China Virus" went viral: Racially charged coronavirus coverage and trends in bias against Asian Americans. *Health Educ Behav.* 2020;47(6):870–879. doi:10.1177/1090198120957949
162. Nguyen TT, Criss S, Dwivedi P, et al. Exploring US shifts in Anti-Asian sentiment with the emergence of COVID-19. *Int J Environ Res Public Health.* 2020;17(19):7032. doi:10.3390/ijerph17197032
163. Bullard RD, Mohai P, Saha R, Wright B. Toxic wastes and race at twenty: Why race still matters after all of these years. *Environ Law.* 2008;38(2):371–411. Accessed April 7, 2025. https://www.jstor.org/stable/43267204
164. Pellow D, Park LS. *Silicon Valley of Dreams: Immigrant Labor, Environmental Injustice, and the High-Tech Global Economy.* New York University Press; 2002.
165. Gordon L, Payne-Sturges D, Gee G. Environmental health disparities: Select case studies related to Asian and Pacific Islander Americans. *Environ Justice.* 2010;3(1):21–26. doi:10.1089/env.2009.0019
166. Chen M, Bacong AM, Feng C, et al. Asthma heterogeneity among Asian American children: The California Health Interview Survey. *Ann Allergy Asthma Immunol.* 2023;132(3):368–373.e2. doi:10.1016/j.anai.2023.10.030
167. Acoba J, Chen SA, Miller CF, Okazaki I. Understanding & improving lung cancer treatment in Asian Americans & Pacific Islanders in the community setting. Association of Community Cancer Centers. 2016. Accessed April 2, 2025. https://www.accc-cancer.org/docs/projects/pdf/LungCancerTools/aapi-whitepaper
168. Becerra BJ, Scroggins CM, Becerra MB. 2014. Association between asthma and obesity among immigrant Asian Americans, California Health Interview Survey, 2001–2011. *Prev Chronic Dis.* 2014;11:140333. doi:10.5888/pcd11.140333
169. Yang Z, Song Q, Li J, Zhang Y. Air pollution as a cause of obesity: Micro-level evidence from Chinese cities. *Int J Environ Res Public Health.* 2019;16(21):4296. doi:10.3390/ijerph16214296
170. Flores K. Long Beach is addicted to fossil fuel money: Schools. *FORTHE.* March 21, 2022. Accessed April 7, 2025. https://forthe.org/journalism/long-beach-is-addicted-to-fossil-fuel-money-schools
171. Robinson CJ. *Cedric J. Robinson: On Racial Capitalism, Black Internationalism, and Cultures of Resistance.* Pluto Press; 2019.
172. Suzara A. Reflections: A Filipina's perspective. *Race Poverty Environ.* 2003;10(1):18. Accessed April 8, 2025. https://www.jstor.org/stable/41554363
173. Hill JJ. The overlooked tragedy of the pandemic: How media coverage of the COVID-19 pandemic has led to an increase in anti-Asian bias and xenophobia. *Asian Pac Am Law J.* 2021;25(1):125–143. doi:10.5070/P325157463
174. Ong P, Cheng A, Ong J. Asian American businesses: The impacts of anti-Asian racism, 2021. UCLA Center for Neighborhood Knowledge. November 2021. Accessed April 8, 2025. https://escholarship.org/uc/item/1x62v28m
175. Ong P, Comandom A, DiRago N, Harper L. COVID-19 impacts on minority businesses and systemic inequality. UCLA: Center for Neighborhood Knowledge. October 2020. Accessed April 8, 2025. https://escholarship.org/uc/item/5jz7c4vd
176. Huang JT, Krupenkin M, Rothschild D, Lee Cunningham J. The cost of anti-Asian racism during the COVID-19 pandemic. *Nat Hum Behav.* 2023;7(5):682–695. doi:10.1038/s41562-022-01493-6

177. de Mena C, Zhang J, Qin S. The labor market impact of Covid-19 on Asian Americans. *Econ Persp.* 2024;February(1). Accessed April 30, 2025. https://www.chicagofed.org/publications/economic-perspectives/2024/1
178. Ong P, Pech C, Medrano D. COVID-19 pandemic employment impacts on Asian Americans. UCLA Asian American Studies Center. February 2023. Accessed April 8, 2025. https://www.aasc.ucla.edu/aapipolicy/reports_feb10/ong-pech-medrano_report.pdf
179. Oberg C, Hodges HR, Gander S, Nathawad R, Cutts D. The impact of COVID-19 on children's lives in the United States: Amplified inequities and a just path to recovery. *Curr Probl Pediatr Adolesc Health Care.* 2022;52(7):101181. doi:10.1016/j.cppeds.2022.101181
180. Ong P, Pech C. COVID-19 pandemic impacts on Asian American housing. UCLA Asian American Studies Center. February 2023. Accessed April 8, 2025. https://www.aasc.ucla.edu/aapipolicy/reports_feb10/Ong-Pech_report.pdf
181. Cainkar L, Maira S. Targeting Arab/Muslim/South Asian Americans: Criminalization and cultural citizenship. *Amerasia J.* 2005;31(3):1–28. doi:10.17953/amer.31.3.9914804357124877
182. Bathija P. Advocating for the Asian American community during the COVID-19 pandemic and beyond. American Hospital Association blog. May 24, 2021. Accessed April 7, 2025. https://www.aha.org/news/blog/2021-05-24-advocating-asian-american-community-during-covid-19-pandemic-and-beyond
183. Yellow Horse AJ, Chen T, Bhalla K, Choi C, Finkle C. Two years and thousands of voices: What community-generated data tells us about anti-AAPI hate. Stop AAPI Hate. 2022. Accessed April 8, 2025. https://stopaapihate.org/wp-content/uploads/2022/07/Stop-AAPI-Hate-Year-2-Report.pdf
184. Jeung R, Yellow Horse A, Chen T, et al. Anti-Asian hate, social isolation, and mental health among Asian American elders during COVID-19. STOP AAPI Hate. May 2022. Accessed April 7, 2025. https://stopaapihate.org/wp-content/uploads/2022/05/SAH-Elder-Report-526.pdf
185. Li L, Kang J, Ho M, et al. Anti-Asian hate and the health of older Asian individuals. *JAMA Intern Med.* 2024;184(7):838–840. doi:10.1001/jamainternmed.2024.1090
186. Jeung R, Yellow Horse A, Lau A, et al. Stop AAPI hate youth report. Stop AAPI Hate. 2021. Accessed April 8, 2025. https://stopaapihate.org/wp-content/uploads/2021/04/Stop-AAPI-Hate-Report-Youth-Incidents-200917.pdf
187. Patchin JW, Hinduja S. Cyberbullying among Asian American youth before and during the COVID-19 pandemic. *J Sch Health.* 2023;93(1):82–87. doi:10.1111/josh.13249
188. Yam K. Anti-Asian hate crimes increased 339 percent nationwide last year, report says. *NBC News.* January 31, 2022. Updated February 14, 2022. Accessed April 8, 2025. https://www.nbcnews.com/news/asian-america/anti-asian-hate-crimes-increased-339-percent-nationwide-last-year-repo-rcna14282
189. Lu Y, Baumler E, Wood L, Le VD, Guillot-Wright SP, Temple JR. Racial discrimination and interpersonal violence in Asian American adolescents during the COVID-19 pandemic. *J Adolesc Health.* 2024;74(2):246–251. doi:10.1016/j.jadohealth.2023.09.016
190. Huynh J, Chien J, Nguyen AT, et al. The mental health of Asian American adolescents and young adults amid the rise of anti-Asian racism. *Front Public Health.* 2023;10:958517. doi:10.3389/fpubh.2022.958517
191. The Asian American Foundation. Annual survey reveals 1 in 2 Asian Americans feel unsafe; nearly 80% do not fully feel they belong and are accepted in the US. STAATUS Index 2023:

Attitudes Towards Asian Americans and Pacific Islanders. May 2, 2023. Accessed April 7, 2025. https://www.taaf.org/news/staatus-index-23-press-release
192. Artiga S, Hill L, Corallo B, Tolbert J. Asian immigrant experiences with racism, immigration-related fears, and the COVID-19 pandemic. Kaiser Family Foundation. June 18, 2021. Accessed April 2, 2025. https://www.kff.org/coronavirus-covid-19/issue-brief/asian-immigrant-experiences-with-racism-immigration-related-fears-and-the-covid-19-pandemic
193. Wu TY, Hsieh HF, Chow CM, Yang X, Resnicow K, Zimmerman M. Examining racism and firearm-related risks among Asian Americans in the United States during the COVID-19 pandemic. *Prev Med Rep*. 2022;27:101800. doi:10.1016/j.pmedr.2022.101800
194. Griffiths J. "We belong to Hong Kong": Thousands gather at solidarity events in 64 cities worldwide. *South China Morning Post*. October 1, 2014. Accessed April 7, 2025. https://www.scmp.com/news/hong-kong/article/1607584/we-belong-hong-kong-thousands-gather-solidarity-events-64-cities
195. Omatsu G. The 'four prisons' and the movements of liberation: Asian American activism from the 1960s to the 1990s. In: Wu JYWS, Chen T, eds. *Asian American Studies Now: A Critical Reader*. Rutgers University Press; 2010:298-330.
196. Miyazato C. Dear Muslim Americans: We see you, and we hear you. From, a Japanese American in solidarity. *The 'F' Word*. Medium. December 12, 2016. Accessed April 8, 2025. https://medium.com/gender-justice-feminism/dear-muslim-americans-we-see-you-and-we-hear-you-from-a-japanese-american-in-solidarity-16d2449a6410
197. Wang FKH. Muslim Americans read "letters from camp" to WWII-incarcerated Japanese Americans. *NBC News*. May 24, 2016. Accessed April 8, 2025. https://www.nbcnews.com/news/asian-america/muslim-americans-read-letters-camp-formerly-incarcerated-japanese-americans-n578961
198. Cho S. Roundtable II: Beyond #StopAsianHate: Criminalization, gender, & Asian abolition feminism. *J Asian Am Stud*. 2022;25(3):431–44. doi:10.1353/jaas.2022.0035
199. Yam K. Why over 85 Asian American, LGBTQ groups opposed the anti-Asian hate crimes bill. *NBC News*. May 14, 2021. Accessed April 8, 2025. https://www.nbcnews.com/news/asian-america/why-over-85-asian-american-lgbtq-groups-opposed-anti-asian-n1267421
200. Lee SJ, Xiong CP, Pheng LM. "Asians for Black lives, not Asians for Asians": Building Southeast Asian American and Black solidarity. *Anthropol Educ Q*. 2020;51(4):405–421. doi:10.1111/aeq.1235.
201. Kim CJ. *Asian Americans in an Anti-Black World*. Cambridge University Press; 2023.
202. Robinson G. *After Camp: Portraits in Midcentury Japanese American Life and Politics*. University of California Press; 2012.
203. Fujino DC, Rodriguez RM, eds. *Contemporary Asian American Activism: Building Movements for Liberation*. University of Washington Press; 2022.
204. Joshi K. *White Christian Privilege: The Illusion of Religious Equality in America*. New York University Press; 2020.
205. Yam K. Illinois becomes first state to require teaching Asian American history in schools. *NBC News*. July 12, 2021. Accessed April 8, 2025. https://www.nbcnews.com/news/asian-america/illinois-becomes-first-state-require-teaching-asian-american-history-schools-n1273774

206. Kramer G. Multicultural K-12 education bill introduced in Ohio House by AAPI women's group. *Ideastream Public Media*. May 15, 2023. Accessed April 8, 2025. https://www.ideastream.org/government-politics/2023-05-15/multicultural-k-12-education-bill-introduced-in-ohio-house-by-aapi-womens-group
207. Penaia CS, Morey BN, Thomas KB, et al. Disparities in Native Hawaiian and Pacific Islander COVID-19 mortality: A community-driven data response. *Am J Public Health*. 2021;111(suppl 2):S49–S52. doi:10.2105/AJPH.2021.306370
208. Morey BN, Penaia CS, Tulua A, et al. Democratizing Native Hawaiian and Pacific Islander data: Examining community accessibility of data for health and the social drivers of health. *Am J Public Health*. 2024;114(supp 1):S103–S111. doi:10.2105/AJPH.2023.307503
209. Office of Minority Health. Advancing equity for Asian American, Native Hawaiian, and Pacific Islander communities in COVID-19 response efforts: An introduction. US Dept of Health and Human Services. 2023. Accessed August 10, 2025. https://www.federalregister.gov/documents/2021/06/03/2021-11792/advancing-equity-justice-and-opportunity-for-asian-americans-native-hawaiians-and-pacific-islanders

Appendix 2A

Table 2A-1. Anti-Asian Racism and Asian American Resistance Throughout US History

Anti-Asian Racism Throughout US History	Asian American Responses, Mobilization, and Resistance
19th century: Chinese Americans faced violence, discrimination, and segregation in schools and other spheres of public life.	<ul><li>1883: Journalist and activist Wong Chin Foo published *The Chinese American* newspaper and used the press to push back against anti-Chinese racism.</li><li>1885: The Tape family successfully challenged racial segregation in San Francisco public schools by pursuing legal action in *Tape v Hurley* and advocacy in the press.</li><li>1886: In *Yick Wo v Hopkins*, Chinese American business owners successfully challenged laws that were applied in a discriminatory fashion.</li></ul>
Late 19th and early 20th century: US government restricted and excluded Chinese women (then men) and all other Asian people from immigrating, most notably with the 1882 Chinese Exclusion Act and the 1924 Johnson-Reed Act.	<ul><li>1889: In *Chae Chan Ping v United States*, Chinese Americans challenged laws that excluded Chinese laborers from the United States.</li><li>1892: Chinese Americans formed the Chinese Equal Rights League and advocated against Chinese exclusion laws.</li><li>1893: In *Fong Yue Ting v United States*, Chinese Americans challenged the Geary Act, which renewed Chinese exclusion and required Chinese immigrants to carry passes.</li><li>1910–1940: Chinese immigrants detained, interrogated, and inspected at Angel Island immigration station expressed their resistance by carving poetry into the walls.</li></ul>
18th through mid-20th century: The US government excluded Asian people from citizenship, including those in US colonies who fought for the US. Early 20th century: California passed Alien Land Laws in 1913 and 1920 to prevent Asian (especially Japanese Americans) from owning land and property so Asian Americans would not settle permanently.	<ul><li>1898: Wong Kim Ark challenged the denial of his entry into the United States and insisted that he was a citizen; the Supreme Court case *United States v Wong Kim Ark* affirmed birthright citizenship.</li><li>1915: Chinese Americans formed the Chinese American Citizens Alliance, the first national Asian American civil rights organization.</li><li>1922: In *Ozawa v United States*, Takao Ozawa argued that Japanese immigrants were eligible for naturalized citizenship.</li><li>1923: In *United States v Thind*, Bhagat Singh Thind argued that Indian immigrants were eligible for naturalized citizenship.</li><li>1929: Japanese Americans formed the Japanese American Citizens League.</li><li>1980s: The Filipino-American Association sought citizenship for Filipino veterans who fought for the United States during wartime after their status as US nationals was taken away in 1946.</li></ul>
1940s: The US government mass incarcerated Japanese Americans during the WWII without due process of law.	<ul><li>1944: In *Korematsu v US*, Japanese Americans challenged the constitutionality of Executive Order 9066, which led to Japanese American incarceration.</li><li>1970s–1980s: Japanese Americans advocated for reparations and a formal apology from the US government. Their efforts resulted in the Civil Liberties Act of 1988.</li></ul>

(Continued)

Table 2A-1. (Continued)

Anti-Asian Racism Throughout US History	Asian American Responses, Mobilization, and Resistance
1950s-1990s: With mid-century immigration reforms, Asian immigrants migrated to the US in larger numbers and increased the Asian American population. However, they continued to face racism, violence, discrimination, and exploitation. Asian American experiences were shaped by geopolitical circumstances, such as the Cold War, and American foreign relations with Asian nations.	• 1940s-1960s: Larry Itliong led a campaign to strike against agribusiness's exploitation of workers. Committed to working in coalition to ensure safer working conditions, he worked with Cesar Chavez to organize joint labor actions with Mexican American and Filipino American farmworkers. These efforts helped forge the United Farm Workers. • 1960s: Asian American activists launched the Asian American movement and the Yellow Power movement, which protested racism, imperialism, and US wars in Southeast Asia. The movement also called for interracial solidarity and an end to patriarchy and misogyny, including that of Asian cultural nationalists. • 1965: Congress passed the Voting Rights Act, which required translated ballots and language assistance. • 1969: A multiracial/multiethnic student movement, which included Asian Americans, organized demonstrations calling for Ethnic Studies in their curriculum. As a result of these efforts, UC Berkeley and San Francisco State College offered the first Asian American studies classes. • 1970s: Chinese American parents successfully sued the San Francisco Unified School District to provide bilingual education for their children in *Lau v Nichols*. • 1971: UCLA began publishing *Amerasia* journal, reflecting the emerging discipline of Asian American studies. • 1978: The East Coast Asian American Student Union was formed. • 1979: The Association for Asian American Studies was formed. • Late 1970s: Mutual assistance associations and community organizations such as the Southeast Asia Resource Action Center were formed to support Southeast Asian refugees resettling and building communities throughout the US. • 1979-2012: The weekly newspaper *AsianWeek* was published. With a circulation of 58,000, it provided coverage of Asian American community political, social, and cultural events. • 1969-1974: The student publication *Gidra* became a highly influential radical Asian American newspaper. • 1972: The Kearny Street Workshop was established to nurture and promote Asian American multidisciplinary arts. • 1974: *The Big Aiiieeeee!*, the first collection of Asian American literature, was published and helped establish the field of Asian American literature. • 1982: Women garment workers in NYC's Chinatown struck for better wages and benefits.

(Continued)

Table 2A-1. (Continued)

Anti-Asian Racism Throughout US History	Asian American Responses, Mobilization, and Resistance
1980s: Economic competition between the US and Japan and hostility against Asian refugees and immigrants contributed to a rise in anti-Asian violence, most notably the murder of Vincent Chin in Michigan.	• 1970s–1980s: Korean and other Asian Americans created the Committee to Free Chol Soo Lee, a movement to vindicate Korean American Lee, who in 1973 was wrongly accused of murdering a Chinatown gang leader, sent to death row, and incarcerated for a decade. Asian American activism helped secure his release. • 1980s: Asian American activists in Michigan formed American Citizens for Justice, which mobilized efforts to call for justice in the murder of Vincent Chin. • 1980s: South Asian and other Asian American activists called for justice for Navroze Mody, who was murdered in 1987 by the "Dotbuster" gang. • 1980: The National Asian American Telecommunication Association (now Center for Asian American Media) was established to screen and fund independent documentary and fictional films by and about Asian Americans. • 1982: *Chan is Missing*, considered to be the first Asian American feature length dramatic film, was released. • 1986: The US Commission on Civil Rights released a report about racially motivated violence, harassment, and discrimination targeting Asian Americans. • 1986–1987: The Asian and Pacific Islander American Health Forum and Association of Asian Pacific Community Health Organizations were established. They were the first national Asian American and Pacific Islander health organizations to challenge the model minority myth that Asian Americans do not experience health disparities. • 1989: The Harvard Kennedy School began publishing *Asian American Policy Review*. • 1989–2002: *A* magazine was published. Reaching a national circulation of 200,000, it focused on news, entertainment, and culture for young Asian Americans.
1990s: Asian Americans continued to experience racism and discrimination in political, economic, cultural, and social life. Anti-Asian racism and violence gained national attention during prominent events such as the Los Angeles "riots."	• 1990: Filipino Americans organized People's CORE to advocate for environmental justice, veterans' rights, and tenants' rights. • 1990: Congress enacted Pub L No. 102-450, permanently designating May as Asian/Pacific American Heritage Month. • 1990: Asian American artists protested casting of white actors portraying Asians in the Broadway production of *Miss Saigon*. • 1991: Asian Americans Advancing Justice, a civil rights organization, was established. • 1992: The Black-Korean Alliance and the Korean American Coalition's Alternative Dispute Resolution Center were formed in response to the Los Angeles "riots" and the murders of LaTasha Harlins and Korean American merchants. The Koreatown community organized a 30,000-strong Peace March and Rally for justice for both Rodney King and for Korean Americans who demanded state compensation for the government's failure to protect Koreatown.

(Continued)

Table 2A-1. (Continued)

Anti-Asian Racism Throughout US History	Asian American Responses, Mobilization, and Resistance
	<ul><li>1989-1993: Feminist, queer, and labor activists in NYC and Boston formed several organizations to address worker exploitation, patriarchy, and queerphobia in both ethnic and mainstream communities, including the New York Taxi Workers' Alliance, the South Asian Lesbian and Gay Association, and Sakhi for South Asian Women/Domestic Workers Committee/Domestic Violence Project.</li><li>1990s: Radical activists at the UC Santa Barbara established ASIAN! (Asian Sisters for Ideas in Action Now!) to advocate for AAPI women's rights, immigrant rights, and affirmative action policies. Similar organizations that emerged during this time included Asians and Pacific Islanders for Community Empowerment (API FORCE), Asian Left Forum, and the Asian Revolutionary Circle.</li><li>1992: The Asian American Pacific Islander Nurses Association was founded.</li><li>1992: The Asian Pacific American Labor Alliance, AFL-CIO, was formed.</li><li>1994: The Congressional Asian Pacific American Caucus and Asian Pacific Islander American Institute for Congressional Studies was created.</li><li>1994: The National Korean American Service & Education Consortium was established.</li><li>1994-2004: *Yolk* magazine, which focused on fashion and entertainment for young Asian Americans, was published, with a circulation of 50,000.</li><li>1996: A coalition of national AAPI organizations united to form the National Council of Asian Pacific Americans.</li><li>1996: APIA Vote, an organization aimed at promoting Asian American civic engagement, was established.</li><li>1996: The National Asian Pacific American Women's Forum, which emphasized an intersectional approach to addressing racial and gender inequity, was established.</li><li>1998: The Association for Asian American Studies began publishing the *Journal of Asian American Studies*.</li><li>1999: President Bill Clinton issued Executive Order 13125, which established the White House Initiative on AAPIs.</li></ul>
2000s-2010s: The 9/11 attacks and the War on Terror contributed to a rise in anti-Muslim racism, racial profiling, and individual attacks on people suspected of being Muslim—especially South Asian and Arab American people.	<ul><li>2000-2003: Civil rights organizations advocating for South Asian Americans—South Asian Americans Leading Together (SAALT) and the Sikh Coalition—were established.</li><li>2017: The New York Taxi Workers Alliance led a large-scale protest at John F. Kennedy airport against the Trump administration's "Muslim Ban."</li></ul>

(Continued)

Table 2A-1. (Continued)

Anti-Asian Racism Throughout US History	Asian American Responses, Mobilization, and Resistance
2020s: The COVID-19 pandemic and US–China tensions gave rise to a surge in acts of anti-Asian harassment, discrimination, and violence, including against frontline workers.	• 2020: The organization Stop AAPI Hate was founded and began to track incidents of community-reported anti-Asian violence, harassment, and discrimination. • 2020: Asian American community groups organized efforts to mobilize voters and address voter suppression in the 2020 election. • 2021: Illinois passed the TEAACH Act, which required public K–12 schools to teach about Asian American history. • 2021: Asian Americans pressured government officials to address hate crimes against Asian Americans, resulting in Congress passing the COVID-19 Hate Crimes Act. This bill caused controversy among Asian Americans, some of whom refused to support the bill due to their objection to using law enforcement to address anti-Asian violence and their commitment to working in solidarity with Black and Brown communities disproportionately impacted by police violence. • 2023: The first National Strategy to Advance Equity, Opportunity, and Justice for Asian American, Native Hawaiian, and Pacific Islander Communities was issued, with Action Plans from 32 federal departments and agencies.

Note: AAPI = Asian American or Pacific Islander; CORE = Community Organization for Reform and Empowerment; NYC = New York City, New York; UC = University of California; UCLA = University of California, Los Angeles; US = United States; WWII = World War II.

3

Strengthening the Health of Black People in the United States Through Systemic and Structural Change

Micere Keels, PhD, Velma McBride Murry, PhD, MS, Robynn Cox, PhD, MA, Tyson H. Brown, PhD, Wendy Ellis, DrPH, MPH, Chelsea Dorsey, MD, Angela Diaz, MD, PhD, MPH, and Eliseo J. Pérez-Stable, MD

INTRODUCTION

More than a century ago, W. E. B. Du Bois's pioneering research empirically illustrated how structural racism and its associated social conditions—both historical and contemporary—harms the health of Black people.[1] Built upon the fallacious presumption that groups racialized as Black are biologically inferior to those racialized as white, race is a sociopolitical construct that places humans on a hierarchy of value.[2,3] Throughout the history of the United States, this hierarchy of human value structures Black people's overexposure to the negative and underexposure to the positive social determinants of heath; consequently, they have lived sicker and died younger than almost all other racialized groups of Americans.[4,5]

While emancipation provided legal freedom to enslaved Black Americans, the social and economic marginalization brought about by the economic and legal institutions that enabled slavery continued and were reproduced through federal, state, and city policies, as well as neighborhood-level covenants. As Christopher notes, we must "reckon first with the disease of human hierarchy, then treat its symptoms of oppression."[6] Racially inequitable social investments through formal and informal policies and practices are embedded in the fabric of American society and in vestiges of Jim Crow laws that were designed to perpetuate the hierarchy of enslavement by limiting the full social, political, educational, and economic participation of Black Americans, and are evidenced in persistent racial gaps in education, employment, income, wealth, and, for the focus of this chapter, creating and sustaining racial hierarchies of health, morbidity, and mortality.[7-10]

The enforcement of the racial hierarchy was at its apex during the transatlantic slave trade and continues in the *slave health deficit*, a term coined to highlight the need for a historical understanding of present-day racial health disparities.[11,12] The slave health deficit is simultaneously an indictment of the racial hierarchy of human value that enabled acceptance of the middle passage death toll and continued indifference and acceptance of the disparate Black mortality that has persisted on American shores from slavery to today.[13] As Caraballo et al. detail, if Black people had the same mortality rate as white people in the United States, over just 22 years from 1999 to 2020, there would have been 1.63 million fewer Black deaths.[14]

This racial hierarchy of human value played an important role in the scientific and medical history of the United States. *American polygeny*, the belief that human races stem from different species, was an important (pseudo)scientific theory that garnered international recognition for American scientists and further cemented the idea of racial hierarchy in health.[8,15,16] This legacy of racial hierarchy pseudoscience lingers in medical training, guidelines, and algorithms applied in diagnostic testing, treatment, varying technology platforms, and consequently in the attitudes and beliefs of present-day health care providers.[17] For example, racial disparities in current pain management practices have been associated with racial stereotypes about biological differences in pain thresholds between Black and white populations, as well as perceptions that Black patients are at greater risk for opioid misuse than white patients and may be exaggerating or making up pain to obtain opioids.[18] Philosophers, scientists, slave owners, and physicians used these beliefs to defend the cruel treatment of enslaved Black people and they continue to impact their descendants (and Black immigrants) through every aspect of the health care system, from unethical research experimentation to biased provision of lifesaving care.[18]

SHIFTING ATTENTION FROM RACE TO RACISM

There is no shortage of reports detailing Black health disparities, such as the 1985 Department of Health and Human Services Report of the Secretary's Task Force on Black and Minority Health, the 2013 Centers for Disease Control and Prevention Health Disparities and Inequities Report, and 20 years of annual National Health Care Quality and Disparities Reports. No shortage of government agencies and think tanks focused on narrowing the gap, such as the National Institutes of Health Office of Research on Minority Health, the National Medical Association's Health Policy Institute, and others. Additionally, over the past 50 years, government and philanthropic organizations have granted billions of dollars to initiatives aimed at closing health disparities. However, despite this attention on disparities and improvements in overall population health, large Black–white gaps persist, and new ones have widened as technologies improve.[19]

Racial health disparities persist because research and interventions have focused on race and largely target proximate rather than system-structural determinants of health, attributing population-level disparities to the lifestyles of individuals within subpopulations.[20] This includes individual-level factors such as health behaviors, education, employment, income, wealth, social support, nutritious foods, and exposure to health risks, while dismissing structural oppression and interpersonal discrimination that create chronic, mundane stressors and foster maladaptive coping.[21] Although these proximate determinants are key pathways through which racism "gets under the skin" and undermines the health of Black people, this focus has not appreciably narrowed racial health disparities. It has instead diverted attention and resources away from structural-system level upstream drivers of the unequal distribution of the social determinants of health.[22-26]

By contrast, attending to racism moves our gaze upstream to focus on formal legislative, legal, other public sector, and private sector policies and practices, as well as informal social structures and social interactions that create and perpetuate discrimination and marginalization that culminate in the disadvantaged health of Black people.[1,27] These structural problems require system-level solutions.[22,28] We aim to further the shift to identifying systemic, population-level change levers that are grounded in the understanding that racism is a fundamental cause of health disparities.[29,30] As previously discussed in the introduction to this book, examining racism's drivers of health inequities requires studying the root causes of racial inequities in health.[4,20]

Many manifestations of structural racism have been so long-standing across generations that they have become invisible—perceived to be the natural order and operation of societal systems. In this paper, place-based systems, criminal legal systems, and health care systems are examined to make visible many of the ways that structural racism affects the health of Black people. First, structural racism embedded in place-based systems has been associated with Black people's overexposure to health-deteriorating factors and underexposure to health-promoting factors, due in large part to the persistence of residential segregation.[31-33] Second, structural racism embedded in criminal legal systems leads to Black people experiencing disproportionately high risks of police brutality, stops, arrests, charges, and convictions—and ultimately it undermines their health.[34,35] Lastly, structural racism embedded in health care systems creates large group inequities in access, quantity, and quality of care, which exacerbates racial health disparities.[36-38]

RACISM, STRESS, AND ITS HEALTH EFFECTS ACROSS THE LIFE COURSE

As discussed in the introduction to this book, a life course perspective is needed because racial health disparities exist across multiple systems with persistent consequences across multiple generations. These patterns have been associated with disproportionate stress and weathering due to overexposure to negative social determinants of heath.[39] A comprehensive understanding of the associations between structural racism and health requires looking back in history and across multiple systems and institutions, because health builds and is maintained across generations and across an individual's life course.

Combining intergenerational and life course frameworks aids our understanding of the stability of racial health disparities despite changes in exposure and expression of health risk in disease trends over time.[32,40] The incorporation of a cumulative disadvantage framework within the life course approach recognizes that the many collateral effects of racism are systematic and compound disadvantage over time.[41]

Geronimus' weathering framework posits that repeated experiences of racism-related stress and threats to one's identity give rise to racism-based traumatic symptoms that, over time, disrupt the body's stress-response systems.[42,43] Racism-related stress includes much more than interpersonal discrimination; it also includes the numerous ways that racism and discrimination cause Black people to experience higher levels of household and neighborhood poverty, including redlining, mass incarceration, land devaluation, and more.[44] As Heard-Garris et al. detail, it is difficult to overstate the negative effects of poverty on health. Racism weathers Black people because it creates numerous forms of chronic stress that change psychological, psychobiological, and behavioral processes.[45-47] Weathering, undergirded by the science of stress and allostatic load, is a dominant and longstanding framework for understanding how social factors affect all aspects of health.[48]

Racism-related stress and weathering are pernicious and cumulative across the life course and have been associated with elevated risk for chronic systemic inflammation, leading to higher rates of heart disease, stroke, diabetes, obesity, cancer, and other diseases.[49] Studies in epigenetics, for example, illustrate that exposure to unrelenting stress over the life course not only changes one's DNA but also changes DNA that is transmitted from one generation to the next.[50] The low relative life expectancy for Blacks across all socioeconomic status levels is congruent with an environment filled with stressors that quite literally "get under the skin."

Population-level divergence starts early, as reflected in Black children's early exposure to structural racism in the form of childhood adversity. Approximately 45% of Black children will be exposed to one adverse childhood experience by their first birthday, but not until their 10th birthday will 43% of white children be exposed to one adverse childhood experience. The unrelenting effects of intergenerational poverty are associated with increased neurohormonal dysregulation early in the life course and greater risk for numerous immune, cardiovascular, and psychiatric diseases.[51-53] From the earliest stages of life, poverty has negative effects on brain development, behavioral disorders, anemia, height for age, and childhood epilepsy.

As Black people age, the effects of structural racism accumulate and result in them being placed at higher risk for numerous metabolic disorders.[54] As individuals age, poverty is associated with maternal depression, obesity, increased incidence of strokes, and dementia.[55-58] Amaro et al.[59] highlight that the direct and indirect effects of racism have been linked to higher allostatic load,[60] accelerated cellular aging,[61] poor pregnancy-related outcomes in Black women,[62-64] chronic illnesses and mortality,[64-66] and substance use initiation and misuse.[64,67] This is not an exhaustive list of the many accumulating negative health effects.

Illustrated in the remainder of this paper are some of the ways that the societal systems that organize our lives are deeply affected by systemic racism, which creates racially disparate exposure to stress and stress relief coping resources. Societal systems matter because individual health behaviors can be highly constrained or enabled by one's environmental resources and circumstances.[68–70] As noted by Amaro et al., all organisms engage in actions to relieve the physiological and psychological distress that is created by experiencing stressful events,[59] and "the motivation for and availability to engage in poor health behaviors as stress-coping or self-regulation strategies is influenced by social structures and contexts . . . and that these social structures are in turn differentially distributed across racial groups."[69(p83)]

PLACE-BASED SYSTEMS

Associations Between Place-Based Systems and Rising Black Youth Suicide

The extent to which the alarming increase in the rate of suicide among Black youth is associated with systemic racism warrants in-depth examination, given the recent dramatic increase. Rates of suicide among Black youth aged 10 to 24 years increased by 37%, rising from 8.2 per 100,000 in 2018 to 11.2 per 100,000 in 2021. No other racial or ethnic group has experienced such an alarming increase in suicide. While explanations are often relegated to race-based individual psychosocial factors, the root cause may be maladaptive coping responses to systemic societal and neighborhood ecological stressors that elevate Black youths' risk for suicide.[71] Black children are further harmed by racial disparities in access to mental health care in general and access to culturally competent care in particular.[72] Their resulting negative experiences in health care settings can dissuade help seeking.

Black and white Americans continue to largely live in separate and unequal neighborhoods, and in recent generations, many predominantly Black neighborhoods, already failing due to racially biased redlining, were harmed further when they were bisected by major roadways, lost their walkability, experienced rising rates of violence, and lost the health-protective sense of belonging when their deep sense of place was disrupted. These conditions were created and maintained by discriminatory policies and practices throughout the 20th and 21st centuries.[31,32,73–76] Neighborhood conditions, often a byproduct of poverty and disinvestment in Black communities, not only elevate risk for childhood chronic conditions, including early onset diabetes, asthma, obesity, attention deficit disorder, and a variety of genetic and birth defects, but have also been associated with mental health and behavioral disorders.[77]

Even under ideal conditions, the developmental stage of youth presents a host of challenges and is replete with many physical, cognitive, and social-emotional changes.[78] These challenges are often exacerbated for Black youth when they grow up in contexts where structural poverty prevents their families from providing the experiences, resources, and services that are essential for them to thrive and grow into healthy, productive adults.[79] From early childhood through the end of the life course, the chronic stressors associated with systemic racism can disrupt healthy development of brain architecture, particularly the structures that regulate executive function, memory, and the adrenal system.[80,81] This has been shown to have devastating effects on psychological, emotional, and behavioral functioning that can present as learning disorders, anxiety, or depression and suicidal ideation.[80,82,83] Many of these mental health effects of racism often go undetected and untreated in a society and health care system that does not recognize the experience of structural racism as a stressor.[23,84]

The social determinants of mental health are manifested in social, economic, political, and environmental policies and practices that strip youth of opportunities to reach their optimal potential. Black youth are six times more likely than white youth to live in high poverty, resource-scarce neighborhoods.[85] As studies have shown, residing in economically stressed communities with high exposure to violence is often associated with the vestiges of redlining and interstate highway construction that locked Black families into high-poverty residential areas. Borofsky et al. noted that community violence exposure has cascading vulnerability effects including psychological symptoms, decreased connectedness to school, and overall compromised academic achievement.[86] Community violence has been linked to elevated psychological distress, often manifested as feelings of helplessness and fear, creating trauma that can lead to posttraumatic stress disorder and other internalizing symptoms, including anxiety, rage, aggression, and increased suicidal vulnerability.

The legacy of disinvestment in Black communities has negative implications for youth social and emotional development through the sense of hopelessness and depression that may be experienced as one witnesses lost opportunities to successfully complete stage-salient developmental tasks.[87] Not completing critical milestones—such as achieving higher education, obtaining employment, or forming intimate relationships as one ages, or seeing missed opportunities to do so—may lead to substance use to manage disappointments or increasing depression and anxiety, which often co-occur, placing one at greater risk for suicide. The behavioral and mental health of Black youth need to be understood through this place-based lens that attends to the historical vestiges of structural policies and practices that significantly advantaged white communities over Black communities.

As noted throughout this chapter, societal systems interact and intersect to amplify racial disparities. For example, educational systems often replicate and reinforce societal oppression. School personnel routinely address mental health and behavioral concerns for Black children through punitive discipline that begins as early as preschool.[88] Continued infractions can result in referral to juvenile detention centers rather than efforts to identify and address the upstream social determinants.[89] Approaches to conduct concerns or low academic achievement may be quite different if educators associated children's behavior with larger systems that affect students' home, neighborhood, and school environments, which manifest in experiences such as food insecurity, medical and pharmaceutical deserts, unsafe common spaces, and polluted communities.[71]

Associations Between Place-Based Systems, Public Education, and Health

Racial disparities in educational opportunity are a critical source of racialized health disparities that are believed to operate through at least three major pathways: (1) direct provision of skills, abilities, and knowledge, including health literacy; (2) determining the professional and thereby workplace health hazards and economic conditions in which one works and lives; and (3) increasing or reducing the psychosocial stressors and resources that impact well-being.[90] Additionally, at every level of educational attainment, Black people report poorer health compared with white people, which suggests that the race, education, and health disparities nexus is about not just quantity but also quality of educational experiences, and the extent to which racism undermines the benefits of schooling.[91] As Sentell, Zhang, and Ching note, "providing years of inadequate education to meet a benchmark is unlikely to provide the health benefits . . . if current inequity in educational quality remains by race/ethnicity."[90(p246)]

As discussed throughout this chapter, many Black families live in areas of concentrated poverty, not by choice, but rather because legacies of federal policy and lending practices created and maintain place-based systems of inequity.[92] High levels of segregation by race and poverty generally produce highly segregated and underresourced neighborhood public schools for Black students.[93] Even with increasing options for school choice through voucher programs, charter schools, and school transfer programs, 73% of the nation's children attend neighborhood schools that rely heavily on local funding.[94] While federal housing and banking policy created a foundation for place-based inequity, state education funding policy often exacerbates inequity by reinforcing the concentration of education dollars to low-poverty areas rather than promoting expansion of educational opportunity based on place-based need.[94] Consequently, neighborhoods of concentrated poverty also contain underfunded schools that are often in poor condition, with limited supplies and higher rates of student dropout and teacher turnover.[95] Underfunded and underresourced schools consistently under-deliver for many of the nation's Black school children who arguably are most in need of the buffer that a quality education can provide across the life span.[96]

More than half of the children attending the nation's public schools live below the federal poverty level, which results in higher levels of childhood adversity concentrated in woefully underresourced school settings.[97] In public school settings, 83% of Black children attend high-poverty schools compared with 53% of poor white children.[98] Racial and economic segregation in America's public schools continues to be largely uncontested and produces an inferior education for many Black schoolchildren.[99] Black students who attend higher-poverty, underfunded schools are less competitive in the college application process and workforce because diplomas from these neighborhoods' schools are less valued in the marketplace, contributing to a vicious cycle of poverty and loss of human potential.[100]

As the United States transitioned into being a knowledge economy, the gradient in health outcomes by educational attainment has steepened, with death rates declining among the most educated Americans accompanied by steady or increasing death rates among the least educated.[101] Research shows that schooling is an effective target of intervention for narrowing population-level health disparities because the physical and mental health of people who experienced childhood socioeconomic disadvantage benefit more from each year of education than for members of socially advantaged groups.[102] Investing in strengthening the quality of schools serving Black students would have multiplicative effects by positively impacting health across generations.

CRIMINAL LEGAL SYSTEMS

Associations Between the Criminal Legal System and Racial Disparities in Maternal Health

A quarter of the way through the 21st century and 160 years after emancipation, the Black maternal mortality rate is 2.5 times higher than the white rate.[103,104] This disparity represents only the tip of the iceberg of severe maternal morbidity.[105] An estimated 16.3 per 1,000 Black birthing people experienced a life-threatening pregnancy-related outcome compared with 8.4 per 1,000 white birthing people.[106] Analysis of the disparities indicates that compared with white birthing people, Black birthing people are at 70% increased risk of experiencing severe maternal morbidity antepartum, 40% increased risk intrapartum, and 18% increased risk postpartum, after adjusting for potential demographic, behavioral, hospital, insurance, and clinical confounders.[107]

Research using novel measures of the association between structural racism and health, specifically, how the criminal legal system (CLS) contributes to racial disparities in maternal health, advances our ability to see the far-reaching effects of systemic disparities.[108,109] Recent conceptualization of the American CLS as a social determinant of health is one of the ways that public health researchers are responding to the need to identify systemic drivers of disparities.[110,111] Incarceration is much more than an individual experience; its costs are borne collectively. This means examining how mass incarceration and mass police surveillance go far beyond directly affecting the health of individuals with CLS contact to having spillover effects that harm the health of romantic partners and their infants and older children.

As recently as 1950, only 175 per 100,000 individuals were incarcerated, compared with 680 per 100,000 in 2021.[111,112] The burden of this rise in incarceration is disproportionately borne by Black people, especially Black men with less than a high school diploma.[113] Approximately 57% of Black men without a high school diploma who were born in the late 1960s spent time in prison by their 30s, compared with approximately 10% of similar white men. Because incarcerated individuals are missing from health surveillance data, we have large gaps in our understanding of Black men's health and health care needs.[114]

Conway provides an informative list of the ways that incarceration functions as a traumatic stressor that disrupts social and financial resources at the household and community levels in ways that disproportionately place pregnant people and infants at higher risk for adverse outcomes.[115] Some of these stressors include the direct stress of removing the father and/or mother from the infant's life and the increased family, financial, and caregiving strain when one parent is removed. Because of residential segregation, the mass incarceration of Black people means there is a doubly disadvantaged concentration of these stressors at the household and neighborhood level, such that families strained by incarceration have fewer community, social, and economic resources they can turn to for help.

From this lens of collateral effects among extended family members and communities, it is seen how quickly the mass incarceration of Black men can create subpopulation disparities. In addition to disparate exposure, research also shows that the negative effects of incarceration are stronger for Black versus white people in the United States.[116] In addition to the indirect health effects that Black women experience from male incarceration, the dramatic rise in female incarceration that has disproportionately affected Black women has direct negative effects for their and their children's health. Some call this increasing incarceration of women the "criminalization of trauma" because the overwhelming majority have a history of traumatic experiences.[117,118]

Because 80% of incarcerated women are mothers and 5% are pregnant while incarcerated,[119,120] the rise in incarceration of Black women has disturbing implications for the intergenerational transmission of trauma and poor health. First, incarceration disrupts/harms parent–child bonding and harms maternal mental health in ways that place their children at disproportionate risk for abuse when reunited. Second, the high rate of Black male incarceration means that the children of incarcerated Black women with a same-race partner are disproportionately placed at risk for entering foster care. Third, because Black mothers are significantly more likely to be sole providers, the economic effects of mass incarceration that extend long after release place their children at disproportionate risk for abuse when reunited.[114]

Associations Between the Criminal Legal System and Racial Disparities in Cognitive Impairment

Cognitive impairment such as Alzheimer's and other dementias are some of the most expensive diseases to treat, with an estimated cost of $345 billion in 2021.[121] There are large racial disparities in the prevalence of cognitive impairment between Black and white people that are greater during midlife than at an older age.[122-125] Specifically, the prevalence of cognitive impairment among Black Americans aged 85 years or older is roughly 2 times that of their white counterparts, but it is 4 times greater for Black versus white Americans aged 55–64.[125] Cognitive impairment and Alzheimer's disease and related disorders provide a clear example of the cumulative and compounding effects of structural racism on health.

Differences between Black and white people in cognitive impairment are largely explained by factors that influence cognitive reserve, which is a functional concept that emphasizes how the efficiency of neural networks can serve as a protective factor against dementia.[126-128] This hypothesis purports that individuals with high levels of cognitive reserve can better endure age-related changes to the brain, which allows them to have greater tolerance for disease, leading to a delay in the onset of dementia. This provides a direct link to how the impact of racism on material resources at the individual and community level can impact the resilience of the brain to cognitive impairment. Richards and Deary propose a life course framework for cognitive reserve by placing a central focus on premorbid cognitive ability, which can be strengthened or, presumably, weakened over the life course.[129] The overwhelmingly negative direct and indirect effects of racism can compound early life disadvantages disproportionately experienced by Black Americans, resulting in higher stress, lower cognitive reserve, and a higher prevalence of early-onset cognitive impairment.

The stress-coping model helps us understand how the environmental effects of racial and ethnic discrimination such as segregation can result in greater access to unhealthy coping mechanisms and limited access to resources that encourage healthy coping and brain health. This makes it more likely for minoritized populations to use negative health behaviors to manage chronic stress through choices that offer immediate relief. For example, low-income Black neighborhoods tend to have higher concentrations of liquor stores and other alcohol outlets, which is associated with greater susceptibility to risky alcohol use.[130] In the long run, these unhealthy coping mechanisms may indirectly cause cognitive impairment by increasing the likelihood of chronic conditions (e.g., diabetes) associated with cognitive impairment.

Racial disparity in incarceration is an indicator that captures many of the disadvantages that result from structural racism because incarcerated individuals are disproportionately Black, less educated, poorer, and suffer from greater mental and physical illnesses than the general population.[34] The imprisonment rate of Black people has increased to the point that a Black male born in 2001 has a 1 in 3 chance of going to prison in his lifetime.[131] Moreover, Black men are imprisoned at rates six times that of their white counterparts. In a relatively sizable nationally representative survey of middle-aged men and women between the ages of 46 and 60 years, Cox and Wallace found the unadjusted prevalence of cognitive impairment and early-onset dementia among formerly incarcerated men and women was at least two times the prevalence among those with no reported incarceration.[132] The results suggest that incarceration could be affecting cognitive impairment through its effects on human capital factors such as educational attainment, physical and mental health, and net worth. That said, incarceration could also affect premorbid cognition and educational attainment through its timing (see Aizer and Doyle[133] for the link between juvenile detention, educational attainment, and later incarceration).

Incarceration likely compounds disadvantage over the life course, leading to early cognitive decline. Cox and Wallace found cognitive impairment differences between incarcerated and nonincarcerated people were explained by a combination of factors, including race, gender, health, net worth, and premorbid cognitive functioning.[132] Nonetheless, differences for dementia were independently explained by premorbid cognitive functioning (measured by Armed Forces Qualification Test [AFQT] scores) and education. AFQT scores significantly influenced early-onset dementia above and beyond its effect through education (i.e., holding constant education levels). Finally, the authors found a relatively robust association between a prior diagnosis of an emotional disorder or depression and cognitive impairment. Given the link between chronic stress and mental health, this highlights the role of stress in cognitive impairment.[132]

These findings align with research investigating the cognitive reserve hypothesis.[134-137] Consistent with prior studies,[136,138] Cox and Wallace found that premorbid measures of cognitive functioning such as AFQT scores were consistently important in explaining cognitive impairment.[132] Given that AFQT scores are also a reflection of environmental and socioeconomic factors,[139,140] their findings highlight the importance of modeling cognitive impairment within a life course framework, as adverse experiences throughout one's life will affect cognitive reserve and, therefore, cognition later in life. Finally, Cox and Wallace found that differences in cognitive impairment between Black and white adults was persistent, holding other factors constant (including premorbid cognition and incarceration), suggesting that discrimination and barriers to social opportunities play a role in disparities in the early onset of cognitive impairment.[132] It should be noted that incarceration impacts not only those directly exposed to an incarceration, but also family members who experience indirect exposure to a loved one's incarceration.[141,142]

Racially disparate contact with CLS causes elevated incidence of chronic and infectious diseases, as well as mortality, through several mechanisms, including stress, stigma, financial hardships, violence, and family instability.[111,143] Moreover, studies show that vicarious CLS exposure via family, friends, and the broader community context undermines the health of Black people.[75,142] Consequently, policies and interventions focused on CLS are essential for achieving racial health equity.[111,144-147] For example, more flexible criminal legal policies at the state level are associated with lower rates of all-cause mortality.[148]

HEALTH CARE SYSTEMS

Associations Between the Health Care System and Racial Disparities in the Cancer Continuum

In middle adulthood, the impact of Black people's overexposure to health-deteriorating factors often manifests in alarming ways, including the disproportionate prevalence of severe health conditions such as cancer. According to the American Cancer Society, Black people have the shortest survival and highest death rate of any racial or ethnic group in the United States for the majority of cancers.[149,150] A prime example of this disparity is seen with breast cancer, from which Black women are 41% more likely to die than white women, despite having a lower incidence of the disease.[151] Similarly, Black men have the highest incidence of prostate cancer (73% higher than white men) and have a 2.2-fold higher risk of death when compared with white men.[152]

Similar to the other health disparities discussed in this chapter, racial disparities in the cancer continuum, which includes prevention, screening, diagnosis, treatment, and survival, are associated with a multitude of structural disparities in racialized access to the social determinants of health.[153] For example, housing insecurity (or the fear of not having safe, affordable, and stable housing) can have a significant impact on patients as they move through the cancer continuum.[152,154] Racial disparities in housing security are alarmingly large; 1 in 6 Black people compared with 1 in 21 white people in the United States are likely to experience homelessness.[155] As previously discussed, many of these present-day racial gaps result from generations of discriminatory housing policies that created and maintain significant inequities in access to the wealth that is generated by homeownership.[154]

The negative effects of disparities in access to the social determinants of health are often exacerbated by the ways the health care system has created systematic barriers for Black people to receive high-quality and timely health care.[12,156] Research reveals stark historical and contemporary anti-Black discrimination in terms of access to care, doctor–patient interactions, racial composition of the health care workforce, adequate prescribing and treatment plans, and experimentation without consent.[36,157-159] Consistent with this, the American Medical Association's assessment of racial inequities in quality of care states that "despite the improvements in the overall health of the country, racial and ethnic minorities experience a lower quality of health care—they are less likely to receive routine medical care and face higher rates of morbidity and mortality than non-minorities."[160]

These systemic disparities in care are illustrated in research on the associations between health insurance and disparities in the diagnosis and treatment of cancer, which shows the cumulative effect of being uninsured (or underinsured) with less access to high-quality and timely cancer screening, diagnostic evaluation, and treatment.[161] For example, Black people are overrepresented in states that have not expanded Medicaid, which creates barriers to care because they are also significantly less likely to have employer-sponsored insurance.[161]

These and other access issues have direct impacts on increasing Black people's likelihood of late-stage cancer diagnosis, which is often harder to treat and carries with it a greater financial cost to the patient and health care system. Black people who screen positive for cancer generally have the lowest proportion of localized-stage cancer and the highest proportion of distant-stage cancer, except for in prostate cancer.[162] Once detected, health system factors like being uninsured and underinsured mean that Black patients are more likely to experience delays in treatment and less likely to receive the recommended treatment.[163] All these factors contribute to creating a system in which Black people have the lowest overall 5-year survival rate and lowest stage-specific survival rate.[162]

The low prevalence of Black doctors is also a health risk because racial concordance is a factor that improves physician–patient experiences and health outcomes, including cancer treatment and outcomes.[164,165] A study of lung cancer patients found that when there was racial concordance, physician communication was experienced as more supportive, more partnering, and more informative, which was associated with greater trust in physicians.[166] Charlot et al. found that concordance also matters for health navigators; Black women with either breast or cervical cancer screening abnormalities had timelier resolution of those screening abnormalities when they were paired with race-concordant navigators compared with those with race-discordant navigators.[167]

Associations Between the Health Care System and Racial Disparities in Maternal and Infant Mortality

Even though overall maternal mortality has decreased over the past 100 years, the Black–white maternal mortality gap has increased. This painfully illustrates that improvements in health and well-being are not equitably distributed, and, often, as population health improves, so too does the gap in racial disparities.[13] For example, the precipitous drop in overall maternal mortality from the 1930s to the 1950s was associated with a corresponding rise in the Black–white disparity in maternal mortality. These are not new truths; there is an abundance of research on the Black–white gap in maternal mortality, yet the gaps persist.[168] These gaps persist because much of the health care research and intervention has focused on individual health behaviors that are correlated with race[169] rather than the foundational causes, such as how structural differences in Black and white women's access to maternity leave and insurance that covers postnatal care are associated with mortality during the 12 months after giving birth.[170,171]

This well-documented persistence of racial disparities in maternal mortality reminds us that knowledge of the problem does not equate to the political will to solve the problem. As Khiara Bridges details in her analysis of the 2018 Preventing Maternal Deaths Act, "race" does not appear anywhere in the text of the statute, which provides US states 12 million dollars annually for five years to fund maternal mortality review commissions.[172] This presents a quandary that has no easy answer, because as Bridges notes, "erasing race" from the text of the act was likely essential to passing the act and getting much-needed resources for maternal health. However, research suggests that obtaining resources to prevent maternal mortality may have no effect on narrowing racial disparities unless disparities are an explicit part of the utilization of resources.[173]

For example, a 2020 report from nine maternal mortality review committees that disaggregated data by race found that there were significant racial differences in the causes of pregnancy-related deaths.[174] Imagine what could be possible at the population level if the 2018 Preventing Maternal Deaths Act instructed all maternal mortality review committees to disaggregate data by race and ethnicity and ensure that interventions aligned with subpopulation needs. To create meaningful change, these committees also need to be instructed to examine morbidity, because there are about 1,200 maternal deaths per year, but a much greater 60,000 annual cases of severe morbidity.[175]

Improved health outcomes based on concordance between the race of the provider and patient is one of many instances where representation has a significant impact on the outcomes for Black versus white people. For example, research has shown that having greater proportions of Black doctors in a county leads to longer life expectancy among Black people.[176] Moreover, a recent study based on 1.8 million hospital births showed that Black infant mortality was reduced by 50% when Black newborns were cared for by Black physicians, compared with those cared for by white physicians.[36] These protective effects of newborn–physician racial concordance among Blacks are especially strong for more complex births and in hospitals where more Black babies are delivered. It is important to note that this effect was not found for white newborns, whose mortality is the same regardless of whether the physician is white or Black.

Physician–patient racial concordance improves health outcomes by ameliorating outgroup prejudices, improving communication, and fostering trust.[36] The low percentage of doctors who are Black (5.7%) relative to the percentage of Black people in the United States (13.6%) is a systemic problem that is rooted in a racially inequitable prekindergarten, elementary, and high school education system. The underrepresentation of Black doctors is the long-term outcome of underresourced schools that do not provide Black children with the foundational educational experiences that would enable them to succeed in college and medical school.[177,178] It is also due to the legacy of systematically underfunding and closing Black medical schools while simultaneously excluding Black students from white medical schools.[179,180] Adequate representation of Black doctors throughout the entire American medical training and care provision system is needed to improve the continuum of care for all health outcomes.

CONCLUSION

As detailed throughout this chapter, the effects of the racial hierarchy of human value persist from crib to coffin; structural racism increases the risk for being exposed to and experiencing systems, policies, and practices that create and sustain circumstances that compromise health.[181] The interaction between public and private systems in the United States creates reinforcing and vicious cycles that are responsible for disparities in health, wealth, and well-being.[182] The intentional design of public policies that establish and rely upon a racial hierarchy to ensure white supremacy in social and political outcomes is evident upon examination of major social, place, voting, economic, and legal policies. From the affirmation of enslavement in the US Constitution, to Black Codes restricting economic and social mobility of Black people prior to the Civil War, to the enforcement of Jim Crow laws during Reconstruction, to mass incarceration of Black people after the enactment of Civil Rights legislation, the social construct of race has served to limit the ability of Black people to achieve the highest levels of health.

Research has shown that systems of oppression are interconnected, and often one system facilitates the operation of another.[26,28] The only way to address racism's many tentacles and the systematic nature of racial oppression is to move upstream from individual health behaviors and examine how systems differentially enable and constrain the health of whole communities that are often segregated by both race and income. There are numerous opportunities for interventions targeting the educational, criminal legal, economic, health care, political, and other systems. Given the interconnected and cascading effects of system-level policies and practices, systemic-change policies and practices need to be bundled across systems, jurisdictions, and institutions to simultaneously address the interconnectivity and upstream impact of structural racism.[28,183,184]

Along with identifying and rooting out the ways that structural racism embedded in each individual system harms the health of Black people, we must maintain attention to the fact that all are rooted in the ways that residential segregation enables the spatial allocation of resources. As stated by Dr. David Williams, "one of America's best-kept secrets is how residential segregation is the secret sauce that creates racial inequality in the United States … there is not even one city where whites live under equal conditions to blacks."[185] Systems of residential segregation buttress systems of economic oppression, creating the unique Black experience of racial and economic hyper-segregation.[1,186] This brings us to one overarching recommendation that can narrow population-level health disparities: place-based economic repair(ations), which is defined as intentional economic investment in predominantly Black neighborhoods.

Effectively translating the idea of place-based economic repair(ations) into implemented initiatives requires that we broaden our conceptualization of what counts as a health intervention. Blankenship et al. identify community organizing to strengthen collective action as a systemic intervention that can create population-level health outcomes.[187] Organizing is a precursor to health equity because segregation impedes coalition building across racial and ethnic groups and encourages economic disinvestments in predominantly Black communities. As they state, "collectivization represents a structural intervention in itself, because through mobilizing themselves, marginalized groups alter the structures of power that keep them oppressed. It also has been an important strategy for demanding structural interventions."[192(p62)] Consistent with this, research on the political determinants of health has made visible the fact that the right to health and the unequal distribution of the social determinants of health are political choices that can only be changed through political action.[188,189]

Narrowing population-level health disparities requires restyling with and reversing disparities in the place-based allocation of resources. For example, interventions aimed at narrowing obesity disparities by targeting individual-level actions, such as diet, nutrition, and physical activity are largely ineffective and have a high failure rate.[190] This is because system-level drivers hinder behavioral health change for individuals living in food deserts and unsafe neighborhoods. Both of those place-based structural barriers are consequences of the ways that racial segregation concentrates poverty and its ill effects for Black people and concentrates wealth and its salubrious effects for White people.

Systemic interventions in place-based systems can narrow health disparities by investing in reducing racial disparities through equipping neighborhoods with equitable access to a high density of positive social determinants of health.[32,184,191] The most comprehensive of these interventions fall under the category of place-based, multisector, equity-oriented interventions that aim for neighborhood-wide coverage of a range of simultaneous interventions that make equity-oriented change in the quality and quantity of services provided to members of underserved communities.[26] Purpose Built Communities, established in 2009, is illustrative of what can be achieved through this approach.

Regarding CLS, the lynchpin role of residential segregation is exemplified in that it is the existence of place-based multipliers that concentrates race with other measures of (dis)advantage that facilitates CLS in deploying racially targeted aggressive policing and disproportionate incarceration with little fear of political repercussions.[192–194] This in turn increases economic, social, and political marginalization by removing large numbers of Black adults from their communities, and for some, permanently removing their voting rights.[195] These are all factors that researchers are beginning to measure and model as novel indicators of structural racism to determine their effect on health.[196] Cox et al. find that segregation causes an increase in Black homicides and Black imprisonment rates, in large part because of decreased investment in factors that deter crime, such as community economic and social development, and high-quality school and out-of-school programs.[31]

Place-based economic repair(ations) in CLS means shifting spending from the numerous forms of detention and incarceration to strengthening preschool programs and public schools. Kurgan examined CLS spending in New York City, New York and found "million-dollar blocks"—single-census blocks in inner-city neighborhoods where the government spends over a million dollars each year to imprison primarily Black residents from those blocks.[197] A similar examination of corrections spending in Chicago found that, over a five-year period, the Illinois Department of Corrections spent over one million dollars per city block incarcerating mostly Black people.[198] It is estimated that including spending from all the other federal, state, and local branches of CLS would change some of Chicago's predominantly Black blocks from million- to billion-dollar blocks. A very different outcome would be possible if CLS funding were invested in educating the predominantly Black children on those same city blocks, given that approximately 70% of male inmates don't have a high school diploma.[177] As Porter notes, investing in detaining and incarcerating instead of educating nonviolent offenders has become very a profitable business in America.[199] Mapping differential spending on factors that contribute to the positive versus the negative social determinants of health enables us to see that it is not lack of funding but lack of political will that prevents the United States from cultivating the health of Black Americans.

Structural interventions, even when initiated within health care systems and by health care providers, aim to change factors that extend far beyond health care settings. For example, standard medical visits should include formal screenings to evaluate patients' social risk and actively facilitate strategies to address their needs.[200] An innovative example is the Health Opportunities Pilot implemented by University of North Carolina Cecil G. Sheps Center for Health Services Research, through funding from Section 1115 of the Social Security Act. They found that embedding nonmedical interventions, such as providing fresh produce and safe housing to Medicaid beneficiaries in health care services, can improve health outcomes and reduce health care costs. Results demonstrated increases in healthy eating, reduction in medication use, lowered A1C and cholesterol, and fewer incidences of asthmatic episodes. In addition, establishing multisector collaboration between the state, primary health care providers, health care systems, and community organizing is needed to address health inequities among underserved populations.[201]

Another example of how health systems can further place-based economic repair(ations) is a health care–initiated intervention aimed at addressing the fact that poverty is a fundamental cause of disease. Gómez et al. conducted a randomized trial study that examined the efficacy of providing financial coaching for parents of infants in a pediatric primary care setting.[202] The financial coaches, who also had backgrounds in social work, were trained by a national nonprofit that works to break intergenerational cycles of poverty. Parents and children in the intervention group had half the rate of missed primary care pediatric visits compared with those in the control group and were 26% more likely to be up to date with immunizations at each visit, with fewer missed vaccinations overall by the end of the six-month visit period. Additionally, parents who received financial coaching reported increased monthly household income relative to when they enrolled in the program. Targeting poverty, a social determinant of health, rather than parents' beliefs about the importance of pediatric appointments, directly improved not only medical appointment adherence and vaccine uptake but also the underlying structural issue of intergenerational poverty.

The call for place-based economic repair(ations) at all levels of government as a health equity intervention is in line with growing evidence that racial health equity can be advanced from policies and interventions that create societal–systemic change.[28,191] For example, Kemp et al. found that civil rights laws and policies passed between 1993 and 2016 were associated with improved physical health outcomes for Black people.[148] Similar to the crosscutting nature of civil rights laws, reparations for Black people who are the descendants of enslaved Black Americans are imperative in the fight for racial equity. Reparations are not solely about repairing the harm from slavery, but about ongoing protectionist policies and practices that were implemented to bolster white socioeconomic status and wealth at the exclusion and detriment of Black prosperity and health. For example, Francis et al. document that from 1875 to 1910, Black families acquired 16 million acres of land but lost roughly 90% of this land between 1910 and 1997 due to discriminatory policies and outright plunder.[203] They estimate the value of the land loss to be roughly $326 billion. There are many such atrocities over the course of American history that need to be itemized when determining the cost of reparations. Darity et al. propose to measure the intergenerational and cumulative value of white oppression on existing descendants of slaves using the racial wealth gap.[9]

We close by emphasizing that interventions and policies aimed at narrowing population-level health disparities will be most effective when they are upstream and preventive. While individual factors such as creating a nurturing home environment may be protective against negative environments, it is going to take local and national policies to address the root cause of racial disparities in health. This includes policies that address racial disparities in employment, wealth, access to quality education, public goods (e.g., green spaces and parks), environmental health, CLS, and access to quality health care needed to close health gaps.[204] An important caveat is that all efforts to narrow health disparities will be limited without simultaneously addressing how racial segregation in housing enables inequitable investment in place. Segregation is characterized as the lynchpin of structural racism because of its spillover effects on many aspects of life, schools, jobs, crime, health care, wealth, and social and human capital.[184] Refer to the Chapter 8 for a broad range of evidence-based, systems-level interventions.

REFERENCES

1. Du Bois, W. E. B. *The Philadelphia Negro: A Social Study*. University of Pennsylvania Press; 1899.
2. Golash-Boza T. A critical and comprehensive sociological theory of race and racism. *Sociol Race Ethn*. 2016;2(2):129–141. doi:10.1177/2332649216632242
3. Omi M, Winant H. *Racial Formation in the United States*. 3rd ed. Routledge; 2014.
4. Braveman P, Egerter S, Williams DR. The social determinants of health: Coming of age. *Annu Rev Public Health*. 2011;32(1):381–398. doi:10.1146/annurev-publhealth-031210-101218
5. Lavizzo-Mourey RJ, Besser RE, Williams DR. Understanding and mitigating health inequities—Past, current, and future directions. *N Engl J Med*. 2021;384(18):1681–1684. doi:10.1056/NEJMp2008628
6. Christopher GC. Commission on Security and Cooperation in Europe (Helsinki Commission): Briefing on truth, reconciliation, and healing toward a unified future, Thursday, July 18, 2019. *Health Equity*. 2021;5(1):662–667. doi:10.1089/heq.2021.29007.chr
7. Collins WJ, Wanamaker MH. African American intergenerational economic mobility since 1880. *Am Econ J Appl Econ*. 2022;14(3):84–117. doi:10.3386/w23395
8. Cox R. Overcoming social exclusion: Addressing race and criminal justice policy in the United States. In: *Vision 2020*. Washington Center for Equitable Growth; 2020. Accessed April 8, 2025. https://equitablegrowth.org/overcoming-social-exclusion-addressing-race-and-criminal-justice-policy-in-the-united-states
9. Darity W Jr, Mullen AK, Slaughter M. The cumulative costs of racism and the bill for Black reparations. *J Econ Persp*. 2022;36(2):99–122. doi:10.1257/jep.36.2.99
10. Baradaran M. *The Color of Money: Black Banks and the Racial Wealth Gap*. Harvard University Press; 2017.
11. Byrd WM, Clayton LA. The 'slave health deficit'. Racism and health outcomes. *Health PAC Bull*. 1991;21(2):25–28.
12. Byrd WM, Clayton LA *An American Health Dilemma: Race, Medicine, and Health Care in the United States 1900-2000*. Routledge; 2002.
13. Jackman MR, Shauman KA. The toll of inequality: Excess African American deaths in the United States over the twentieth century. *Du Bois Rev*. 2019;16(2):291–340. doi:10.1017/S1742058X20000028
14. Caraballo C, Massey DS, Ndumele CD, et al. Excess mortality and years of potential life lost among the Black population in the US, 1999-2020. *JAMA*. 2023;329(19):1662–1670. doi:10.1001/jama.2023.7022
15. Gould SJ. *Mismeasure of Man*. W. W. Norton; 1996.
16. Keel TD. Charles V. Roman and the spectre of polygenism in progressive era public health research. *Soc Hist Med*. 2015;28(4):742–766. doi:10.1093/shm/hkv035
17. Vyas DA, Eisenstein LG, Jones DS. Hidden in plain sight—Reconsidering the use of race correction in clinical algorithms. *N Engl J Med*. 2020;383(9):874–882. doi:10.1056/NEJMms2004740
18. Hoffman KM, Trawalter S, Axt JR, Oliver MN. Racial bias in pain assessment and treatment recommendations, and false beliefs about biological differences between Blacks and Whites. *Proc Natl Acad Sci USA*. 2016;113(16):4296–4301. doi:10.1073/pnas.1516047113

19. Timmermans S, Kaufman R. Technologies and health inequities. *Annu Rev Sociol.* 2020;46:583–602. doi:10.1146/annurev-soc-121919-054802
20. Krieger N. Structural racism, health inequities, and the two-edged sword of data: Structural problems require structural solutions. *Front Public Health.* 2021;9:655447. doi:10.3389/fpubh.2021.655447
21. Murry VM, Butler-Barnes ST, Mayo-Gamble TL, Inniss-Thompson MN. Excavating new constructs for family stress theories in the context of everyday life experiences of Black American families. *J Fam Theory Rev.* 2018;10(2):384–405. doi:10.1111/jftr.12256
22. Woolf SH, Chin MH, Murry VM, Gee GC. The plight of marginalized populations in 2025: The assault on health equity through a systems lens. *Am J Public Health.* 2025 July 31:e1–e6. doi:10.2105/AJPH.2025.308221. Epub ahead of print.
23. Murry VM, Nyanamba JM, Hanebutt R, et al. Critical examination of resilience and resistance in African American families: Adaptive capacities to navigate toxic oppressive upstream waters. *Dev Psychopathol.* 2023;35(5):2113–2131. doi:10.1017/S0954579423001037
24. Brown TH, Lee HE, Hicken MT, Bonilla-Silva E, Homan P. Conceptualizing and measuring systemic racism. *Annu Rev Public Health.* 2025;46(1):69–90. doi:10.1146/annurev-publhealth-060222-032022
25. Williams DR, Lawrence JA, Davis BA, Vu C. Understanding how discrimination can affect health. *Health Serv Res.* 2019;54(suppl 2):1374–1388. doi:10.1111/1475-6773.13222
26. Bailey ZD, Krieger N, Agénor M, Graves J, Linos N, Bassett MT. Structural racism and health inequities in the USA: evidence and interventions. *Lancet.* 2017;389(10077):1453–1463. doi:10.1016/S0140-6736(17)30569-X
27. Jones-Eversley SD, Dean LT. After 121 years, it's time to recognize W. E. B. Du Bois as a founding father of social epidemiology. *J Negro Educ.* 2018;87(3):230. doi:10.7709/jnegroeducation.87.3.0230
28. Brown TH, Homan P. The future of social determinants of health: Looking upstream to structural drivers. *Milbank Q.* 2023;101(suppl 1):36–60. doi:10.1111/1468-0009.12641
29. Phelan JC, Link BG. Is racism a fundamental cause of inequalities in health?. *Annu Rev Sociol.* 2015;41:311–330. doi:10.1146/annurev-soc-073014-112305
30. Weinstein JN, Geller A, Negussie Y, Baciu A, eds. *Communities in Action: Pathways to Health Equity.* National Academies Press; 2017.
31. Cox R, Cunningham JP, Ortega A, Whaley K. Black lives: The high cost of segregation. Washington Center for Equitable Growth working papers. May 2022. Accessed April 8, 2025. https://equitablegrowth.org/working-papers/black-lives-the-high-cost-of-segregation
32. Gee GC, Ford CL. Structural racism and health inequities: Old issues, new directions. *Du Bois Rev.* 2011;8(1):115–132. doi:10.1017/S1742058X11000130
33. Williams DR, Collins C. Racial residential segregation: a fundamental cause of racial disparities in health. *Public Health Rep.* 2001;116(5):404–416. doi:10.1093/phr/116.5.404
34. Cox R. Mass incarceration, racial disparities in health, and successful aging. *Generations.* 2018;42(2):48–55. Accessed April 8, 2025. https://www.jstor.org/stable/26556360
35. Alexander M. *The New Jim Crow: Mass Incarceration in the Age of Colorblindness.* New Press; 2010.

36. Greenwood BN, Hardeman RR, Huang L, Sojourner A. Physician-patient racial concordance and disparities in birthing mortality for newborns. *Proc Natl Acad Sci USA*. 2020;117(35):21194–21200. doi:10.1073/pnas.1913405117
37. Hardeman RR, Murphy KA, Karbeah J, Kozhimannil KB. Naming institutionalized racism in the public health literature: A systematic literature review. *Public Health Rep*. 2018;133(3):240–249. doi:10.1177/0033354918760574
38. Smedley, BD, Stith Butler A, Bristow LR; Institute of Medicine Committee on Institutional and Policy-Level Strategies for Increasing the Diversity of the US Healthcare Workforce. *In the Nation's Compelling Interest: Ensuring Diversity in the Health-Care Workforce*. National Academies Press; 2004.
39. Forde AT, Crookes DM, Suglia SF, Demmer RT. The weathering hypothesis as an explanation for racial disparities in health: A systematic review. *Ann Epidemiol*. 2019;33:1–18.e3. doi:10.1016/j.annepidem.2019.02.011
40. Lynch J, Smith GD. A life course approach to chronic disease epidemiology. *Annu Rev Public Health*. 2005;26(1):1–35. doi:10.1146/annurev.publhealth.26.021304.144505
41. Dannefer D. Cumulative advantage/disadvantage and the life course: Cross-fertilizing age and social science theory. *J Gerontol B Psychol Sci Soc Sci*. 2003;58(6):S327–S337. doi:10.1093/geronb/58.6.s327
42. Geronimus AT. The weathering hypothesis and the health of African-American women and infants: evidence and speculations. *Ethn Dis*. 1992;2(3):207–221. Accessed April 8, 2025. https://www.jstor.org/stable/45403051
43. Simons RL, Lei MK, Klopack E, Beach SRH, Gibbons FX, Philibert RA. The effects of social adversity, discrimination, and health risk behaviors on the accelerated aging of African Americans: Further support for the weathering hypothesis. *Soc Sci Med*. 2021;282:113169. doi:10.1016/j.socscimed.2020.113169
44. Heard-Garris N, Boyd R, Kan K, Perez-Cardona L, Heard NJ, Johnson TJ. Structuring poverty: How racism shapes child poverty and child and adolescent health. *Acad Pediatr*. 2021;21(suppl 8):S108–S116. doi:10.1016/j.acap.2021.05.026
45. Brondolo E, Gallo LC, Myers HF. Race, racism and health: Disparities, mechanisms, and interventions. *J Behav Med*. 2009;32(1):1–8. doi:10.1007/s10865-008-9190-3
46. McEwen BS. Neurobiological and systemic effects of chronic stress. *Chronic Stress (Thousand Oaks)*. 2017;1:2470547017692328. doi:10.1177/2470547017692328
47. Mezuk B, Rafferty JA, Kershaw KN, et al. Reconsidering the role of social disadvantage in physical and mental health: stressful life events, health behaviors, race, and depression. *Am J Epidemiol*. 2010;172(11):1238–1249. doi:10.1093/aje/kwq283
48. Turner RJ. Understanding health disparities: The promise of the stress process model. In: Avison WR, Aneshensel CS, Schieman S, Wheaton B, eds. *Advances in the Conceptualization of the Stress Process: Essays in Honor of Leonard I. Pearlin*. Springer; 2010:3–21.
49. Brody GH, Yu T, Chen E, Miller GE, Barton AW, Kogan SM. Family-centered prevention effects on the association between racial discrimination and mental health in black adolescents: Secondary analysis of 2 randomized clinical trials. *JAMA Netw Open*. 2021;4(3):e211964. doi:10.1001/jamanetworkopen.2021.1964

50. Berens A, Jenson S, Nelson C. Biological embedding of childhood adversity: From physiological mechanisms to clinical implications. *BMC Med.* 2017;15(1):135. doi:10.1186/s12916-017-0895-4
51. Jenkins LM, Chiang JJ, Vause K, et al. Subcortical structural variations associated with low socioeconomic status in adolescents. *Hum Brain Mapp.* 2020;41(1):162–171. doi:10.1002/hbm.24796
52. Hyde LW, Gard AM, Tomlinson RC, Burt SA, Mitchell C, Monk CS. An ecological approach to understanding the developing brain: Examples linking poverty, parenting, neighborhoods, and the brain. *Am Psychol.* 2020;75(9):1245–1259. doi:10.1037/amp0000741
53. Council on Community Pediatrics. Poverty and child health in the United States. *Pediatrics.* 2016;137(4):e20160339–e20160339. doi:10.1542/peds.2016-0339
54. Ford JL, Williams KP, Kue JK. Racism, stress, and health. *Nurs Res.* 2021;70(suppl 5):S1–S2. doi:10.1097/NNR.0000000000000534
55. Beatty K, Egen O, Dreyzehner J, Wykoff R. Poverty and health in Tennessee. *South Med J.* 2020;113(1):1–7. doi:10.14423/smj.0000000000001055
56. Maalouf M, Fearon M, Lipa MC, Chow-Johnson H, Tayeh L, Lipa D. Neurologic complications of poverty: The associations between poverty as a social determinant of health and adverse neurologic outcomes. *Curr Neurol Neurosci Rep.* 2021;21(7). doi:10.1007/s11910-021-01116-z
57. Schmeer KK, Piperata BA. Household food insecurity and child health. *Matern Child Nutr.* 2016;13(2):e12301. doi:10.1111/mcn.12301
58. Smith MV, Mazure CM. Mental health and wealth: Depression, gender, poverty, and parenting. *Annu Rev Clin Psychol.* 2021;17(1):181–205. doi:10.1146/annurev-clinpsy-071219-022710
59. Amaro H, Sanchez M, Bautista T, Cox R. Social vulnerabilities for substance use: Stressors, socially toxic environments, and discrimination and racism. *Neuropharmacology.* 2021;188:108518. doi:10.1016/j.neuropharm.2021.108518
60. Zilioli S, Imami L, Ong AD, Lumley MA, Gruenewald T. Discrimination and anger control as pathways linking socioeconomic disadvantage to allostatic load in midlife. *J Psychosom Res.* 2017;103:83–90. doi:10.1016/j.jpsychores.2017.10.002
61. Rewak M, Buka S, Prescott J, et al. Race-related health disparities and biological aging: Does rate of telomere shortening differ across blacks and whites?. *Biol Psychol.* 2014;99:92–99. doi:10.1016/j.biopsycho.2014.03.007
62. Alio AP, Richman AR, Clayton HB, Jeffers DF, Wathington DJ, Salihu HM. An ecological approach to understanding Black–white disparities in perinatal mortality. *Matern Child Health J.* 2010;14(4):557–566. doi:10.1007/s10995-009-0495-9
63. David RJ, Collins JW Jr. Differing birth weight among infants of US-born Blacks, African-born Blacks, and US-born whites. *N Engl J Med.* 1997;337(17):1209–1214. doi:10.1056/NEJM199710233371706
64. Turner RJ. Understanding health disparities: The promise of the stress process model. In: Avison WR, Aneshensel CS, Schieman S, Wheaton B, eds. *Advances in the Conceptualization of the Stress Process: Essays in Honor of Leonard I. Pearlin.* Springer; 2009:3–21.
65. Chae DH, Clouston S, Hatzenbuehler ML, et al. Association between an internet-based measure of area racism and Black mortality. *PLoS One.* 2015;10(4):e0122963. doi:10.1371/journal.pone.0122963

66. Jackson JS, Knight KM, Rafferty JA. Race and unhealthy behaviors: chronic stress, the HPA axis, and physical and mental health disparities over the life course. *Am J Public Health*. 2010;100(5):933–939. doi:10.2105/AJPH.2008.143446
67. Gilbert PA, Zemore SE. Discrimination and drinking: A systematic review of the evidence. *Soc Sci Med*. 2016;161:178–194. doi:10.1016/j.socscimed.2016.06.009
68. Jackson JS, Knight KM. Race and self-regulatory health behaviors: The role of the stress response and the HPA axis in physical and mental health disparities. In: Schaie KW, Carstensen LL, eds. *Social Structures, Aging, and Self-Regulation in the Elderly*. Springer; 2006:189–239.
69. Mezuk B, Abdou CM, Hudson D, et al. "White box" epidemiology and the social neuroscience of health behaviors: The environmental affordances model. *Soc Ment Health*. 2013;3(2). doi:10.1177/2156869313480892
70. Rothstein MA. Structural challenges of precision medicine. *J Law Med Ethics*. 2017;45(2):274–279. doi:10.1177/1073110517720655
71. Cohen DR, Lindsey MA, Lochman JE. Applying an ecosocial framework to address racial disparities in suicide risk among black youth. *Psychology Sch*. 2022;59(12), 2405–2421. doi:10.1002/pits.22588
72. Murry VM, Heflinger CA, Suiter SV, Brody GH. Examining perceptions about mental health care and help-seeking among rural African American families of adolescents. *J Youth Adolesc*. 2011;40(9):1118–1131. doi:10.1007/s10964-010-9627-1
73. Cutler DM, Glaeser EL. Are ghettos good or bad?. *Q J Econ*. 1997;112(3):827–872. doi:10.3386/w5163
74. Elbers B. Trends in US residential racial segregation, 1990 to 2020. *Socius*. 2021;7:237802312110539. doi:10.1177/23780231211053982
75. Sewell AA, Jefferson KA. Collateral damage: The health effects of invasive police encounters in New York City. *J Urban Health*. 2016;93(suppl 1):42–67. doi:10.1007/s11524-015-0016-7
76. Massey DS, Denton NA. *American Apartheid: Segregation and the Making of the Underclass*. Harvard University Press; 1993.
77. Kneeshaw-Price S, Saelens BE, Sallis JF, et al. Children's objective physical activity by location: Why the neighborhood matters. *Pediatr Exerc Sci*. 2013;25(3):468–486. doi:10.1123/pes.25.3.468
78. Bonnie RJ, Backes EP, eds. *The Promise of Adolescence: Realizing Opportunity for All Youth*. National Academies Press; 2019.
79. Malat J, Oh HJ, Hamilton MA. Poverty experience, race, and child health. *Public Health Rep*. 2005;120(4):442–447. doi: 10.1177/003335490512000411
80. Assari S, Moghani Lankarani M, Caldwell CH. Discrimination increases suicidal ideation in Black adolescents regardless of ethnicity and gender. *Behav Sci (Basel)*. 2017;7(4):75. doi:10.3390/bs7040075
81. Barlow JN. Restoring optimal black mental health and reversing intergenerational trauma in an era of Black Lives Matter. *Biography*. 2018;41(4):895–908. doi:10.1353/bio.2018.0084
82. Atkins-Loria S, Macdonald H, Mitterling C. Young African American men and the diagnosis of conduct disorder: The neo-colonization of suffering. *Clin Soc Work J*. 2015;43(4):431–441. doi:10.1007/s10615-015-0531-8
83. Myers HF, Wyatt GE, Ullman JB, et al. Cumulative burden of lifetime adversities: Trauma and mental health in low-SES African Americans and Latino/as. *Psychol Trauma*. 2015;7(3):243–251. doi:10.1037/a0039077

84. Bath E. Black and blue: Understanding stigma and diagnostic barriers to increase treatment receipt for African American youth with depression and anxiety disorders. *JAACAP Open.* 2019;58(10):S61–S62. doi:10.1016/j.jaac.2019.07.950
85. Benzow A, Fikri K. The expanded geography of high-poverty neighborhoods: How the economic recovery from the Great Recession failed to change the landscape of poverty in the United States. Economic Innovation Group. May 2020. Accessed April 8, 2025. https://eig.org/wp-content/uploads/2020/04/Expanded-Geography-High-Poverty-Neighborhoods.pdf
86. Borofsky LA, Kellerman I, Baucom B, Oliver PH, Margolin G. Community violence exposure and adolescents' school engagement and academic achievement over time. *Psychol Violence.* 2013;3(4):381–395. doi:10.1037/a0034121
87. Prelow HM, Danoff-Burg S, Swenson RR, Pulgiano D. The impact of ecological risk and perceived discrimination on the psychological adjustment of African American and European American youth. *J Community Psychol.* 2004;32(4):375–389. doi:10.1002/jcop.20007
88. Gilliam WS, Maupin AN, Reyes CR, Accavitti M, Shic F. Do early educators' implicit biases regarding sex and race relate to behavior expectations and recommendations of preschool expulsions and suspensions?. Yale University Child Study Center. September 28, 2016. Accessed April 8, 2025. https://files-profile.medicine.yale.edu/documents/75afe6d2-e556-4794-bf8c-3cf105113b7c
89. Wald J, Losen DJ. Defining and redirecting a school-to-prison pipeline. *New Dir Youth Dev.* 2003;2003(99):9–15. doi:10.1002/yd.51
90. Sentell T, Zhang W, Ching LK. Insights in public health: The importance of considering educational inequity and health literacy to understand racial/ethnic health disparities. *Hawaii J Med Public Health.* 2015;74(7):244–247.
91. Zajacova A, Lawrence EM. The relationship between education and health: Reducing disparities through a contextual approach. *Annu Rev Public Health.* 2018;39:273–289. doi:10.1146/annurev-publhealth-031816-044628
92. Kimble J. Insuring inequality: The role of the Federal Housing Administration in the urban ghettoization of African Americans. *Law Soc Inq.* 2007;32(2):399–434. doi:10.1111/j.1747-4465.2007.00064.x
93. Rothstein R. The racial achievement gap, segregated schools, and segregated neighborhoods: A constitutional insult. *Race Soc Probl.* 2014;7(1):21–30. doi:10.1007/s12552-014-9134-1
94. Baker BD, Corcoran SP. The stealth inequities of school funding: How state and local school finance systems perpetuate inequitable student spending. Center for American Progress. September 19, 2012. Accessed April 8, 2025. https://www.americanprogress.org/article/the-stealth-inequities-of-school-funding
95. Chyn E, Katz LF. Neighborhoods matter: Assessing the evidence for place effects. *J Econ Persp.* 2021;35(4):197–222. doi:10.1257/jep.35.4.197
96. Ostrander RR. School funding: Inequality in district funding and the disparate impact on urban and migrant school children. *BYU Educ Law J.* 2015;2015(1):9. Accessed August 11, 2025. https://digitalcommons.law.byu.edu/elj/vol2015/iss1/9
97. Southern Education Foundation. A new majority: Low income students now a majority in the nation's public schools. Research bulletin. 2015. Accessed April 8, 2025. https://eric.ed.gov/?id=ED555829

98. Garcia E. Schools are still segregated, and Black children are paying a price. Economic Policy Institute. February 12, 2020. Accessed August 11, 2025. https://www.epi.org/publication/schools-are-still-segregated-and-black-children-are-paying-a-price
99. Reardon SF. School segregation and racial academic achievement gaps. *RSF*. 2016;2(5):34–57 doi:10.7758/RSF.2016.2.5.03
100. Kucsera J, Orfield G. New York State's extreme school segregation: Inequality, inaction and a damaged future. March 26, 2014. Accessed April 8, 2025. http://www.escholarship.org/uc/item/5cx4b8pf
101. Zimmerman E, Woolf SH. Understanding the relationship between education and health. Discussion Paper, Institute of Medicine. 2014. doi:10.31478/201406A
102. Vable AM, Cohen AK, Leonard SA, Glymour MM, Duarte CDP, Yen IH. Do the health benefits of education vary by sociodemographic subgroup? Differential returns to education and implications for health inequities. *Ann Epidemiol*. 2018;28(11):759–766.e5. doi:10.1016/j.annepidem.2018.08.014
103. Joseph KS, Boutin A, Lisonkova S, et al. Maternal mortality in the United States: Recent trends, current status, and future considerations. *Obstet Gynecol*. 2021;137(5):763–771. doi:10.1097/AOG.0000000000004361
104. Jang CJ, Lee HC. A Review of Racial Disparities in Infant Mortality in the US. *Children (Basel)*. 2022;9(2):257. doi:10.3390/children9020257
105. Manuck TA. Racial and ethnic differences in preterm birth: A complex, multifactorial problem. *Semin Perinatol*. 2017;41(8):511–518. doi:10.1053/j.semperi.2017.08.010
106. Leonard SA, Main EK, Scott KA, Profit J, Carmichael SL. Racial and ethnic disparities in severe maternal morbidity prevalence and trends. *Ann Epidemiol*. 2019;33:30-36. doi:10.1016/j.annepidem.2019.02.007
107. Liese KL, Mogos M, Abboud S, Decocker K, Koch AR, Geller SE. Racial and ethnic disparities in severe maternal morbidity in the United States. *J Racial Ethn Health Disparities*. 2019;6(4):790–798. doi:10.1007/s40615-019-00577-w
108. Mehra R, Boyd LM, Ickovics JR. Racial residential segregation and adverse birth outcomes: A systematic review and meta-analysis. *Soc Sci Med*. 2017;191:237–250. doi:10.1016/j.socscimed.2017.09.018
109. Gadson A, Akpovi E, Mehta PK. Exploring the social determinants of racial/ethnic disparities in prenatal care utilization and maternal outcome. *Semin Perinatol*. 2017;41(5):308–317. doi:10.1053/j.semperi.2017.04.008
110. Roberts D. *Torn Apart: How the Child Welfare System Destroys Black Families—And How Abolition Can Build a Safer World*. Basic Books; 2022.
111. Wildeman C, Wang EA. Mass incarceration, public health, and widening inequality in the USA. *Lancet*. 2017;389(10077):1464–1474. doi:10.1016/S0140-6736(17)30259-3
112. Carson EA, Kluckow R. Correctional populations in the United States, 2021—Statistical tables. Office of Justice Programs, US Dept of Justice. February 2023. Accessed August 11, 2025. https://www.ojp.gov/ncjrs/virtual-library/abstracts/correctional-populations-united-states-2021-statistical-tables
113. Western B, Wildeman C. The Black family and mass incarceration. *Ann Am Acad Pol Soc Sci*. 2009;621(1):221–242. doi:10.1177/0002716208324850

114. Nowotny KM, Rogers RG, Boardman JD. Racial disparities in health conditions among prisoners compared with the general population. *SSM Popul Health*. 2017;3:487–496. doi:10.1016/j.ssmph.2017.05.011
115. Conway JM. Mass incarceration and children's health: A state-level analysis of adverse birth outcomes and infant, child, and teen mortality. *Fam Community Health*. 2021;44(3):194–205. doi:10.1097/FCH.0000000000000295
116. Pager D. The mark of a criminal record. *Am J Sociol*. 2003;108(5):937–975. doi:10.1086/374403
117. Sered SS, Norton-Hawk M. *Can't Catch a Break: Gender, Jail, Drugs and the Limits of Personal Responsibility*. University of California Press; 2014.
118. Nowotny KM, Belknap J, Lynch S, DeHart D. Risk profile and treatment needs of women in jail with co-occurring serious mental illness and substance use disorders. *Women Health*. 2014;54(8):781–795. doi:10.1080/03630242.2014.932892
119. Clarke JG, Simon RE. Shackling and separation: motherhood in prison. *Virtual Mentor*. 2013;15(9):779–785. doi:10.1001/virtualmentor.2013.15.9.pfor2-1309
120. McCampbell SW. The gender-responsive strategies project: Jail applications. April 2005. National Institute of Corrections, US Dept of Justice. Accessed August 11, 2025. https://www.urban.org/sites/default/files/2015/02/19/mccampbellnicpaper.pdf
121. Nandi A, Counts N, Bröker J, et al. Cost of care for Alzheimer's disease and related dementias in the United States: 2016 to 2060. *NPJ Aging*. 2024;10(1):13. doi:10.1038/s41514-024-00136-6
122. Mayeda ER, Glymour MM, Quesenberry CP, Whitmer RA. Inequalities in dementia incidence between six racial and ethnic groups over 14 years. *Alzheimers Dement*. 2016;12(3):216–224. doi:10.1016/j.jalz.2015.12.007
123. Schwartz BS, Glass TA, Bolla KI, et al. Disparities in cognitive functioning by race/ethnicity in the Baltimore Memory Study. *Environ Health Perspect*. 2004;112(3):314–320. doi:10.1289/ehp.6727
124. Sloan FA, Wang J. Disparities among older adults in measures of cognitive function by race or ethnicity. *J Gerontol B Psychol Sci Soc Sci*. 2005;60(5):242–250. doi:10.1093/geronb/60.5.p242
125. Lines LM, Wiener JM. Racial and ethnic disparities in Alzheimer's disease: A literature review. January 31, 2014. US Dept of Health and Human Services. Accessed August 12, 2025. https://aspe.hhs.gov/reports/racial-ethnic-disparities-alzheimers-disease-literature-review-0
126. Peterson R, Butler EA, Fain MJ, Ehiri JE, Carvajal SC. The role of social status and chronic stress for racial disparities in cognitive aging. *Alzheimer's Dementia* 2019;15(suppl 7):P1571–P1571. doi:10.1016/j.jalz.2019.08.185
127. Peterson RL, Butler EA, Ehiri JE, Fain MJ, Carvajal SC. Mechanisms of racial disparities in cognitive aging: An examination of material and psychosocial well-being. *J Gerontol B Psychol Sci Soc Sci*. 2021;76(3):574–582. doi:10.1093/geronb/gbaa003
128. Weuve J, Rajan KB, Barnes LL, Wilson RS, Evans DA. Secular trends in cognitive performance in older Black and white US adults, 1993–2012: Findings from the Chicago Health and Aging Project. *J Gerontol B Psychol Sci Soc Sci*. 2018;73(suppl 1):S73–S81. doi:10.1093/geronb/gbx167
129. Richards M, Deary IJ. A life course approach to cognitive reserve: A model for cognitive aging and development?. *Ann Neurol*. 2005;58(4):617–622. doi:10.1002/ana.20637

130. Theall KP, Drury SS, Shirtcliff EA. Cumulative neighborhood risk of psychosocial stress and allostatic load in adolescents. *Am J Epidemiol.* 2012;176(suppl 7):S164–S174. doi:10.1093/aje/kws185
131. Bonczar TP. Prevalence of imprisonment in the US population, 1974–2001. Bureau of Justice Statistics, US Dept of Justice. August 2003. Accessed August 11, 2025. https://bjs.ojp.gov/content/pub/pdf/piusp01.pdf
132. Cox RJA, Wallace RB. The role of incarceration as a risk factor for cognitive impairment. *J Gerontol B Psychol Sci Soc Sci.* 2022;77(12):e247–e262. doi:10.1093/geronb/gbac138
133. Aizer A, Doyle JJ. Juvenile incarceration, human capital, and future crime: Evidence from randomly assigned judges. *Q J Econ.* 2015;130(2):759–803. doi:10.1093/qje/qjv003
134. Greenfield EA, Akincigil A, Moorman SM. Is college completion associated with better cognition in later life for people who are the least, or most, likely to obtain a bachelor's degree?. *J Gerontol B Psychol Sci Soc Sci.* 2020;75(6):1286–1291. doi:10.1093/geronb/gbz132
135. Meng X, D'Arcy C. Education and dementia in the context of the cognitive reserve hypothesis: A systematic review with meta-analyses and qualitative analyses. *PLoS One.* 2012;7(6):e38268. doi:10.1371/journal.pone.0038268
136. Schmand B, Smit JH, Geerlings MI, Lindeboom J. The effects of intelligence and education on the development of dementia. A test of the brain reserve hypothesis. *Psychol Med.* 1997;27(6):1337–1344. doi:10.1017/s0033291797005461
137. Stern Y. Cognitive reserve in ageing and Alzheimer's disease. *Lancet Neurol.* 2012;11(11):1006–1012. doi:10.1016/S1474-4422(12)70191-6
138. Valenzuela MJ, Sachdev P. Brain reserve and cognitive decline: A non-parametric systematic review. *Psychol Med.* 2006;36(8):1065–1073. doi:10.1017/S0033291706007744
139. Cordero-Guzmán HR. Cognitive skills, test scores, and social stratification: The role of family and school-level resources on racial/ethnic differences in scores on standardized tests (AFQT). *Rev Black Polit Econ.* 2001;28(4):31–71. doi:10.1007/s12114-001-1008-2
140. Rodgers M, Spriggs WE. The effect of federal contractor status on racial differences in establishment-level employment shares: 1979–1992. *Am Econ Rev.* 1996;86(2):290–293. Accessed August 11, 2025. https://www.jstor.org/stable/2118139
141. Cox R, Wallace S. Identifying the link between food security and incarceration. *South Econ J.* 2016;82(4):1062–1077. doi:10.1002/soej.12080
142. Lee H, Wildeman C. Assessing mass incarceration's effects on families. *Science.* 2021;374(6565):277–281. doi:10.1126/science.abj7777
143. Massoglia M, Pridemore WA. Incarceration and health. *Annu Rev Sociol.* 2015;41:291–310. doi:10.1146/annurev-soc-073014-112326
144. Homan PA, Brown TH. Sick and tired of being excluded: Structural racism in disenfranchisement as a threat to population health equity. *Health Aff (Millwood).* 2022;41(2):219–227. doi:10.1377/hlthaff.2021.01414
145. Johnson RC, Raphael S. The effects of male incarceration dynamics on acquired immune deficiency syndrome infection rates among African American women and men. *J Law Econ.* 2009;52(2):251–293. doi:10.1086/597102
146. Lee H. How does structural racism operate (in) the contemporary US criminal justice system? *Annu Rev Criminol.* 2024;7:233–255. doi:10.1146/annurev-criminol-022422-015019

147. Turney K, Wildeman C, Schnittker J. As fathers and felons: Explaining the effects of current and recent incarceration on major depression. *J Health Soc Behav.* 2012;53(4):465–481. doi:10.1177/0022146512462400
148. Kemp B, Grumbach JM, Montez JK. US state policy contexts and physical health among midlife adults. *Socius.* 2022;8:10.1177/23780231221091324. doi:10.1177/23780231221091324
149. Singh GK, Jemal A. Socioeconomic and racial/ethnic disparities in cancer mortality, incidence, and survival in the United States, 1950–2014: Over six decades of changing patterns and widening inequalities. *J Environ Public Health.* 2017:2819372. doi:10.1155/2017/2819372
150. Zhao J, Han X, Zheng Z, et al. Racial/ethnic disparities in childhood cancer survival in the United States. *Cancer Epidemiol Biomarkers Prev.* 2021;30(11):2010–2017. doi:10.1158/1055-9965.EPI-21-0117
151. Jatoi I, Sung H, Jemal A. The emergence of the racial disparity in US breast-cancer mortality. *N Engl J Med.* 2022;386(25):2349–2352. doi:10.1056/NEJMp2200244
152. Rebbeck TR. Prostate cancer disparities by race and ethnicity: From nucleotide to neighborhood. *Cold Spring Harb Perspect Med.* 2018;8(9):a030387. doi:10.1101/cshperspect.a030387
153. Bona K, Keating NL. Addressing social determinants of health: Now is the time. *J Natl Cancer Inst.* 2022;114(12):1561–1563. doi:10.1093/jnci/djac137
154. Fan Q, Nogueira L, Yabroff KR, Hussaini SMQ, Pollack CE. Housing and cancer care and outcomes: A systematic review. *J Natl Cancer Inst.* 2022;114(12):1601–1618. doi:10.1093/jnci/djac173
155. Fowle MZ. Racialized homelessness: A review of historical and contemporary causes of racial disparities in homelessness. *Hous Policy Debate.* 2022;32(6):940–967. doi:10.1080/10511482.2022.2026995
156. Yearby R. Racial disparities in health status and access to healthcare: The continuation of inequality in the United States due to structural racism. *Am J Econ Sociol.* 2018;77(3–4):1113–1152. doi:10.1111/ajes.12230
157. Garcia MA, Homan PA, García C, Brown TH. The color of COVID-19: Structural racism and the disproportionate impact of the pandemic on older Black and Latinx adults. *J Gerontol B Psychol Sci Soc Sci.* 2021;76(3):e75–e80. doi:10.1093/geronb/gbaa114
158. Paradies Y, Truong M, Priest N. A systematic review of the extent and measurement of healthcare provider racism. *J Gen Intern Med.* 2014;29(2):364–387. doi:10.1007/s11606-013-2583-1
159. Feagin J, Bennefield Z. Systemic racism and US health care. *Soc Sci Med.* 2014;103:7–14. doi:10.1016/j.socscimed.2013.09.006
160. American Medical Association. Reducing disparities in health care. October 23, 2023. Accessed April 8, 2025. https://www.ama-assn.org/delivering-care/patient-support-advocacy/reducing-disparities-health-care
161. American Cancer Society. Cancer facts & figures for African American/Black people 2022–2024. Accessed April 8, 2025. https://www.cancer.org/research/cancer-facts-statistics/cancer-facts-figures-for-african-americans.html
162. Islami F, Guerra CE, Minihan A, et al. American Cancer Society's report on the status of cancer disparities in the United States, 2021. *CA Cancer J Clin.* 2022;72(2):112–143. doi:10.3322/caac.21703
163. Gorin SS, Heck JE, Cheng B, Smith SJ. Delays in breast cancer diagnosis and treatment by racial/ethnic group. *Arch Intern Med.* 2006;166(20):2244–2252. doi:10.1001/archinte.166.20.2244

164. Frakes MD, Gruber J. Racial concordance and the quality of medical care: Evidence from the military. National Bureau of Economic Research. December 2022. doi:10.3386/w30767
165. Crown, A, Joseph KA. Addressing breast cancer disparities by improving diversity of the oncology workforce. *Curr Breast Cancer Rep.* 2022;14(4):162–167. doi:10.1007/s12609-022-00456-0
166. Gordon HS, Street RL Jr, Sharf BF, Kelly PA, Souchek J. Racial differences in trust and lung cancer patients' perceptions of physician communication. *J Clin Oncol.* 2006;24(6):904–909. doi:10.1200/JCO.2005.03.1955
167. Charlot M, Santana MC, Chen CA, et al. Impact of patient and navigator race and language concordance on care after cancer screening abnormalities. *Cancer.* 2015;121(9):1477–1483. doi:10.1002/cncr.29221
168. Wang E, Glazer KB, Howell EA, Janevic TM. Social determinants of pregnancy-related mortality and morbidity in the United States: A systematic review. *Obstet Gynecol.* 2020;135(4):896–915. doi:10.1097/AOG.0000000000003762
169. El-Sayed AM, Finkton DW Jr, Paczkowski M, Keyes KM, Galea S. Socioeconomic position, health behaviors, and racial disparities in cause-specific infant mortality in Michigan, USA. *Prev Med.* 2015;76:8–13. doi:10.1016/j.ypmed.2015.03.021
170. Taylor JK. Structural racism and maternal health among Black women. *J Law Med Ethics.* 2020;48(3):506–517. doi:10.1177/1073110520958875
171. Howell EA. Reducing disparities in severe maternal morbidity and mortality. *Clin Obstet Gynecol.* 2018;61(2):387–399. doi:10.1097/GRF.0000000000000349
172. Bridges KM. Racial disparities in maternal mortality. *NYU Law Rev.* 2020;95(5):1229–1318. Accessed April 8, 2025. https://nyulawreview.org/issues/volume-95-number-5/racial-disparities-in-maternal-mortality
173. Davidson C, Denning S, Thorp K, et al. Examining the effect of quality improvement initiatives on decreasing racial disparities in maternal morbidity. *BMJ Qual Saf.* 2022;31(9):670–678. doi:10.1136/bmjqs-2021-014225
174. Building US Capacity to Review and Prevent Maternal Deaths. Report from Nine Maternal Review Committees. 2018. Accessed April 8, 2025. https://www.cdcfoundation.org/sites/default/files/files/ReportfromNineMMRCs.pdf
175. Admon LK, Winkelman TNA, Zivin K, Terplan M, Mhyre JM, Dalton VK. Racial and ethnic disparities in the incidence of severe maternal morbidity in the United States, 2012–2015. *Obstet Gynecol.* 2018;132(5):1158–1166. doi:10.1097/AOG.0000000000002937
176. Snyder JE, Upton RD, Hassett TC, Lee H, Nouri Z, Dill M. Black representation in the primary care physician workforce and its association with population life expectancy and mortality rates in the US. *JAMA Netw Open.* 2023;6(4):e236687. doi:10.1001/jamanetworkopen.2023.6687
177. Darling-Hammond L. Inequality in teaching and schooling: How opportunity is rationed to students of color in America. In: Smedley BD, Stith AY, Colburn L, Evans CH, eds. *The Right Thing to Do, The Smart Thing to Do: Enhancing Diversity in the Health Professions.* National Academies Press; 2001:208–233.
178. Gándara P. Lost opportunities: The difficult journey to higher education for underrepresented minority students. In: Smedley BD, Stith AY, Colburn L, Evans CH, eds. *The Right Thing to Do, The Smart Thing to Do: Enhancing Diversity in the Health Professions.* National Academies Press; 2001:234–259.

179. Harley EH. The forgotten history of defunct Black medical schools in the 19th and 20th centuries and the impact of the Flexner Report. *J Natl Med Assoc.* 2006;98(9):1425–1429.
180. Bullock SC, Houston E. Perceptions of racism by black medical students attending white medical schools. *J Natl Med Assoc.* 1987;79(6):601–608.
181. D'Amico EJ, Ellickson PL, Collins RL, Martino S, Klein DJ. Processes linking adolescent problems to substance-use problems in late young adulthood. *J Stud Alcohol.* 2005;66(6):766–775. doi:10.15288/jsa.2005.66.766
182. Ellis W, Dietz WH, Chen KD. Community resilience: A dynamic model for public health 3.0. *J Public Health Manag Pract.* 2022;28(suppl 1):S18–S26. doi:10.1097/PHH.0000000000001413
183. Michener J, Ford TN. Racism and health: Three core principles. *Milbank Q.* 2023;101(suppl 1):333–355. doi:10.1111/1468-0009.12633
184. Ray R, Lantz PM, Williams D. Upstream policy changes to improve population health and health equity: A priority agenda. *Milbank Q.* 2023;101(suppl 1):20–35. doi:10.1111/1468-0009.12640
185. Williams D. How racism makes us sick. TEDMED. November 2016. Accessed April 8, 2025. https://www.ted.com/talks/david_r_williams_how_racism_makes_us_sick
186. Massey DS, Denton NA. Hypersegregation in US metropolitan areas: Black and Hispanic segregation along five dimensions. *Demography.* 1989;26(3):373–391. doi:10.2307/2061599
187. Blankenship KM, Friedman SR, Dworkin S, Mantell JE. Structural interventions: Concepts, challenges and opportunities for research. *J Urban Health.* 2006;83(1):59–72. doi:10.1007/s11524-005-9007-4
188. Dawes DE. *The Political Determinants of Health.* Johns Hopkins University Press; 2020.
189. Kickbusch I. The political determinants of health—10 years on. *BMJ.* 2015;350:h81. doi:10.1136/bmj.h81
190. Brown AF, Ma GX, Miranda J, et al. Structural interventions to reduce and eliminate health disparities. *Am J Public Health.* 2019;109(suppl 1):S72–S78. doi:10.2105/AJPH.2018.304844
191. Williams DR, Mohammed SA. Racism and health I: Pathways and scientific evidence. *Am Behav Sci.* 2013;57(8). doi:10.1177/0002764213487340
192. Ananat EO, Washington E. Segregation and black political efficacy. *J Public Econ.* 2009;93(5-6):807–822. doi:10.1016/j.jpubeco.2009.02.003
193. Derenoncourt E. Can you move to opportunity? Evidence from the Great Migration. *Am Econ Rev.* 2022;112(2):369–408. doi:10.1257/aer.20200002
194. Gordon D. The police as place-consolidators: The organizational amplification of urban inequality. *Law Soc Inq.* 2020;45(1):1–27. doi:10.1017/lsi.2019.31
195. Uggen C, Larson R, Shannon S, Stewart R, Lueder C. The denial of voting rights to people with criminal records. In: Budd KM, Lane DC, Muschert GW, Smith JA, eds. *Beyond Bars: A Path Forward from 50 Years of Mass Incarceration in the United States.* Policy Press; 2023:73–85.
196. Chambers BD, Erausquin JT, Tanner AE, Nichols TR, Brown-Jeffy S. Testing the association between traditional and novel indicators of county-level structural racism and birth outcomes among Black and White women. *J Racial Ethn Health Disparities.* 2018;5(5):966–977. doi:10.1007/s40615-017-0444-z
197. Kurgan L. *Close Up at a Distance: Mapping, Technology, and Politics.* Zone Books; 2013.

198. Chicago's Million Dollar Blocks. Accessed April 8, 2025. https://chicagosmilliondollarblocks.com/#section-1
199. Porter TR. The school-to-prison pipeline: The business side of incarcerating, not educating, students in public schools. *Ark Law Rev.* 2015;68:55-81. Accessed April 8, 2025. https://law.uark.edu/alr/PDFs/68-1/alr-68-1-55-81Porter.pdf
200. Bradywood A, Leming-Lee TS, Watters R, Blackmore C. Implementing screening for social determinants of health using the Core 5 screening tool. *BMJ Open Qual.* 2021;10(3):e001362. doi:10.1136/bmjoq-2021-001362
201. Berkowitz SA. Health care's new emphasis on social determinants of health. *NEJM Catalyst.* 2023;4(4). doi:10.1056/cat.23.0070
202. Gómez A, Karimli L, Holguin M, Chung P, Szilagyi P, Schickedanz A. Bills, babies, and (language) barriers: Associations among economic strain, parenting, and primary language during the newborn period. *Fam Relat.* 2022;71(1):352-370. doi:10.1111/fare.12587
203. Francis DV, Hamilton D, Mitchell TW, Rosenberg NA Stucki BW. Black land loss: 1920-1997. *AEA Papers and Proceedings.* 2022;112:38-42. doi:10.1257/pandp.20221015
204. Harrell CJP, Burford TI, Cage BN, Nelson TM, Shearon S, Thompson A, Green S. Multiple pathways linking racism to health outcomes. *Du Bois Rev.* 2011;8(1):143-157. doi:10.1017/S1742058X11000178

4

Examining the Impacts of the Interrelated Systems of Education, Employment, and Health Care on the Life Course and Well-Being of Latino Populations

Ruth Enid Zambrana, PhD, MSW, José E. Rodríguez, MD, José A. Pagán, PhD, Angela Diaz, MD, PhD, MPH, Lenny López, MD, MPH, MDiv, and Antonia M. Villaruel, PhD, RN

INTRODUCTION

The Latino population is a significant and growing population, making up 19.1% (63.7 million) of the US population in 2022.[1] By 2060, the Latino population is projected to increase to 26.9% (97.7 million) of the US population.[2] The largest Latino subgroups are Mexicans/Mexican Americans (58.9%) and Puerto Ricans (9.3%).[3] The remaining Latino subgroups, from over 20 other Latin American countries, represent 30% of the total Latino population (see Table 4-1).[3–6]

The terms *Hispanic* and *Latino*, used by the US Census Bureau (or *Latinx, Latine*), are widely disputed terms (see Table 4-2; see also Table 4A-1 in Appendix 4A).[7–12] The US Census definition is not an accurate classification, as not all Hispanics are of Spanish ancestry (e.g., large European-descended populations migrated to South America after World Wars I and II). Notably, many Brazilians and Haitians self-identify as Latinos in surveys while many Spanish immigrants see themselves as European Americans but are aggregated under Hispanic ethnicity.[10] The original US Office of Management and Budget (OMB) term *Hispanic* was used to refer to populations that were historically Spanish speaking or from countries colonized by Spain. Neither *Hispanic* nor *Latino* as terms adequately describe the heterogeneity of Latino populations, nor the multiplicative interactions of historic, ethno-racial, socioeconomic, and health factors on Latino groups.[13,14] Because these terms are commonly used in research and academic literature, unless noted, we use the terms *Hispanic* and *Latino* interchangeably regardless of gender, ethnicity, and race.

For Mexican and Puerto Rican populations with a rich and mixed ancestry and multiple social statuses, the intersections of education, employment, and health care are historically linked to group experiences that have blocked access to opportunity structures

Table 4-1. Socioeconomic and Educational Profile by Hispanic Background: United States, 2020–2022

	Population (Thousands)	Hispanic Population (%)	Median Age (Y)	≤High School Education[a] (%)	≥Bachelor's Degree[b] (%)	Median Household Income[c] ($)	Median Household Net Worth[c] ($)	Living in Poverty (%)	English Proficient[d] (%)	Foreign Born (%)	US Citizens[e] (%)	Homeowners[f] (%)	Without Health Insurance (%)
All Hispanics	62,650	100	30	56	20	59,000	52,190	18	72	32	81	51	18
Mexican	37,236	59.5	28	61	15	59,200	52,650	18	74	29	81	53	20
Puerto Rican	5,798	9.3	31	47	24	52,000	35,770	21	83	2	99	34	8
Salvadoran	2,474	4.0	30	68	13	61,000	30,600	17	56	53	66	46	24
Cuban	2,400	3.8	40	47	30	58,700	92,700	14	64	53	82	56	12
Dominican	2,394	3.8	30	52	22	50,000	9,430	20	61	50	78	31	10
Guatemalan	1,772	2.9	27	72	11	52,000	NA	23	51	58	58	34	34
Colombian	1,402	2.2	36	36	38	69,000	141,200	12	66	57	79	53	13
Honduran	1,148	1.8	27	67	14	50,000	NA	26	47	63	51	31	40
Spanish	996	1.6	34	28	40	74,000	NA	13	95	12	95	63	7
Ecuadorian	813	1.3	33	48	27	65,000	NA	13	61	54	73	45	17
Peruvian	721	1.1	38	34	36	69,000	NA	11	65	59	79	56	12
Venezuelan	660	1.0	36	20	57	65,000	NA	13	56	76	51	39	15
Nicaraguan	457	0.7	34	45	27	66,000	NA	13	65	52	78	46	17
Argentine	297	0.5	39	30	46	80,000	NA	7	78	54	78	62	10
Panamanian	238	0.4	33	27	38	64,300	NA	12	87	36	90	54	8
Chilean	188	0.3	35	27	42	65,000	NA	12	76	49	80	54	11
Costa Rican	188	0.3	34	35	38	76,000	NA	8	80	45	79	53	12

Source: Based on data from Moslimani et al.,[3] Statista,[3] Sherer and Mayol García,[5] and IPUMS.[6]

Note: NA = not available. Data pertain to Latinos in the 50 US states and Washington, DC. Persons living in US territories are not included, so the Puerto Rican population is significantly undercounted in these data.

[a] Aged ≥25 years. Includes those who have attained a high school diploma or equivalent, such as a General Educational Development (GED) certificate.
[b] Aged ≥25 years.
[c] Data from 2021 American Community Survey (1% IPUMS). Due to how IPUMS assigns poverty values, this data will differ from US Census Bureau data.
[d] Of those aged ≥5 years, those who speak only English at home or who speak English very well.
[e] By birth or naturalization.
[f] Household heads living in owner-occupied homes.

Table 4-2. Definition of Terms

Term	Definition
Hispanic and Latino	Hispanic was introduced for the 1980 US census to refer to populations that were historically Spanish speaking or colonized by Spain. Hispanic and Latino are uniquely employed in the US and are contested terms. OMB defines *Hispanic* or *Latino* as a group that "includes individuals of Mexican, Puerto Rican, Salvadoran, Cuban, Dominican, Guatemalan, and other Central or South American or Spanish culture or origin."[7] Before 2024, the Census collected 2 ethnicities (Hispanic or Latino and non-Hispanic or non-Latino) but this was changed in 2024 when the questions for race and ethnicity were combined into 1 question.
Latino	Latino was created to encapsulate the diverse Latin American origins present in the US. *Latino* describes any person with ancestry in Latin America, a politically defined region unified by the predominance of Romance languages. This definition includes Portuguese-speaking Brazil and French-speaking Haiti but excludes Spain.[8-11]
Latinx and Latine	Recent debate has ensued on the need to develop gender-neutral terms, including *Latinx* and *Latine*. Both are used as gender-neutral alternatives to Latina/Latino to be more inclusive. *Latinx* as a nonbinary form of Latino/Latina started being used in the early 2000s and is used more frequently by academics, students, and the LGBTQ+ community. In Spanish-speaking countries, the term *Latine* with the suffix "-e" is circulating as an alternative to the -o/-a binary and is preferred to Latinx, primarily because of its better adherence to Spanish grammar.[8-12]

Note: LGBTQ+ = lesbian, gay, bisexual, transgender, queer, and questioning; OMB = US Office of Management and Budget.

and societal resources, coupled with mistreatment in society.[15-19] This chapter primarily focuses on two Latino subgroups—Mexicans and Puerto Ricans (68.2% of all Latinos)—because they are integral to the national landscape of the United States and have historically contributed to its economic, social, and cultural strengths. Yet these groups have disproportionately experienced long-standing, intergenerational life course disadvantages due to US policies and laws that have limited upward mobility and created a significant wealth gap. The impact of historic policies differs substantially from the opportunity structures available to many Latino immigrant groups in the United States.[20-24] While we recognize there are considerable political, economic, and social issues related to the immigrant populations, particularly from Central America and the Caribbean, Hispanic immigration and immigrant studies are beyond the scope of this chapter. Nonetheless, we acknowledge that structural inequities profoundly impact the lives of recent immigrants, particularly Indigenous Central Americans and Afro-Caribbeans. Some comparisons are noted to identify inequity in opportunity structures among select immigrant groups.

This chapter discusses the intersecting impacts of the educational, employment, and health care systems on the life course opportunities of predominantly low-income Mexican-origin individuals and Puerto Ricans. Persistent educational and employment disadvantages emphasize how structural inequity contributes to intergenerational, disproportionate, adverse social and economic outcomes. The connected systems operate in the following way: low-resourced K–12 educational systems contribute to the lower likelihood of attending college and employment in lower-paying service jobs that dampen opportunities for upward mobility, professional pathways, wealth and asset accumulation, and increase health care disparities. We address two questions: (1) What are the social determinants (demographic, educational, and economic indicators) associated with adverse life course and health outcomes? (2) What are actionable strategies that can be implemented to improve the health and well-being of Mexican- and Puerto Rican–origin groups? How might these apply to other Latino subgroups? Our methods to address these questions include four approaches: (1) a scanning of interdisciplinary and multidisciplinary bodies of literature on Latinos in the three systems of interest; (2) presenting demographics of the Latino population by race and subgroup; (3) inclusion of the epidemiology of prominent health conditions among adults and children; and (4) descriptive case studies employing composites of individuals to illustrate the lived experiences of predominantly Mexican-origin and Puerto Rican individuals.

Underlying this narrative review are three significant bodies of scholarly work: (1) critical race history of how historic incorporation produced inequities that are codified in current customs, practices, governance, and policies in the United States[25–28]; (2) the constructs of *social determinants of health (SDOH)* and *intersectionality*[29,30]; and (3) institutional discriminatory policies or *political determinants of health* (i.e., government policies of disinvestment of resources that shape SDOH) across the life course.[31,32] These analyses describe salient and pressing issues about how Mexican-origin and Puerto Rican people are differentially impacted by historical incorporation and structural inequities, and how these patterns of experiences impact the contours of their present and future well-being.

Current data have many limitations, since information about Latinos is often presented in aggregated form with a disregard for ethnicity, education level, class, ancestry, race, and colorism. Much of the contemporary data on Latinos makes it difficult to identify disparities and disallows comparisons across diverse social contexts (e.g., urban/rural, state/community) that impact employment, educational, and health disparities by subgroup. In this chapter, we present data from these important indicators as available.

The following section is informed by existing bodies of knowledge on historic policies and laws, institutional policies in education, employment, and health care systems, adverse impacts of these systems on the life course outcomes of Mexican-origin and Puerto Rican groups, and actionable strategies to address structural inequity.

HETEROGENEITY OF LATINOS: HISTORY, RACE, AND OPPORTUNITY

Mexicans and Puerto Ricans in the United States: Intersections of History, Law and Policy

Although a robust body of historical and contemporary scholarship has been produced on the Mexican-origin story in the United States[15–17] and Puerto Rico's colonial status,[33,34] the resistance to the inclusion of the plight of the original inhabitants and intentional erasure of the history and involuntary incorporation of original peoples on US land muddles the discourse on historicism, oppression and inequality.

In Table 4A-2 (see Appendix 4A), we provide an overview of laws and policies on land repossession, immigration policy (with a focus on Mexican groups), and the harms of medical abuse practices, including violation of women's reproductive health rights such as birth control experimentation and nonconsensual sterilization.[35-38] The timeline (1848–present) shows legislation and events that profoundly impacted the human and civil rights of Mexican Americans and Puerto Ricans passed from 1911 to 2012.

For Mexican-origin peoples, long-standing immigration legislation and border crossing enforcement have blocked access to the US opportunity structure with tenacious and harmful impacts, while opening doors to many other immigrant groups. Mexican-origin peoples originally resided in what is now the US Southwest and West. In 1848, México ceded about 55% of its northern lands to the United States to end the Mexican–American War, and in 1898, Spain ceded the island of Puerto Rico to the United States to end the Spanish–American War.[39,40] Thus, Mexicans who have familial and ancestral roots in the northern lands that were once México are now denied entry. Mexican-origin peoples have a long and sordid history with the US Immigration and Naturalization Service that speaks to their distinct and deleterious relationship and the negative treatment of both Mexican US citizens and Mexican immigrants.[17-19] The impact of these histories is widely described in other publications.[17,41-43]

Events encapsulating the experience of Puerto Ricans and Mexican Americans include the 1917 Jones–Shafroth Act (Puerto Ricans gained US citizenship), *Mendez v Westminster* in 1946 (banned segregation of Mexican American children in schools), and California's Proposition 187 in 1994 and *Arizona v United States* in 2012 (hyper-policing of Latinos). Mexican Americans and Puerto Ricans in the United States share unique historical conditions and distinct characteristics as US citizens and as former subjects of medical experimentation (birth control trials and sterilization) in the 1940s and 1950s.[36,38] Although affirmative action legislation aimed to remedy the barriers to access to social and economic opportunities for Mexican-origin, Puerto Rican, African American, and American Indian or Alaska Native people, its goals to promote increased representation in higher education and professional integration have not been attained.[44] Unexpectedly, the Civil Rights Act (1964) and affirmative action (1973) were an impetus to increased immigration (1965 Hart–Celler Act) and the initiation of a demographic shift in the US Latino population.

The circumstances and conditions of Mexican immigrants and citizens and Puerto Ricans in the United States must be distinguished from South American or Cuban immigrants, who arrived in the United States for educational or professional opportunities or as economic and political refugees. For example, in the 1960s to the 1980s, Cubans were granted asylum and refugee status with access to health and social resources that assisted their integration into US society (Cuban Refugee Program, 1960–1970; Cuban Adjustment Act, 1966). Simultaneously, the passage of the 1965 Hart–Celler Act marked the largest welcoming in US history of European, Asian, and other professional immigrants and was a turning point in US immigration policy. These historically significant policy changes paved the way for significant immigration from South America in 2000 and an influx of Central American immigrants in the 1980s to 1990s, made possible through changes such as the creation of *temporary protected status* in 1990 (Immigration Act of 1990).[45,46] These diasporic waves of South and Central American immigrants have produced a considerable demographic shift by socioeconomic status (class), education, ancestry, ethnicity, and race[47] and an urgency to examine the meaning of the terms *Hispanic* and *Latino*.

Who Are Latinos, Hispanics, and Afro-Latinos?

Hispanic/Latino is an ethnicity, not a race, and includes many national and ancestral ethnic groups that may be white, Black, Mestizo, Asian, or Indigenous.[48] Although often ignored, race among Latino populations does matter significantly. Latinos are extremely heterogeneous with respect to race, colorism, and mixed race in the United States.[13,49] Mexicans and Puerto Ricans have historically been deeply affected by the policies and practices associated with race, ethnicity, indigeneity, and mixed-race identities, including Afro-Latinos.[50–54] Racialization due to history, phenotype, and skin color are key determinants of treatment in the United States for those groups where colonization and land takeover occurred.

We define the Mexican-origin population to include both immigrants and US born people. US-born and foreign-born Mexicans (23% of all US immigrants in 2022) do not differ significantly in median household income, home ownership, or social and economic mobility in spite of differences in educational attainment, nativity, and citizenship.[3,22] Among the Mexican population, 18% of US-born Mexicans live in poverty, as do 17% of foreign-born Mexicans; rates of homeownership are 54% for the US-born and 53% for foreign-born. Among Mexicans aged 25 and older, the US-born are more likely than the foreign-born to have a bachelor's degree or higher (21% vs. 9%). Although 62% of foreign-born Mexicans have been in the United States for over 20 years, only 35% of foreign-born Mexicans are US citizens. Among full-time, year-round workers, Mexicans earn about $40,000. The Mexican-origin population has historically had an economic push-and-pull relationship with the United States and continues to play a key role in the US agricultural industry.[55]

For Mexican-origin peoples, racialization (although the census previously classified Mexicans as white) and phenotype play a key role in their exclusion from economic opportunity, including lower levels of education, concentration in lower-paying jobs, and continued identification not just as foreigners but as "undesirable immigrants." These racial biases have engendered hostility and exploitation of members of the Mexican-origin community—adults and children, citizens and noncitizens—and recently, Central American communities. The last decade has yielded a flourishing corpus of work on Latinos and Blackness and a call for a space in the race debate.[53,56]

Recent estimates suggest that 6 million US Latino adults, or about 10% of the population, identify as Afro-Latino and that one in seven Afro-Latinos identify as Hispanic; 29% of Afro-Latino adults are of Puerto Rican descent, and 23% are of Mexican descent.[56] Similar patterns of the linked *white race advantage*, higher education, and wealth among light-skinned or white-presenting Latinos are observed among South and Central Americans who are referred to as "honorary whites."[50,57] South and Central American and Caribbean self-identified Latinos are racially, ethnically, culturally, ancestrally, linguistically, and socioeconomically diverse, representing over 20 countries across the Americas with various phenotypes, mixed-race statuses, and citizenship statuses. Many of the more educated Latin American groups with European ancestry have experienced high integration into professional spheres, including participation in the health care workforce.[3,58]

Striking demographic differences and residential concentration patterns are evident by subgroup.[3] A few data highlights (see Table 4-1) include the following: Mexican-origin groups are concentrated in nine states (California, Texas, Arizona, New Mexico, Colorado, and Illinois), while Puerto Ricans are more likely to reside in New York, Connecticut, Massachusetts, New Jersey, and Florida. Citizenship and English language proficiency are highest among Puerto Ricans, Spaniards, Panamanians, Cubans, and Mexicans. Mexican Americans and Puerto Ricans, despite their English language proficiency, remain at high rates in low-paying positions and experience disproportionately lower intergenerational social and economic mobility.[24] In 2020, Hispanics had a poverty rate of 17.0%, Blacks had a poverty rate of 19.5%, while American Indians/Alaska Native groups had the highest poverty rate (25.4%) and Asians (8.1%) the lowest.[59] However, poverty rates have hovered at 20% to 30% for Mexican Americans and Puerto Ricans for the last four decades and vary by state.[60] Poverty is strongly associated with educational level, a major factor in social mobility. Cubans (30%), Argentines (46%), Venezuelans (57%), and Spanish (40%) have 2 to 3 times the college graduation rates of Mexicans (15%) and Puerto Ricans (24%). A review of net worth, which is strongly associated with educational level, shows that native-born Mexicans ($52,650), Mexican immigrants ($47,530), and Puerto Ricans ($35,770) have a significantly lower net worth compared with, for example, Cubans ($92,700) and Colombians ($141,200).[5]

Although a disproportionate number of Latinos as an aggregate are reported to have high rates of employment, Mexican-origin people and Puerto Ricans tend to be concentrated in low-wage and informal service sectors. Employment in service sectors is highly associated with low rates of education, lack of health insurance coverage, higher medical debt, and lower wealth accumulation.[61] These interrelationships are illustrated by the following data: non-Hispanic white householders had a median household wealth of $187,300 and Asian householders $206,400, compared with $14,100 for Black householders and $31,700 for Hispanic householders. Households with members without health insurance for all or part of the year had dramatically lower median wealth ($21,550) than households in which all members had coverage for the full year ($156,600). Those without health insurance were almost twice as likely as fully insured households to hold medical debt (27.9% and 14.6%, respectively).[20,62]

In sum, Mexican-origin and Puerto Rican subgroups are most likely to speak English, be US citizens, earn the lowest salaries, live in socially segregated and structurally disadvantaged neighborhoods (e.g., food deserts, lack of green space), and have multiple chronic health conditions. These two subgroups are, proportionally speaking, the least likely to have health insurance and/or more likely to be underinsured and are the least likely to have completed high school or college. Although Latinos as a whole experience material hardship at double the rate of non-Latinos, Mexican-origin people and Puerto Ricans experience these hardships at quadruple the rate of non-Latinos.[5]

Despite these major subgroup differences by race, education, and employment, Latinos are considered a monolithic population in most health research. Immigration status, nativity, and educational level are often ignored. Although the Hispanic Community Health Study/Study of Latinos has a large sample size, 79% of its respondents are immigrants, which is not representative of the US Latino population.[63] The aggregation of very different population groups has contributed to the myth of the *Hispanic paradox*, the *healthy immigrant effect,* and has skewed education, employment, and health data, constructing a false portrait of health and well-being across subgroups.[64,65] Historical incorporation, medical reproductive rights abuses, and discriminatory immigration policies contribute to significant differences between Mexican-origin people and Puerto Ricans and other subgroups on SDOH, educational and economic opportunities, and health life course experiences and outcomes. Although beyond the scope of this chapter, an extensive body of literature is available on the harms of historic and contemporary US immigration policy on poor immigrants from in México and Central America.[51,66]

Discriminatory patterns in access to quality educational systems, protected employment systems, and health care as well as immigration regulation and surveillance continue to play a significant role in the lives of less educated, mixed-race, and poor immigrants from México and Central America. Central Americans experience barriers to entry to the United States, associated with their intersecting characteristics of race (Black and/or Indigenous), low education, and poverty. Currently, many undocumented Latinos from México (64%) and Central America (26%) reside in five states (California, Texas, Florida, New York, and Illinois).[67] The untoward negative effects of personal and institutional immigrant discrimination have an adverse effect on documented and US-born Mexican-origin people as all Mexican-origin people are often perceived as undocumented immigrants.[22,68] Historic exclusion and mistreatment across the life course manifest in intergenerational wage and education gaps and minimal progress in social and economic mobility. The study of Latino subgroups requires the contextualization of demographics, SDOH, state of residence, and political determinants to produce a reliable and accurate understanding of outcomes.

Intersectional approaches argue that individual and group demographic markers are influenced and shaped by multiple dimensions of inequality, including historical incorporation and the confluence of numerous factors.[32,69] This approach acknowledges the notion of *simultaneity*. This means "an account of an individual's experiences of oppression will be a cluster of persistent, domain-crossing, and interlinking injustices that reflect the overall complexity of an individual's (or group's) social positions."[70(p237)] For example, community educational resources and schools' dependency on local real estate taxes or policing practices and prison terms in poor neighborhoods have disenfranchised many individuals, thwarting social and economic mobility.[71-76]

New ways of thinking about structural racism and intersecting racial, ethnic, and socioeconomic status differences and their impact on education, employment, and health outcomes, including social position, are central to understanding Latino subgroup differences. We argue for disaggregating Latino subgroups by race (mixed race, Indigenous, and Black), education, nativity, and immigrant status, and European ancestry subgroup (US citizens and immigrants) to inform actionable strategies to promote structural and racial equity. We now turn to a discussion of the systems of education, employment, and health and the structural barriers that work against quality education, living-wage jobs, stable and affordable housing, and quality health care for Mexicans/Mexican Americans, Puerto Ricans, and other poor Latinos.[16,47]

EDUCATION AND EMPLOYMENT: LEVERS OF INEQUALITY

SDOH range from neighborhood context and social and economic resources to structural racism in access to health and medical resources. Population health research often omits key systems and contextual intersections of history, race and ethnicity, and institutional power, reducing the importance of social and political determinants and the accumulation of disadvantages over the life course.[26,28,77,78] These factors have deep roots in unequal access to quality education and employment that impact socioeconomic status and opportunity structures, such as lack of a living wage,[79] discriminatory police surveillance policies, and limited access to community health resources like healthy food markets, employment opportunities, and quality schools.[51]

Poor-quality schools disadvantage low-income groups throughout the life course and are a powerful factor in adversely affecting professional workforce development pathways. Unequivocally disproportional low-quality schools in low-income Mexican/Mexican American and Puerto Rican communities frequently have limited resources in K–12 schools, such as unlicensed teachers, few Latino teachers, and limited college counselors who encourage and work with these students to seek college opportunities. A strong body of work illustrates the extraordinary impact of low expectations and low preparation for college attendance among these K–12 students that contributes to low college attendance and graduation rates. In addition, in public schools, academic resources, such as science and math courses, advanced placement courses, technology, and college-bound resource information are often absent.[74,80–82] Stereotypic representations of low intelligence for Mexican-origin and Puerto Rican children and adolescents and low expectations of counselors discourage these groups from pursuing academic education.[73] Negative experiences in schooling and the inability to pursue occupations and careers to achieve social and economic mobility contribute to adverse health behaviors, mental health issues, and suicide, especially among Latina girls.[83] Although a minority of low-income Mexican-origin and Puerto Rican youth experience success due to the few teachers who recognize their abilities and intelligence and support their educational goals, these experiences are relatively rare. Education systems in low-income communities contribute to producing high concentrations of less-educated people in low-paying service sector jobs.

Inadequately resourced school systems coupled with unfair employment practices and lack of health care access stifle access to an opportunity structure of stable employment, family economic stability, and intergenerational mobility. These political determinants wield power to shape how society is organized, how groups are treated, and how government values and ideologies, as reflected in policy, differentially structured systems (see case studies in Marmot and Allen[27] and Shapiro[31]). Differences in employment options and opportunities for economic mobility vary by state, enforcement of worker protection laws, and where the minimum wage is a living wage. These factors are associated with the multilayered identities of race, ethnicity, class, education, and location and profoundly affect lifetime earnings, benefits, and outcomes of specifically Mexican and Puerto Rican groups.[25,31,51]

Whereas the Latino adult population generally comprises a large racial/ethnic service workforce (see Table 4-1), Mexicans and Puerto Ricans (and notably mixed-race and poor Central Americans and Afro-Caribbeans) are concentrated in semi-skilled, unskilled, or informal work sectors that seldom offer employer-based health insurance coverage.[84] Predictably, the COVID-19 pandemic hit the low-income, less-educated Latino workforce hard because they are overrepresented in the service industries,[85] representing those jobs first to be cut.[86] Although the United States has a federal guaranteed minimum wage ($7.25/hour), Latino subgroups are often paid far less than non-Latinos, a phenomenon also known as *wage theft*, meaning they are paid less than the full wages to which they are legally entitled.[87] Minimum-wage laws are variable among states and do not apply to all business settings, particularly day work, farm work, and other seasonal employment. Disproportionate concentrations of Mexicans and poor Indigenous Central American groups are employed in about five to six informal service sectors, namely, construction, drivers/sales workers and truck drivers, grounds maintenance work, chefs and cooks, and agricultural workers, compared with other Latino and racial/ethnic groups.[43,88,89] In these sectors, the lack of protections such as state and federal laws, surveillance, and enforcement of employment practices facilitates worker abuse among low-income Mexicans, Puerto Ricans, and Central Americans with minimal education.

By contrast, Mexican-origin people and Puerto Ricans are underrepresented in all professional sectors. Mexican adults are the least likely to hold professional positions and/or business financial positions. Table 4-3 shows the percentage of health care providers and health service providers by race and ethnicity.[90-92] Low-educated Latino subgroup members are underrepresented in all health care provider roles and overrepresented in low-paying health care service roles. Mexican Americans and Puerto Ricans are proportionally underrepresented among health care professionals and overrepresented in the health service sector, while Cuban Americans are overrepresented among health care professionals. While about 20% of the US population identifies as Latino, representation in health diagnosing and training professions for Mexican Americans ranges from 1.56% (pharmacists) to 1.77% (physicians). Health care support and personal care professions range from 7.9% (licensed practical nurses) to 8.9% (personal aides).[58] In addition, only 4% of medical school leaders and 2% of hospital leaders are Latino.[93] The importance of racially/ethnically concordant providers who are knowledgeable and demonstrate a commitment to serve underserved and under-resourced communities is critically important in decreasing medical bias and increasing the overall health and well-being of disadvantaged Latino and racial/ethnic groups.[94-96]

HEALTH SYSTEMS AS POLITICAL DETERMINANTS OF SOCIAL INEQUALITY

Health systems are governed by goals, values, and practices that shape the delivery of health care services and access by privileging those with employment that offers health insurance and those who can pay for private health insurance.[26] For example, states determine access to Medicaid funding and Affordable Care Act coverage; federal policies determine access to programs based on immigration status, refugee status, or any status that is deemed appropriate by the federal government. Moreover, eligibility for premium-free Medicare Part A—hospital insurance for adults aged 65 years and older—depends on working and paying Medicare taxes for 10 years. As such, many Mexicans and Puerto Ricans who have worked in informal sectors and service sectors may not have access to Medicare Part A benefits.[97]

Table 4-3. Health Occupations by Race/Ethnicity: United States, 2022

Occupation	NH White (%)	NH Black/African American (%)	NH Asian (%)	Hispanic or Latino (%)
Community and Social Service Occupations				
Substance abuse and behavioral disorder counselors	74.6	16.3	3.4	15.9
Mental health counselors	82.4	14.9	1.1	10.6
Child, family, and school social workers	61.3	30.5	6.2	11.1
Health care social workers	69.3	23.5	5.8	13.9
Health Care Practitioners				
Active MD residents[a]	48.8	6.1	21.6	8.1
Chiropractors	80.9	9.0	7.3	1.5
Dentists	76.9	7.7	14.0	7.1
Dietitians and nutritionists	74.9	18.1	3.1	9.6
Pharmacists	68.1	10.6	18.7	6.9
Respiratory therapists	79.4	12.8	6.6	12.7
Registered nurses	73.6	14.5	8.9	8.1
Health Care Technical Occupations				
Clinical laboratory technologists and technicians	69.0	12.0	14.9	13.5
Dental hygienists	91.4	2.5	5.6	12.7
Emergency medical technicians	82.4	9.1	5.3	15.6
Psychiatric technicians	61.0	31.6	4.2	19.8
Surgical technologist	70.2	22.6	2.1	13.1
Dietetic technicians and ophthalmic medical technicians	66.5	23.2	3.1	11.8
Service Occupations				
Home health aides	52.5	32.5	11.1	28.9
Personal care aides	60.8	26.2	8.0	21.0
Nursing assistants	55.4	36.0	5.6	15.3
Orderlies and psychiatric aides	56.7	30.0	3.7	18.6
Dental assistants	77.5	9.8	9.0	28.3
Medical assistants	75.7	15.7	5.6	32.9
Phlebotomists	59.0	22.0	7.9	20.2
Personal Care and Service Occupations				
Childcare workers	77.6	13.5	3.7	23.9
Total employment of persons aged ≥16 years	62.0	62.2	64.5	66.3

Source: Based on US Bureau of Labor Statistics[97,98] and Association of American Medical Colleges.[99]
Note: NH = non-Hispanic; MD = medical doctor.
[a] Active US-citizen MD residents in 2021-2022. Other distribution includes 0.6% American Indian or Alaska Native and 0.2% Native Hawaiian or Pacific Islander. 18% of active MD residents were non-US citizens in 2021-2022.

Understanding the development, structure, and operation of health systems is essential to gain insight into how long-term lack of insurance for the poor, access to health insurance coverage, and quality of health care (including medical bias, medical errors and denial of care) exacerbate disparities and inequities in health care access and produce adverse outcomes for disproportionately poor Latinos over the life course. Data from the 2021 American Community Survey show that 17.6% of Latinos are uninsured compared with 9.6% of Blacks, 5.8% of Asians, and 5.7% of non-Hispanic whites.[61] National data mask the reality of highly concentrated communities of poverty as geographic locations of higher levels of disparity. For example, about 10.9 million uninsured Latinos live in the United States—3.3 million in Texas, 1.8 million in California, and about 1 million in Florida. Approximately 28% of Latinos in Texas are uninsured, compared with 17.2% of Latinos in Florida and 11.7% of Latinos in California. The percentage of uninsured Latinos varies from 31.2% in Tennessee to 4.2% in Vermont.[98]

Mexican and Puerto Rican populations are largely concentrated in service sector jobs that offer no or limited choices of employer-sponsored health insurance coverage.[89] Health insurance coverage options vary by state and when available are inaccessible due to the high cost of buying a policy in the non-group market, qualification rules that exclude those that earn more than what is required to qualify for Medicaid and other government programs, or are not eligible for health insurance coverage due to their immigration status. About 27% of Latino adults report having employer-sponsored health insurance coverage compared with 53% of non-Latino white adults.[99] A negative consequence of being employed in service sector jobs, aside from the lack of insurance, is medical debt. For example, 35% of Latino adults had trouble paying medical bills since the COVID-19 shutdown in February 2020; about 11% of Latino adults lost health insurance coverage during this same period.[100]

Challenges during COVID-19 were compounded by the fact that unemployment increased in Latino-heavy service and hospitality sectors during the recession. Latinos made up 22% of the 16 million workers in the leisure and hospitality industry before COVID-19. Eight million jobs were lost during the first two months of COVID-19, and many of these jobs may never come back.[101] According to the US Bureau of Labor Statistics, the speed of recovery post-pandemic varies between racial groups, and Black and Latino workers are recovering more slowly than the total labor market.[102,103] For example, in 2020, 43.5% of Latinas (~700,000) lost their jobs in leisure and hospitality.[104] Two important findings are associated with job losses and inequality: Latinas experienced the greatest job losses, and the declining value of the federal minimum wage over time has contributed to growth in US income inequality.[105]

Minimum-wage jobs, lack of job security, and low or no benefits exacerbate health care access in communities and states with a high proportion of uninsured populations.[88] Uninsured population rates have significant consequences for health care access and quality for all Latinos, not just uninsured Latinos. Almost half of Latino adults (48%) say limited access to quality health care is a significant reason for poor health outcomes.[106] Access and quality of health care services explain about 20% of health outcomes.[107] Often quality care is compromised by Latino experiences of explicit and implicit (unconscious or unintentional) biases.[108,109] Clinics and hospitals serving communities with high uninsured populations face a substantial financial burden because they provide uncompensated or charity care to uninsured populations. These facilities are not fully compensated by the local, state, or federal governments for providing these services and, as a result, pass on this cost to others in those communities.[110] What is more relevant is that the low rates of health insurance coverage at the local level mean that clinics and hospitals are not able to provide preventive and primary care services that should be accessible to everyone, and the quality of these services is likely to be lower. In other words, in communities of high Mexican and Puerto Rican concentration, the high numbers of uninsured impact the ability of all others in those communities to access high-quality health care while raising the cost of care.

The triple epidemic of inadequate employment and educational systems, structural racism, and a failing health care system, jointly with observations and evidence-based scholarship about intergenerational and life course consequences of poverty on the physical, emotional, and social health of low-income Mexican-origin and Puerto Rican children and families, calls for more equitable, actionable solutions. This includes increased medical and health care workforce leadership, representation, and higher political participation to make progress on health and health care issues of importance to the significant proportion of low-income Mexicans and Puerto Ricans and other economically disadvantaged Latino populations.[111] For example, a compelling body of evidence documents the importance of racial/ethnic workforce development, patient–provider concordance, and colocated community-based health care services.[96,112–115] Racial/ethnic patient–provider concordance has been associated with improved health outcomes, decreased medical bias, and lower health care costs.[94,98]

Redressing shortcomings in the health care system is bolstered by a clear actionable solution that health care *teams*, not individual providers, be reimbursed for health care. These teams include physicians, nurses, medical assistants, pharmacists, social workers, nurse case managers, and front office staff.[116] While health care teams should include staff representatives of the communities they serve at all levels of the organization, there is a wide gap. Equitable access must include health insurance coverage and financial investments in colocated, comprehensive, community-based public health centers that can serve both insured and uninsured Latinos. Expanding the number and quality of community-based health care facilities that serve predominately underserved Mexican-origin, Puerto Rican, Central American, and Afro-Caribbean communities is an important first step to making sure that these low-income communities receive the primary and specialized care they need. This care requires delivery in environments that are affordable, responsive, and appropriate to their needs, in the language of their preference, and with a health workforce (nurses, doctors, and staff) that provide welcoming, high-quality service.[60,117]

INTERSECTIONS OF SOCIAL DETERMINANTS OF HEALTH AND THEIR IMPACT ON LATINOS ACROSS THE LIFE COURSE

In 2018, the estimated economic burden of racial and ethnic health inequities was between $421 billion and $451 billion, and the estimated burden of low education–related health inequities was between $940 billion and $978 billion.[21] For Latinos, most of the economic burden was attributable to excess medical care costs and lost labor market productivity. Although an important study, the data analyses masked Latino subgroup education and socioeconomic differences by aggregating Latinos into one group. Low-income Latinos are more likely to experience adverse life events (SDOH) such as material hardship, food insecurity, poverty, low education, violence, and fear of crime or deportation throughout their life course, which takes a toll on their family life, health, and mental well-being. A brief overview of the mutually reinforcing interrelationships among SDOH, health conditions, mental health, stressful life events, and its intergenerational impact on life course is presented with illustrative examples.

Latino Children and Health

SDOH critically impact the health and well-being of low-income Latinos from childhood to adulthood. Berkman et al. offer a life course health framework that emphasizes three relationships that have particular salience to low-income Latino children: (1) the embeddedness of children's lives in historical times and places; (2) the links between children's lives and the lives of their family and community members; and (3) the accumulation of disease risks and exposures over the life course that both mediate and moderate risks from previous developmental periods that can cause illness and poor health in adulthood.[118] Intergenerationally, the negative health effects of chronic stress are primarily concentrated among individuals with parental low education attainment and thus low childhood socioeconomic position (SEP).

Four patterns of interrelationships have existed for Latino children over the decades: (1) a majority of Latino children (55.2%), compared with 23.7% of white, Asian, and Black children, depend on public health insurance, including Medicaid and the Children's Health Insurance Program, which cover primary and preventive health care services.[119] Access to comprehensive pediatric primary and preventive health care services is integral to promoting wellness and reducing disparities.[120–122] (2) Poverty rates increased from an additional 4% to 27.3% for all Latino children during the COVID-19 pandemic and 6% to 42.4% for Latino children whose families are headed by non–US citizens.[123] Low-income Latino children are the least likely to be insured, have a regular source of health care, have received preventive health care in the previous year, be fully immunized, and have a medical home. Compared with non-Latino white children, low-income Latino children are more likely to utilize emergency room services for primary care needs.[60,124,125] (3) Living in under-resourced communities and schools combined with a lack of preventive and primary care at the earliest stages of life has adverse effects across the lifespan, from cognitive deficits, behavioral disorders, and mental health challenges in childhood to increased incidence of mild strokes to severe strokes and dementia as adults.[126,127] (4) Adverse childhood experiences are prevalent among US Latino children and are associated with depressive symptoms, obesity, cancer, coronary heart disease, and chronic obstructive pulmonary disease.[128,129] Perreira and Allen summarize the factors that affect Latino child health:

> For the health and development of Hispanic children, migration is an enduring theme. Although the vast majority of Hispanic children are US-born, 55% have at least one immigrant parent, and an estimated 25%–28% have a parent who was an unauthorized immigrant. Children with two unauthorized parents have worse health than those with only one unauthorized parent, and a mother's nativity and legal status may matter more than a father's for children's health. Thus, ecological and life-course models of Hispanic children's development must also incorporate multiple dimensions of immigration background (i.e., child's nativity, parent's nativity, and legal status) as key components of social stratification.[78(p3)]

Mexican-origin groups, Central American groups, and those that are disproportionately poor and in mixed citizenship–status families experience disproportionate stressful life events (e.g., high rates of poverty, food insecurity, unsafe communities, no health insurance) and are deeply affected more often by adverse health (e.g., obesity, asthma) and mental health outcomes in their lifetime and intergenerationally.[130]

Chronic Health Conditions, Poverty, and Health Care Access in Adulthood

The Centers for Disease Control and Prevention Social Vulnerability Index provides indicators of SDOH for every US county and census tract.[131] The 16 social factors are grouped into four broad themes: (1) socioeconomic status (below poverty level, unemployed, housing cost burden, no health insurance, and no high school diploma); (2) household characteristics (aged ≥65 years, aged ≤17 years, individuals with a disability, single-parent households, and English-language proficiency); (3) racial/ethnic minority status; and (4) housing type and transportation (multiunit structure, mobile home, crowding, group quarters, and no vehicle).

Asthma is one example of a health condition disproportionately affecting Puerto Rican adults living in adverse urban environments that is strongly associated with SDOH. In

2008 to 2011, the overall prevalence of physician-diagnosed asthma among Hispanics was 16.4%, and the prevalence of current asthma was 7.4%.[132] The age- and sex-adjusted prevalence of asthma was highest among Puerto Ricans (36.5%), intermediate among Cubans (21.8%), Dominicans (15.4%), and other or mixed-ancestry groups (17.7%), and lowest among South Americans (9.1%) and Mexicans (7.5%). By contrast, the higher prevalence of chronic obstructive pulmonary disease among Puerto Ricans (14.1%) and Cubans (9.8%) was reflective of higher rates of smoking and the presence of asthma. In general, Latinos who were born in the United States or immigrated as children had a higher asthma prevalence than those who had immigrated as adults (19.6%, 19.4%, and 14.1%, respectively; $p<0.001$). No similar increase associated with US residence was observed among Central and South American immigrants, and asthma rates among Cuban immigrants were lower after relocation. The higher prevalence of asthma among Latino subgroups intersects with poverty, low health literacy, language barriers, and lack of high-quality health services and insurance. These factors contribute to Latinos being less likely to have an asthma action plan or discuss asthma control with their health care provider and having higher rates of emergency department visits and hospitalization for asthma.[133]

Exposure to multiple adverse SDOH has been associated with a cumulative burden of social disadvantage, leading to incrementally higher cardiovascular disease (CVD) mortality.[134] In 2020 and 2021, the leading cause of death for Latino adults was COVID-19, with higher death rates associated with an increasing number of adverse SDOH.[135,136] CVD death rates vary substantially by Latino ancestry group. For example, between 2003 and 2012, Mexicans and Puerto Ricans died younger at the time of CVD death than Cubans and non-Hispanic whites, with nearly 20% of CVD deaths occurring before age 50.[137] Puerto Ricans experienced the highest years of potential life lost (YPLL) for all types of CVD compared with Mexicans and Cuban adults, a disparity that remains unchanged.[138] Puerto Ricans had the highest YPLL for ischemic and hypertensive heart disease, while Mexicans had the highest YPLL for cerebrovascular disease. Upward mobility, through higher education attainment leading to higher SEP, has been demonstrated to mitigate some of the negative cardiovascular effects of childhood disadvantage in Latinos.[139] A higher SEP in parents or their adult offspring strengthens the intergenerational continuum of ideal cardiovascular health behaviors.[140]

The three systems of education, employment, and health are interconnected and, in tandem, produce vulnerability among a significant percentage of educationally and economically disadvantaged Mexican and Puerto Rican groups and reinforce layers of disadvantage in health and mental health outcomes. Place impacts the SDOH; Mexicans and Puerto Ricans are more likely to be concentrated in about nine states alongside poor Central American and Afro-Caribbean Latinos. Often, community resources and child health state policies decrease access to health resources, as shown by higher rates of uninsured and poverty rates associated with more adverse health outcomes.[60] States in the highest (third) tertile of the social vulnerability index had predominantly poor Black and Hispanic populations and higher rates of unemployment and substance use.[141] These individuals also had higher rates of hypertension, diabetes, hyperlipidemia, chronic kidney disease, smoking, and atherosclerotic CVD compared with those living in the first tertile of the social vulnerability index.

CASE STUDIES OF MARGINALIZATION: EMPLOYMENT, EDUCATION, AND HEALTH CARE SYSTEMS

Adverse impacts of US institutional and policy structures are not readily evident. The following case studies are composites of real-life experiences and showcase how the structural systems of employment, educational pathways, and community health care systems adversely impact population health.

Employment Experiences

Families and individuals with multiple intergenerational and citizenship statuses are described to elaborate on the heterogeneity of poor and less educated Mexican-origin people, Puerto Ricans, and other poor Latinos. Multilayered disadvantaged statuses significantly affect personal and economic resources. In these cases, two distinct characteristics can be observed: high levels of discrimination, including impacts of exclusionary immigrant discrimination policies, and low education coupled with low-wage jobs and no health or retirement benefits.

Case 1: Children of First-Generation Parents

This case study describes a family who came from El Salvador and México seeking employment to support their family. José's parents were from a small town outside of San Salvador plagued by violence. His parents, Francisco and Sonia, immigrated to the United States, where José was born. Due to his family's difficulty making rent, José left high school to work in a restaurant as a server. Unable to obtain adequate housing given his income, he lived with his parents. At work, he met Julieta, who was also born in the United States, though her family was from México. They soon started a family, and José worked to pay for his growing family. He later learned that Julieta quit high school for the same reason he did. At $7.25 per hour, he was not paid fairly, but because he worked 60 hours a week, he took home about $400 a week.

After ten years, José became obese and developed diabetes. He still works six days a week, now as a cook and earning $10 per hour. He misses work weekly to see his doctors, and because his job does not provide insurance, he frequently has to choose between getting his medicine and paying his bills. The family now has two children, a 9-year-old daughter and a 3-year-old son. Julieta works as a dishwasher in a different restaurant when José is home, as their combined income does not allow for childcare costs. José Jr.

qualifies for Head Start,* but it is only three days a week until he turns four, when Julieta can work longer hours. Minimum-wage laws are not enough to provide José and Julieta a life free of poverty. At $7.25 an hour, with both adults working full time, they would be $160 above the federal poverty line if they could work every week without vacation. José does not earn a living wage, which is the minimum hourly amount that a full-time worker must earn to afford basic needs where they live and be self-sufficient.[79]

Case 2: Undocumented

This case describes a family who crossed the US border from México without documentation. Julio was 21 years old and looking for work in his small village on the shore of Lake Atitlán, Guatemala. He wanted to come to the United States but learned the waiting list to get an appointment for a visa is two years. His town had no work, and his parents no longer worked due to health problems. He made the four-day trip to Ciudad Juárez, México, where he tried to legally find a way into the United States. Julio found work in Juarez, but the pay was very low. At work, he met María, who convinced him to stay a little longer. María became pregnant, and they married. They hired a "coyote" to take them across the border, and his uncle in California arranged to pick Julio and María up in Texas. They were taken to the border at night and crossed on foot. Although their money was stolen after payment to the coyote, they crossed the border without further assaults. Outside El Paso, his uncle picked them up and drove them to California to start a new life. Julio first worked in his uncle's restaurant but soon left to work in construction, which paid much better. After giving birth, Maria returned to work clearing tables in a restaurant. Because of her additional income, the family moved into a one-bedroom apartment, which they shared with another family. Although switching jobs brought more money into the family, it was hard on Julio's body. Julio fell off a low roof, and his back pain did not subside for several weeks. He saw a doctor, who recommended he take three weeks off from work. Because Julio's job did not provide insurance or paid time off, he took the prescription and returned to work the next day. His pain worsened, so he got more medications, eventually progressing from ibuprofen to oxycodone. This has become problematic because he can no longer see his doctors due to a lack of time off and no insurance and now must obtain the medicines on the street at a very high cost. Without the medications, the pain makes it impossible for him to work.

Low wages, no health insurance, and no benefits, including sick days, ensure poverty now, poverty in retirement, intergenerational cycles of poverty, and limited economic and social mobility for many Latino workers. Gender differences show that low-income Latino women are paid less than other low-income women, which negatively affects their

---

*Head Start is a Department of Health and Human Services program that provides early childhood education, health, nutrition, and parental involvement services to low-income families. See https://headstart.gov for more information.

life expectancy.[87] Poverty continues to negatively affect the less educated and mixed-race Latino population. Citizenship is not a protection against racism, poverty, or low net worth for Mexican Americans and Puerto Ricans.

Educational Experiences Throughout the Life Course

The case studies that follow address the educational experiences of two US citizens. These cases demonstrate patterns of persistent educational, stereotypic discriminatory practices in low-income school districts and discriminatory barriers along the physician career trajectory.[142–145]

Case 3: 11th Generation US Citizen, Mexican American

Jessica Chavez, the oldest of four children, was born in Santa Fe, New Mexico. Her mother Julie is Tiwa and was raised on a reservation in Santa Fe County, near Taos, and learned English as an adult. Her father's family had been there since the initial colonizers came with the Spanish in the early 1600s. His side of the family was granted land by the Spanish government in 1690, and their land was repossessed by the US government when they took over the land from the Spanish. Jessica's family has been in court battles for generations trying to have the land originally deeded to her family returned. Jessica feels a connection to it as it is near the reservation where her mother grew up. Currently, large multinational oil companies own the land and make millions in oil sales. Her father works in grounds maintenance for the local school district, and her mother works as a teachers' aide in the same district. Between her parents' income, the family of six barely stays above the federal poverty line. As the oldest daughter, Jessica has multiple responsibilities at home, including caring for her younger siblings when her parents are at work. Jessica was learning Spanish in high school; her parents speak only English to each other. Her academic achievement was noticed by her Spanish teacher, who was Cuban American. This teacher became a mentor to Jessica and helped her to identify classes for college-bound students, as well as rallied other professionals to assist Jessica in applying for college scholarships and filling out federal financial aid forms. Together, they found enough money for Jessica to live in Albuquerque, New Mexico and attend the University of New Mexico as the first person on either side of the family to attend college. Jessica could not cover the moving costs, so she took a year off, worked, and started at the university the following year.

Case 4: US Citizen, Puerto Rican

María Rodriguez was born in Yabucoa, Puerto Rico, a small town in the western part of the island known as the sugar city. Her parents both lived in New York City, New York as children but dropped out of high school to move back to Puerto Rico to work in the sugar cane factory. María and her family returned to New York City when she was 8 years old when the sugar cane factory finally closed. In the Bronx, María was placed in bilingual education but did not initially learn English. Both her parents spoke Spanish in the home. After completing bilingual classes, María could communicate well in English and the teachers and students learned that she was smart. Even though she had teachers who believed in her, she was unable to take the necessary classes to prepare her for an academic high school. In the Bronx, where most residents are Latino, she was constantly told, "Your people don't go to college." Although teachers were unable to guide her toward a four-year college, María attended Bronx Community College, where she found a community in which she belonged. She found herself at the top of her class and graduated from Bronx Community College and Lehman College, both summa cum laude. She applied to 20 medical schools, obtained a fee waiver for most of those schools, was placed on two wait lists, and was rejected by all others. She was eventually accepted into a bridge postbaccalaureate conditional admission program, and five years later, she graduated from Rosalind Franklin School of Medicine in Chicago, Illinois. She initially wanted to be a surgeon but was discouraged by medical school faculty. María chose family medicine and was accepted to a residency program in social medicine at Montefiore Medical Center in the Bronx. Upon completing residency, she joined the faculty at New York City Medical School and found herself completely isolated with no Latino faculty in the department.

Isolation, racism, devaluing, and lack of educational attention are endemic in the educational pathways of Latino US citizens. These experiences disproportionately occur among Mexican Americans and Puerto Ricans. Their prior life course experiences are often shaped by higher rates of poverty, racialized/Indigenous phenotypes and skin color, living in low-resourced communities, and as a result fewer skills in negotiating privileged environments. Another phenomenon that occurs among many Puerto Rican and Mexican-origin health professionals is that they are disrespected as professionals and viewed only as representatives of diversity.[146,147] The high clinical obligations and excessive diversity work that are near-universal experiences of minority faculty in academic medicine are well documented. These experiences accumulate and persist over time and contribute to the severe underrepresentation of these groups. Low institutional representation of these groups is evident and for those who serve in these capacities, the articulation of community needs often becomes an additional professional burden. However, how and what needs are articulated and for whom vary by immigrant status, nativity, and color.[148] Robust and equitable pathway programs must be developed to ensure that Mexican American and Puerto Rican students (K–20) and early career professionals are socialized and integrated into the pathway early and that structures and policies are put into practice that ensure that students in high school are well-guided and counseled and medical professionals are well mentored, so that they remain motivated to complete a demanding health professions education.[149,150]

Health Care System: Role of Access and Outcomes in a Community Public Health Clinic

The Mount Sinai Adolescent Health Center (MSAHC) in New York City applies a unique model that integrates medical, sexual and reproductive health, health education, behavioral and mental health, nutrition, dental, optical, and legal services. MSAHC also provides specialized care for lesbian, gay, bisexual, transgender, queer, and questioning (LGBTQ+) youth, youth living with or at risk for HIV, pregnant youth, young parents and their children, and survivors of trauma, including a history of childhood abuse and trafficking. All care is confidential and provided at no cost to patients under one roof, making it highly accessible for youth.

Case 5: Free, Community-Based Adolescent Health and Mental Health Care, Mexican American Female

Rachel, a 14-year-old, 5th-generation Mexican American, came to MSAHC when she needed a physical exam for working papers and new eyeglasses for school. She heard she could get care there at no cost, which was an important financial support. Her provider assured her that all care was confidential and learned that while Rachel worked hard in school, she had trouble motivating herself to study. She revealed that she had recently started having sex with her boyfriend, who often called her names and put her down. Rachel talked through her reproductive health needs, including birth control options, with a trained health educator and decided to get an intrauterine device. The provider discussed the importance of dual protection to prevent pregnancy and sexually transmitted infections, and Rachel learned strategies for talking with her boyfriend about safer sex through role play. Her physician also introduced Rachel to a mental health professional with whom she discussed healthy and unhealthy relationships, setting boundaries with her boyfriend, and managing the stress of school. Rachel was diagnosed with attention-deficit/hyperactivity disorder and was introduced to a lawyer who secured her an Individualized Education Program. Psychotherapy and MetroCards were provided at no cost. With this support, she left her unhealthy relationship, her grades improved dramatically, and she is currently starting freshman year of college.

Case 6: Free Wraparound Services, Adolescent Dominican/Puerto Rican Gay Male With a Chronic Condition

Ben, a 16-year-old student, had an asthma attack at school and went to the MSAHC school-based health center. The physician treated and worked with him to devise a plan to manage his asthma. While Ben was born in Puerto Rico, his Dominican mother's visa had expired. She worked multiple jobs to pay the bills and their relationship was strained. Ben, who was gay, was scared to come out to her. He felt overwhelmed with shame and self-hate, and to cope, had turned to alcohol and self-harm. Moreover, he had a run-in with the police for a minor offense but didn't know whether he needed to pay a fine or go to court. Through a social worker, he learned strategies to manage his emotions when he felt overwhelmed. He appreciated the free health care and confidentiality of psychotherapy without the worry that his mother would find out. His therapist introduced him to a lawyer in the clinic, who helped Ben clear his record and connected Ben's mother with immigration specialists. Ben and his mother received family therapy and with the support of his therapist, Ben was able to come out to his mother and quit drinking. He is currently working toward becoming a doctor.

This matrix of access to comprehensive individual and family care, including addressing SDOH and other innovative strategies, helps serve populations who are low-income and below the federal poverty level. Low-income Latinos (US citizens and immigrants) in the United States can benefit from the amplification and replication of these innovative models. In addition, having a patient-centered, culturally relevant service design facilitates access to "whole-person" care and leads to better outcomes. While the cost–benefit of addressing SDOH is well established, such evidence is critical in disseminating and scaling up similar efforts.[151–153] This exemplar of service represents comprehensive, prevention-driven health care. A system of community public health clinics colocated with major hospital facilities is a salubrious solution to increasing access and identifying and responding to basic preventive community needs and primary care conditions. Systemic changes at the state and federal levels are needed to provide legislated funding for systems like MSAHC to support the nation's health at the state and community levels.

ADVANCING ACTIONABLE STRATEGIES: DISMANTLING PATHWAYS OF INSTITUTIONAL RACISM WITH SYSTEMIC CHANGES

The story of Mexican-origin people and Puerto Ricans in US history uncovers the challenges in obtaining full access to its opportunity structures. The structures of opportunity for social and economic mobility are driven by access to high-quality and equitable (fair) educational, employment, and health care systems. Their exclusion from and by these systems is evidenced by their high rates of poverty and severe and disproportionate underrepresentation of Mexican American and Puerto Rican professionals in all professional fields, particularly the health and medical fields. A resolute educational and economic disinvestment represents a denial of equity to these groups who have contributed to the foundation and social, economic, and cultural fabric of US society.

Drawing on the vast interdisciplinary historical, demographic, policy and public health/medical literature on Mexicans and Puerto Ricans in the United States, we conclude that SDOH and political determinants of health (policy and systems) adversely and disproportionately impact the economic and social mobility and healthy outcomes of low-income and less educated (< high school education) Mexican, Puerto Rican and racialized Latinos. We address economic justice in employment and education, educational equity, and health care access and quality. While not an exhaustive list, presented in Table 4-4 are select strategic actionable solutions in education, employment, and health to initiate a process of change to alter intergenerational, institutional patterns of inequity and improve the health and well-being of Mexicans, Puerto Ricans, and other poor, racialized, disadvantaged Latino populations.[86,106,154–166]

Table 4-4. Actionable Strategies in Education, Employment, and Health

Issue	Research Supporting Issue	Policy Proposals & Best Practices
Education		
Childcare	Most Hispanic communities tend to have few childcare providers due to discrimination in accessing small business loans, the wealth gap, and higher existing amounts of debt.[154] Pre-pandemic rules regarding funding for childcare set payment caps that were too low.[155]	Provide for core operational grants that are not restrictive and can be used for a variety of situations that a childcare provider may face.[155]
Community college	Latinos are more likely to attend community colleges when compared with white peers due to cost and accessibility.[156]	Provide scholarships that cover all or almost all of tuition for students, including at community colleges, and allow individuals to apply regardless of immigration status.[157]
Student loan debt	Americans owe >$1.7 trillion in student loan debt, with the average Latino borrower owing $41,700 after a 4-year degree.[158] Broad restructuring efforts at public universities and colleges have also given more power to institutions to set tuition rates, putting students from working-class families at a further disadvantage.[159]	Beyond student loan debt cancellation, double the maximum Pell Grant award, improve income-driven repayment and Public Service Loan Forgiveness terms, extend eligibility for federal financial aid to undocumented students, and pass congressional legislation to meet any unmet needs for Pell Grant-eligible students at public colleges and universities.[159]
Employment		
Paid leave	Hispanics have the lowest level of access to paid leave, including parental leave, maternity/paternity leave, sick leave, leave for elder care, or leave to care for a sick family member.[160,161]	Pass the Healthy Families Act, which would set a national baseline for all employees to receive 7 paid sick days per year.[161] Establish paid leave programs at the state and federal level.
Federal minimum wage	Federal minimum wage has not been raised since 2009 and sits at $7.25/hour, with the purchasing power of this wage level having steadily decreased over the past several decades.[162] On average, Latinos are paid 10%–15% less than whites with similar characteristics.[163]	Raise the federal minimum wage to $15/hour. This would raise pay for 32 million workers, 21% of the US workforce; some areas along the southern borders of TX and NM with large Hispanic populations would see ~50% of workers being impacted.[164]

(Continued)

Table 4-4. (Continued)

Issue	Research Supporting Issue	Policy Proposals & Best Practices
Union membership	Latinos have some of the lowest rates of unionization among any demographic group in the country. Long-standing labor inequities have disproportionately impacted Latino workers and were exacerbated by the COVID-19 pandemic, including unstable employment, stagnant/low wages, and few to no benefits.[86]	Pass the PRO Act, strengthening the ability of federal and state governments to penalize employers and corporations that engage in union-busting activities, implementing a federal jobs guarantee, and reinforcing union protections from the National Labor Relations Act of 1935.[86]
Health Care		
Universal coverage	Hispanic adults overall are less likely to have health insurance and receive preventative medical care, with this largely being due to holding lower-quality jobs, having higher rates of poverty, and existing language and cultural barriers.[106]	Expand Medicaid to include undocumented immigrants and develop a model utilizing *promotores de salud*, or community health workers, to provide health education and outreach services to Latino communities.[164] Pass the Medicare for All Act to establish a universal single-payer national health insurance system out-of-pocket expenses, insurance premiums, deductibles, or co-payments.[165]
FQCHCs	FQCHCs are part of the "safety net" of medically underserved and low-income communities and have shown to be effective for telehealth appointments, substance abuse treatment, and resources relating to housing, food, and transportation.[166]	Increase funding for CHCs and implement policies that support these centers, especially as Medicaid coverage is curtailed.[166]

Note: FQCHC = Federally Qualified Community Health Center; NM = New Mexico; PRO Act = Protecting the Right to Organize Act; TX = Texas.

Economic Justice: Employment and Education

Economic justice, or ensuring a means to a dignified life, eludes the low-income and less educated Mexican-origin and Puerto Rican populations due to their high concentrations in low-paying, minimum-wage jobs (wages are even less among undocumented workers).[89] Many of these jobs do not have retirement plans, health insurance, or disability insurance.[84] Drawing on long-standing employment inequity for less educated groups, policies that link employment and health care benefits, as well as a minimum wage for all service and nonprofessional workers, are essential. These policies represent important steps toward economic justice and equity and reduction of the negative impact of SDOH for all Latinos, although Mexicans and Puerto Ricans as the largest groups are disproportionately impacted.

Educational equity for low-income Latinos is a life course investment that begins with access to high-quality early childhood education: a K–12 experience that prepares students for college careers, postsecondary education, and access to lifelong learning opportunities. The lack of access, outreach, and high rates of disenrollment and dropouts of Mexican and Puerto Rican youth in federal and state education programs calls for increased accountability of funding priorities to ensure equitable access to monetary, recreational, and academic skill-building programs. There is no shortage of policy recommendations or efforts by local, state, and federal governments as well as Latino, education, and higher education advocacy groups.[82] Strategic actions range from ensuring universal access to early childhood education, funding parity for K–12 educational systems throughout the nation, and free tuition at community colleges to providing responsive, quality, and equitably funded Hispanic-serving institutions of higher education and addressing access to broadband internet.

A set of value-driven strategies drawing on the right of high-quality education as an equity lever for all would address not only the disproportionately lower rates of high school and college completion among Mexican and Puerto Rican groups, but also the increasing number of mixed citizenship–status families among Mexican and Central American subgroups, such as Dreamers who benefited from Deferred Action for Childhood Arrivals (DACA). A fair educational policy needs to reconstruct the avenues of funding for our schools (e.g., national funding as part of the tax structure) and our values on a right to education for all.

Health: Social Determinants of Health, Access, and Workforce Representation

Equitable, actionable solutions to decrease medical bias and support good health outcomes among Mexicans and Puerto Ricans and all low-income Latinos include investments addressing SDOH, access to health insurance coverage, and adequate, proportionate, and representative workforce development.[167] Health-related social needs can be identified and coordinated through comprehensive and integrated health care delivery and social services systems. Incentives, such as value-based health care, can be employed to encourage health care systems and social services providers to modify their programs to address the specific needs of the Latino communities they serve. Socioeconomic needs vary across different populations. Integrated interventions and collaboration with community partners are necessary for programs to address biopsychosocial, immigration status issues, and economic needs more effectively.[168]

Health insurance coverage facilitates access to health care services. Reducing the health insurance gap requires that more employers offer health insurance coverage to their workers, as well as expanding Medicaid and other individual non-group market health insurance choices that can make coverage more affordable. Moreover, developing varying options for health care access for all Latinos, including undocumented groups, such as the development of financial assistance programs by safety-net clinics and health systems to provide services to uninsured populations, is a step in the right direction.[169]

Representative workforce development is closely aligned with the need to advocate for the allocation of services and resources to disadvantaged communities. Investments in public health infrastructure and inclusive workforce development practices are the most impactful levers of change. Dismantling pathways of racism and closed opportunity structures across the interrelated systems of education, employment, and health require immediate attention to increase the representation of power brokers who are advocates of change. Latino community members and organizations who are knowledgeable of community interests are critical in advocating for additional resources, fundraising, and developing innovative programs to meet the needs of the different Latino subgroups in different states. Creating opportunity pathways for representatives of the varying Latino subgroups to take on managerial and leadership roles in the different sectors can improve the voice of representative Latinos (Mexican American, Puerto Rican, Salvadoran, or Dominican) in health care positions of leadership—as well as underrepresentation in other key sectors. Caution must be taken not to engage in racial/ethnic "clumping" or aggregation as the heterogeneity of group experiences needs to be acknowledged.[13] Improving educational and employment opportunities, reducing food and housing insecurity, increasing affordable childcare options and making transportation more easily available will go a long way to creating opportunities to improve the health and well-being of Latinos.

CONCLUSION

The foundational history of the United States is best understood within a framework of fairness, opportunity, equity (access to and allocation of resources to those most in need to assure access to equal opportunity), and proportional representation to promote accurate articulation of community needs and knowledgeable and committed engagement within communities. The historical record has shown adverse sociopolitical, policy, and legislative impacts of closing the doors of opportunity for Mexican and Puerto Rican groups who are fundamental in the creation of the US nation. The "hands of government" created policies to block opportunity for historically colonized groups (Mexican-origin, Indigenous, African American with an intergenerational legacy of slavery, and Puerto Ricans) and divested the resources of these communities, which has had persistent impacts on SDOH and therefore health outcomes.[15,17,19,31] These policies included segregation and discrimination, for example, segregated low-resourced schools, public housing, inhumane and unregulated farm labor work and immigration policy for Mexican "trespassers," and corporate tax havens in Puerto Rico (see Act 20 and Act 22 in Table 4A-2 in Appendix 4A). These issues are further compounded by matters of race and immigration status, which increasingly impact poor Indigenous Central Americans, which should be examined in future discourse. Many historic and contemporary proposed policies have adversely impacted Mexican and Puerto Rican wealth, assets, and educational and occupational mobility. These policies and laws further decrease the ability of these groups to represent, advocate, and support their communities—especially as it relates to health and well-being.

Three important lessons are drawn from this narrative review of the impacts of three interrelated systems (education, employment, and health) on the life course and well-being of predominantly Mexican-origin and Puerto Rican population groups. (1) Disaggregated data must be collected by Latino subgroup to identify distinct differences within and across subgroups to properly inform on SDOH and health disparities by ethnic subgroup, socioeconomic status, and race. Race, ancestry, nation, and class intersect and inform SDOH.[170,171] The aggregation of all Latinos into one group erases the impact of historic policies and laws on Mexican-origin and Puerto Rican communities and their economic and health disparities, wealth gaps, and disproportionate professional underrepresentation in US society. (2) These two groups are disproportionately more likely to be mixed race (racialized), Indigenous, and/or Black, less likely to be prepared educationally, and more likely to be employed in service sectors. (3) Significant diasporic immigrant movements over the last 50 years from Latin American countries to the United States have contributed to a demographic shift in who is Latino. South and Central American diasporic movements represent heterogeneous groups of varying socioeconomic statuses, ancestries, and races (white European, Indigenous, and Black). Many of these predominantly South American groups, jointly with Cuban Americans, have higher education levels, more wealth, easier integration and acceptance in US society, and are accorded different privileges and opportunities from those available to Mexican-origin, Puerto Rican, and many Central American and Afro-Latino groups. For example, white European, educated individuals from a Hispanic-identified country or European or Asian immigrants with education and wealth will more easily integrate into US society than less educated, mixed-race Latinos. These lessons highlight that heterogeneity within the "master construct of Latino" does not inform as an aggregate on health conditions, disability, quality of life, and intergenerational social and economic mobility among the distinct ancestral and cultural/ethnic groups included in the term.

This chapter illustrates how some Latino subgroups are deeply impacted by historical policy and maltreatment, race, socioeconomic status, structural inequity in employment, underresourced educational systems, and minimally responsive health care systems (opportunity structures).[172] Without a radical change in quality, access, and accountability in these three systems, the quality of life and the health and mental well-being of Latinos, particularly those subgroups with a historical legacy in the United States (Mexican and Puerto Rican populations), will not considerably improve. Access to opportunity structures requires diminishing the political determinants that adversely impact SDOH.[172] Equity needs to be a shared value among the haves and have-nots; this is often touted as allyship. Vast wealth, assets, and education gaps exist across and within different racial/ethnic groups. The future may provide a roadmap for how the changing immigrant profile of global citizens in the United States over the last five decades will maintain the racial hierarchy or create more equitable opportunity structures for all Americans.

ACKNOWLEDGMENTS

The authors would like to acknowledge Dr. Diana Torres-Burgos and Katherine A. Van Nuys, former research coordinator, for their research assistance and contributions to this chapter.

REFERENCES

1. US Census Bureau. Facts for features: Hispanic Heritage Month: 2023. August 17, 2023. Accessed April 9, 2025. https://www.census.gov/newsroom/facts-for-features/2023/hispanic-heritage-month.html
2. Vespa J, Medina L, Armstrong DM. Demographic turning points for the United States: Population projections for 2020 to 2060. US Census Bureau. Revised February 2020. Accessed August 15, 2025. https://www.census.gov/content/dam/Census/library/publications/2020/demo/p25-1144.pdf
3. Moslimani M, Lopez MH, Noe-Bustamante L. 11 facts about Hispanic origin groups in the US. Pew Research Center. 2022. Accessed April 9, 2025. https://www.pewresearch.org/short-reads/2023/08/16/11-facts-about-hispanic-origin-groups-in-the-us
4. Hispanic population in the US by origin 2021. Statista. 2023. Accessed August 15, 2025. https://www.statista.com/statistics/234852/us-hispanic-population
5. Scherer Z, Mayol-García Y. Half of people of Dominican and Salvadoran origin experienced material hardship in 2020. US Census Bureau. September 8, 2022. Accessed April 7, 2025. https://www.census.gov/library/stories/2022/09/hardships-wealth-disparities-across-hispanic-groups.html
6. Pew Research Center. US Hispanic Population Detailed Tables. Tabulations of the 2000 decennial census (5% IPUMS) and the 2010 and 2021 American Community Surveys (1% IPUMS). Accessed April 7, 2025. https://docs.google.com/spreadsheets/d/1vxtbpCROMbOhemXCb4g8ZukOpGLjWtAv/edit?usp=sharing&ouid=107954968574441737010&rtpof=true&sd=true
7. Marks R, Jones N, Battle K. What updates to OMB's race/ethnicity standards mean for the Census Bureau. US Census Bureau blog. April 8, 2024. Accessed April 7, 2025. https://www.census.gov/newsroom/blogs/random-samplings/2024/04/updates-race-ethnicity-standards.html
8. Campos A. What's the difference between Hispanic, Latino and Latinx? On navigating identity, language and community from a scholarly and first-person perspective. University of California October 6, 2021. Accessed April 17, 2025. https://www.universityofcalifornia.edu/news/choosing-the-right-word-hispanic-latino-and-latinx

9. Yarin S. If Hispanics hate the term "Latinx," why is it still used? *Boston University Today.* October 7, 2022. Accessed April 17, 2025. https://www.bu.edu/articles/2022/why-is-latinx-still-used-if-hispanics-hate-the-term
10. Lopez MH, Krogstad JM, Passel JS. Who is Hispanic? Pew Research Center. September 12, 2024. Accessed April 17, 2025. https://www.pewresearch.org/short-reads/2023/09/05/who-is-hispanic
11. Simón Y. Latino, Hispanic, Latinx, Chicano: The history behind the terms. History.com. September 14, 2020. Accessed April 17, 2025. https://www.history.com/news/hispanic-latino-latinx-chicano-background
12. del Río-González AM. To Latinx or not to Latinx: A question of gender inclusivity versus gender neutrality. *Am J Public Health.* 2021;111(6):1018–1021. doi:10.2105/AJPH.2021.306238
13. Lugo-Lugo CR. "So you are a mestiza": Exploring the consequences of ethnic and racial clumping in the US Academy. *Ethn Racial Stud.* 2008;31(3):611–628. doi:10.1080/01419870701568882
14. Aragones A, Hayes SL, Chen MH, González J, Gany FM. Characterization of the Hispanic or Latino population in health research: A systematic review. *J Immigr Minor Health.* 2014;16(3):429–439. doi:10.1007/s10903-013-9773-0
15. Acuña R. *Occupied America: The Chicano's Struggle Toward Liberation.* Canfield Press; 1972.
16. Barrera M. *Race and Class in the Southwest: A Theory of Racial Inequality.* University of Notre Dame Press; 1979.
17. Gonzalez J. *Harvest of Empire: A History of Latinos in America.* 2nd ed. Penguin Press; 2022.
18. Bender S. *Greasers and Gringos: Latinos, Law, and the American Imagination.* New York University Press; 2003.
19. Dunbar-Ortiz R. *Not "A Nation of Immigrants": Settler Colonialism, White Supremacy, and a History of Erasure and Exclusion.* Beacon Press; 2021.
20. Bennett N, Hays B, Sullivan B. 2019 data show baby boomers nearly 9 times wealthier than millennials. US Census Bureau. August 1, 2022. Accessed April 17, 2025. https://www.census.gov/library/stories/2022/08/wealth-inequality-by-household-type.html
21. LaVeist TA, Pérez-Stable EJ, Richard P, et al. The economic burden of racial, ethnic, and educational health inequities in the US. *JAMA.* 2023;329(19):1682–1692. doi:10.1001/jama.2023.5965
22. Telles EE, Ortiz V. *Generations of Exclusion: Mexican Americans, Assimilation, and Race.* Russell Sage Foundation; 2008.
23. Villarosa L. *Under the Skin: Racism, Inequality, and the Health of a Nation.* Doubleday; 2022.
24. Zong J. A mosaic, not a monolith: A profile of the US Latino population, 2000–2020. UCLA Latino Policy & Politics Institute. October 26, 2022. Accessed April 17, 2025. https://latino.ucla.edu/research/latino-population-2000-2020
25. Flynn A, Warren D, Wong F, Holmberg S. *The Hidden Rules of Race: Barriers to an Inclusive Economy.* Cambridge University Press; 2017.
26. Marmot M. Medical care, social determinants of health, and health equity. *World Med Health Policy.* 2018;10(2):195–197. doi:10.1002/wmh3.261
27. Marmot M, Allen JJ. Social determinants of health equity. *Am J Public Health.* 2014;104(suppl 4):S517–S519. doi:10.2105/AJPH.2014.302200
28. Dawes D. *The Political Determinants of Health.* Johns Hopkins University Press; 2020.

29. Dill BT, Zambrana RE, eds. *Emerging Intersections: Race, Class, and Gender in Theory, Policy, and Practice.* Rutgers University Press; 2009.
30. Weber L, Zambrana RE, Fore ME, Parra-Medina D. Racial and ethnic health inequities: An intersectional approach. In: Batur P, Feagin JR, eds. *Handbook of the Sociology of Racial and Ethnic Relations.* 2nd ed. Springer; 2018:133–160.
31. Shapiro TM. *Toxic Inequality: How America's Wealth Gap Destroys Mobility, Deepens the Racial Divide, and Threatens Our Future.* Basic Books; 2017.
32. Zambrana RE, Parra-Medina D, Butler C. Social determinants of health: Intersectional impact of race, ethnicity, class, and place on life course. In: Scrimshaw S, Lane S, Fisher J, Rubinstein R, eds. *Handbook of Social Sciences in Health and Medicine.* 2nd ed. Sage Publications; 2022:38–59.
33. Denis NA. *War Against All Puerto Ricans: Revolution and Terror in America's Colony.* Public Affairs; 2015.
34. Ramos JGP, Garriga-López A, Rodríguez-Díaz CE. How is colonialism a sociostructural determinant of health in Puerto Rico? *AMA J Ethics.* 2022;24(4):305–312. doi:10.1001/amajethics.2022.305
35. Chavez HL, Partida MG. 1978: Madrigal v. Quilligan. Library of Congress. August 17, 2020. Updated December 14, 2023. Accessed April 18, 2025. https://guides.loc.gov/latinx-civil-rights/madrigal-v-quilligan
36. Gutiérrez E. *Fertile Matters: The Politics of Mexican-Origin Women's Reproduction.* University of Texas Press; 2008.
37. Espino V, Jimenez L, Gutiérrez ER, Chavez-Garcia M. Forced sterilization: Then and now. Presented at: Hammer Museum, UCLA. October 29, 2017. Accessed April 18, 2025. https://hammer.ucla.edu/programs-events/2017/10/forced-sterilization-then-and-now
38. Lopez I. *Matters of Choice: Puerto Rican Women's Struggle for Reproductive Freedom.* Rutgers University Press; 2008.
39. National Archives. Treaty of Guadalupe Hidalgo (1848). Accessed April 18, 2025. https://www.archives.gov/milestone-documents/treaty-of-guadalupe-hidalgo
40. Thurber MD, ed. World of 1898: International perspectives on the Spanish American War. Introduction. Library of Congress. 2022. Updated February 28, 2023. Accessed April 18, 2025. https://guides.loc.gov/world-of-1898
41. MacDonald VM ed. *Latino Education in the United States: A Narrated History from 1513–2000.* Palgrave McMillian; 2004.
42. Zambrana RE. *Latinos in American Society: Families and Communities in Transition.* Cornell University Press; 2011.
43. Sáenz R, Morales MC. *Latinos in the United States: Diversity and Change.* Polity; 2015.
44. Ashkenas J, Park H, Pearce A. Even with affirmative action, Blacks and Hispanics are more underrepresented at top colleges than 35 years ago. *New York Times.* August 24, 2017. Accessed April 18, 2025. https://www.nytimes.com/interactive/2017/08/24/us/affirmative-action.html
45. Chavez HL, Partida MG. A Latinx resource guide: Civil rights cases and events in the United States: Introduction. Library of Congress. August 17, 2020. Updated December 14, 2023. Accessed April 18, 2025. https://guides.loc.gov/latinx-civil-rights
46. US Citizenship and Immigration Services. Temporary Protected Status. Updated April 7, 2025. Accessed April 18, 2025. https://www.uscis.gov/humanitarian/temporary-protected-status

47. Krogstad JM, Passel JS, Moslimani M, Noe-Bustamante L. Key facts about US Latinos for National Hispanic Heritage Month. Pew Research Center. September 22, 2023. Accessed April 18, 2025. https://www.pewresearch.org/short-reads/2023/09/22/key-facts-about-us-latinos-for-national-hispanic-heritage-month
48. González Burchard E, Borrell LN, Choudhry S, et al. Latino populations: A unique opportunity for the study of race, genetics, and social environment in epidemiological research. *Am J Public Health*. 2005;95(12):2161–2168. doi:10.2105/AJPH.2005.068668
49. Amaro H, Zambrana RE. Criollo, mestizo, mulato, LatiNegro, indígena, white, or Black? The US Hispanic/Latino population and multiple responses in the 2000 census. *Am J Public Health*. 2000;90(11):1724–1727. doi:10.2105/ajph.90.11.1724
50. Bonilla-Silva E. *Racism without Racists: Color-Blind Racism and the Persistence of Racial Inequality in the United States*. Rowman & Littlefield; 2017.
51. Chavez L. *The Latino Threat: Constructing Immigrants, Citizens, and the Nation*. 2nd ed. Stanford University Press; 2013.
52. Galdámez M, Gomez M, Perez R. Centering Black Latinidad: A profile of the US Afro-Latinx population and complex inequalities. UCLA Latino Policy and Politics Institute. April 20, 2023. Accessed April 18, 2025. https://latino.ucla.edu/research/centering-black-latinidad
53. López N, Vargas ED, Juarez M, Cacari-Stone L, Bettez S. What's your "street race"? Leveraging multidimensional measures of race and intersectionality for examining physical and mental health status among Latinxs. *Sociol Race Ethn (Thousand Oaks)*. 2018;4(1):49–66. doi:10.1177/2332649217708798
54. Rodríguez C. *Changing Race: Latinos, the Census, and the History of Ethnicity in the United States*. New York University Press; 2000.
55. Villareal MA. US–Mexico economic relations: Trends, issues, and implications. Congressional Research Services Report. June 2020. Accessed April 18, 2025. https://crsreports.congress.gov/product/pdf/RL/RL32934
56. Gonzalez-Barrera A. About 6 million US adults identify as Afro-Latino. Pew Research Center. May 2, 2022. Accessed April 18, 2025. https://www.pewresearch.org/short-reads/2022/05/02/about-6-million-u-s-adults-identify-as-afro-latino
57. Perreira KM, Telles EE. The color of health: Skin color, ethnoracial classification, and discrimination in the health of Latin Americans. *Soc Sci Med*. 2014;116:241–250. doi:10.1016/j.socscimed.2014.05.054
58. Islas IG, Brantley E, Portela Martinez M, Salsberg E, Dobkin F, Frogner BK. Documenting Latino representation in the US health workforce. *Health Aff (Millwood)*. 2023;42(7):997–1001. doi:10.1377/hlthaff.2022.01348
59. Creamer J, Shrider EA, Burns K, Chen F. *Poverty in the United States: 2021*. US Census Bureau; 2022. Accessed August 15, 2025. https://www.census.gov/library/publications/2022/demo/p60-277.html
60. Zambrana RE, Torres-Burgos D, Carvajal DN. Expert perspectives on effective community-based pediatric healthcare for low-income Latino families: Persistent issues over time. *J Racial Ethn Health Disparities*. 2022;9(3):1051–1061. doi:10.1007/s40615-021-01044-1

61. Branch B, Conway D. Health insurance coverage by race and Hispanic origin: 2021. US Census Bureau. November 2022. Accessed April 18, 2025. https://www.census.gov/content/dam/Census/library/publications/2022/acs/acsbr-012.pdf
62. Kochhar R, Moslimani M. Wealth surged in the pandemic, but debt endures for poorer Black and Hispanic families. Pew Research Center. December 4, 2023. Accessed April 18, 2025. https://www.pewresearch.org/race-ethnicity/2023/12/04/wealth-surged-in-the-pandemic-but-debt-endures-for-poorer-black-and-hispanic-families
63. Gallo LC, Penedo FJ, Carnethon M, et al. The Hispanic Community Health Study/Study of Latinos Sociocultural Ancillary Study: Sample, design, and procedures. *Ethn Dis*. 2014;24(1): 77–83. Accessed August 15, 2025. https://ethndis.org/archive/files/ethndis-24-77.pdf
64. Errisuriz VL, Zambrana RE, Parra-Medina D. Critical analyses of Latina mortality: Disentangling the heterogeneity of ethnic origin, place, nativity, race, and socioeconomic status. *BMC Public Health*. 2024;24(1):190. doi:10.1186/s12889-024-17721-9
65. Nicole W. Paradox lost? The waning health advantage among the US Hispanic population. *Environ Health Perspect*. 2023;131(1):12001. doi:10.1289/EHP11618
66. Abrego LJ. *Sacrificing Families: Navigating Laws, Labor, and Love Across Borders*. Stanford University Press; 2014.
67. Millet E, Pavilon J. Demographic profile of undocumented Hispanic immigrants in the United States. Center for Migration Studies of New York. October 14, 2022. Accessed April 18, 2025. https://cmsny.org/publications/hispanic-undocumented-immigrants-millet-pavilon-101722
68. Perreira KM, Pedroza JM. Policies of exclusion: Implications for the health of immigrants and their children. *Annu Rev Public Health*. 2019;40:147–166. doi:10.1146/annurev-publhealth-040218-044115
69. Williams DR, Lawrence JA, Davis BA. Racism and health: Evidence and needed research. *Annu Rev Public Health*. 2019;40:105–125. doi:10.1146/annurev-publhealth-040218-043750
70. Martín A. Intersectionality without fragmentation. *Ethics*. 2024;134(2):214–245. doi:10.1086/727271
71. Contreras F. *Achieving Equity for Latino Students: Expanding the Pathway to Higher Education Through Public Policy*. Teachers College Press; 2011.
72. Contreras F, Contreras GJ. Raising the bar for Hispanic serving institutions: An analysis of college completion and success rates. *J Hispanic High Educ*. 2015;14(2):151–170. doi:10.1177/1538192715572892
73. Contreras F, Rodriguez J, Bybee ER, et al. Investing in educational equity for Latinos: How accountability, access, and systemic inequity shape opportunity. In: Valencia RR, Alemán E, eds. *Handbook of Latinos and Education*. 2nd ed. Routledge; 2022:103–113.
74. Gandara P, Contreras F. *The Latino Education Crisis: The Consequences of Failed Social Policies*. Harvard University Press; 2009.
75. MacDonald VM, Rivera J. History's prism in education: A spectrum of legacies across centuries of Mexican American agency, experience and activism 1600s–2000s. In: Zambrana RE, Hurtado S, eds. *The Magic Key: The Educational Journey of Mexican Americans From K–12 to College and Beyond*. University of Texas Press; 2015:25–52.
76. Rios VM. *Punished: Policing the Lives of Black and Latino Boys*. New York University Press; 2011.

77. Garcia C, Garcia MA, Ailshire JA. Sociocultural variability in the Latino population: Age patterns and differences in morbidity among older US adults. *Demogr Res.* 2018;38:1605–1618. doi:10.4054/DemRes.2018.38.52
78. Perreira KM, Allen CD. The health of Hispanic children from birth to emerging adulthood. *Ann Am Acad Pol Soc Sci.* 2021;696(1):200–222. doi:10.1177/00027162211048805
79. Glasmeier AK. What is a living wage and how is it estimated? Living Wage Calculator. Massachusetts Institute of Technology. 2024. Accessed April 18, 2025. https://livingwage.mit.edu/pages/methodology
80. Galindo C. Taking an equity lens: Reconceptualizing research on Latinx students' schooling experiences and educational outcomes. *Ann Am Acad Pol Soc Sci.* 2021;696(1):106–127. doi:10.1177/00027162211043770
81. Valenzuela A. *Subtractive Schooling: US-Mexican Youth and the Politics of Caring.* State University of New York Press; 2019.
82. Zambrana RE, Hurtado S, eds. *The Magic Key: The Educational Journey of Mexican Americans from K–12 to College and Beyond.* University of Texas Press; 2015.
83. Zayas LH, Gulbas LE. Are suicide attempts by young Latinas a cultural idiom of distress?. *Transcult Psychiatry.* 2012;49(5):718–734. doi:10.1177/1363461512463262
84. Berchick ER, Hood E, Barnett JC. *Health Insurance Coverage in the United States: 2017.* US Census Bureau; 2018. Accessed April 18, 2025. https://www.census.gov/content/dam/Census/library/publications/2018/demo/p60-264.pdf
85. Dubina K. Hispanics in the labor force: 5 facts. US Dept of Labor blog. September 15, 2021. Accessed April 18, 2025. https://web.archive.org/web/20220213234152/http://blog.dol.gov/2021/09/15/hispanics-in-the-labor-force-5-facts
86. González N, Galdámez M. More than solidarity: How labor unions preserved Latino jobs. UCLA Latino Policy & Politics Institute. September 6, 2021. Accessed April 18, 2025. https://latino.ucla.edu/wp-content/uploads/2021/09/More-than-Solidarity-How-Labor-Unions-Preserved-Latino-Jobs-1.pdf
87. Eisenberg-Guyot J, Keyes KM, Prins SJ, et al. Wage theft and life expectancy inequities in the United States: A simulation study. *Prev Med.* 2022;159:107068. doi:10.1016/j.ypmed.2022.107068
88. MacDonald VM. *Latino Education in the United States: A Narrated History From 1513–2000.* Palgrave MacMillan; 2007.
89. Khattar R, Vela J, Roque L. Latino workers continue to experience a shortage of good jobs. Center for American Progress. July 18, 2022. Accessed April 18, 2025. https://www.americanprogress.org/article/latino-workers-continue-to-experience-a-shortage-of-good-jobs
90. US Bureau of Labor Statistics. Labor force characteristics by race and ethnicity, 2022. BLS Reports. November 2023. Accessed April 7, 2025. https://www.bls.gov/opub/reports/race-and-ethnicity/2022
91. US Bureau of Labor Statistics. Civilian labor force participation rate by age, sex, race, and ethnicity. 2022. Accessed April 7, 2025. https://www.bls.gov/emp/tables/civilian-labor-force-participation-rate.htm
92. Association of American Medical Colleges. Report on residents: Table B5. Number of active MD residents, by race/ethnicity (alone or in combination) and GME specialty. 2022. Accessed

September 26, 2023. https://www.aamc.org/data-reports/students-residents/data/report-residents/2022/table-b5-md-residents-race-ethnicity-and-specialty

93. Ramirez AG, Lepe R, Cigarroa F. Uplifting the Latino population from obscurity to the forefront of health care, public health intervention, and societal presence. *JAMA*. 2021;326(7):597–598. doi:10.1001/jama.2021.11997

94. Guillaume G, Robles J, Rodríguez JE. Racial concordance, rather than cultural competency training, can change outcomes. *Fam Med*. 2022;54(9):745–746. doi:10.22454/FamMed.2022.633693

95. Carvajal DN, Reid LD, Zambrana RE. URiMs and imposter syndrome: Symptoms of inhospitable work environments? *Fam Med*. 2023;55(7):433–451. doi.org/10.22454/FamMed.2023.376821.

96. Brown TT, Hurley VB, Rodriguez HP, et al. Shared decision-making lowers medical expenditures and the effect is amplified in racially-ethnically concordant relationships. *Med Care*. 2023;61(8):528–535. doi:10.1097/MLR.0000000000001881

97. US Dept of Health and Human Services. What's the difference between Medicare and Medicaid? Updated December 8, 2022. Accessed April 18, 2025. https://www.hhs.gov/answers/medicare-and-medicaid/what-is-the-difference-between-medicare-medicaid/index.html

98. State Health Access Data Assistance Center. State health compare. University of Minnesota. Accessed April 18, 2025. https://statehealthcompare.shadac.org

99. Keisler-Starkey K, Bunch LN. *Health Insurance Coverage in the United States: 2019*. US Census Bureau; 2020. Accessed April 18, 2025. https://www.census.gov/content/dam/Census/library/publications/2020/demo/p60-271.pdf

100. Noe-Bustamante L, Krogstad JM, Lopez MH. For US Latinos, COVID-19 has taken a personal and financial toll. Pew Research Center. July 15, 2021. Accessed April 18, 2025. https://www.pewresearch.org/race-ethnicity/2021/07/15/for-u-s-latinos-covid-19-has-taken-a-personal-and-financial-toll

101. Klein A, Shiro AG. The COVID-19 recession hit Latino workers hard. Here's what we need to do. The Brookings Institution. October 1, 2020. Accessed April 18, 2025. https://www.brookings.edu/articles/the-covid-19-recession-hit-latino-workers-hard-heres-what-we-need-to-do

102. Brandon MB. In the race from COVID-19, who wins? *Monthly Labor Review*. US Bureau of Labor Statistics. September 2023. Accessed April 18, 2025. https://www.bls.gov/opub/mlr/2023/beyond-bls/in-the-race-from-covid-19-who-wins.htm

103. Borkowski C, Kaynas R, Wilkins M. Unemployment rate inches up during 2023, labor force participation rises. *Monthly Labor Review*. US Bureau of Labor Statistics. May 2024. doi:10.21916/mlr.2024.7

104. Hernández K, Garcia D, Nazario P, Rios M, Domínguez-Villegas R. Latinas exiting the workforce: How the pandemic revealed historic disadvantages and heightened economic hardship. UCLA Latino Policy & Politics Initiative. June 14, 2021. Accessed April 18, 2025. https://latino.ucla.edu/research/latina-unemployment-2020-2

105. Gould E, Perez D, Wilson V. Latinx workers—particularly women—face devastating job losses in the COVID-19 recession. Economic Policy Institute. August 20, 2020. Accessed August 15, 2025. https://www.epi.org/publication/latinx-workers-covid

106. Funk C, Lopez MH. Hispanic Americans' experiences with health care. Pew Research Center. June 14, 2022. Accessed April 18, 2025. https://www.pewresearch.org/science/2022/06/14/hispanic-americans-experiences-with-health-care
107. Hood CM, Gennuso KP, Swain GR, Catlin BB. County health rankings: Relationships between determinant factors and health outcomes. *Am J Prev Med*. 2016;50(2):129–135. doi:10.1016/j.amepre.2015.08.024
108. White RS, Tangel VE, Lui B, Jiang SY, Pryor KO, Abramovitz SE. Racial and ethnic disparities in delivery in-hospital mortality or maternal end-organ injury: A multistate analysis, 2007–2020. *J Womens Health (Larchmt)*. 2023;32(12):1292–1307. doi:10.1089/jwh.2023.0245
109. Jiang W, Chen W, Li D. Racial and ethnic disparities in the incidence, healthcare utilization, and outcomes of retained placenta among delivery hospitalizations in the United States, 2016–2019. *BMC Pregnancy Childbirth*. 2023;23(1):783. doi:10.1186/s12884-023-06097-0
110. Institute of Medicine. *America's Uninsured Crisis: Consequences for Health and Healthcare*. National Academies Press; 2009.
111. Kirby JB, Cohen JW. Do people with health insurance coverage who live in areas with high uninsurance rates pay more for emergency department visits? *Health Serv Res*. 2018;53(2):768–786. doi:10.1111/1475-6773.12659
112. Shen MJ, Peterson EB, Costas-Muñiz R, et al. The effects of race and racial concordance on patient-physician communication: A systematic review of the literature. *J Racial Ethn Health Disparities*. 2018;5(1):117–140. doi:10.1007/s40615-017-0350-4
113. Alsan M, Garrick O, Graziani G. Does diversity matter for health? Experimental evidence from Oakland. *Am Econ Rev*. 2019;109(12):4071–4111. doi:10.1257/aer.20181446
114. Ma A, Sanchez A, Ma M. The impact of patient-provider race/ethnicity concordance on provider visits: Updated evidence from the medical expenditure panel survey. *J Racial Ethn Health Disparities*. 2019;6(5):1011–1020. doi:10.1007/s40615-019-00602-y
115. Takeshita J, Wang S, Loren AW, et al. Association of racial/ethnic and gender concordance between patients and physicians with patient experience ratings. *JAMA Netw Open*. 2020;3(11):e2024583. doi:10.1001/jamanetworkopen.2020.24583
116. Robinson SK, Meisnere M, Phillips RL, Jr., McCauley L, eds.; National Academies of Sciences, Engineering, and Medicine. *Implementing High-Quality Primary Care: Rebuilding the Foundation of Health Care*. National Academies Press; 2021.
117. Sepúlveda MJ, Villarruel AM, Amaro HLA. Achieving Latino equity in medicine, nursing, and dentistry education: Accelerating the path forward. *NAM Perspectives*. National Academy of Medicine. May 9, 2022. doi:10.31478/202205a
118. Berkman LF, Kawachi I, Glymour MM, eds. *Social Epidemiology*. Oxford University Press; 2014.
119. Annie E. Casey Foundation. *2020 Kids Count Data Book: State Trends in Child Well-Being*. 2020. Accessed April 18, 2025. https://www.aecf.org/resources/2020-kids-count-data-book
120. Beck TL, Le TK, Henry-Okafor Q, Shah MK. Medical care for undocumented immigrants: National and international issues. *Physician Assist Clin*. 2019;4(1):33–45. doi:10.1016/j.cpha.2018.08.002
121. Bogard K, Murry VM, Alexander CM, eds. *Perspectives on Health Equity And Social Determinants of Health*. National Academy of Medicine; 2017.

122. Hodgkinson S, Godoy L, Beers LS, Lewin A. Improving mental health access for low-income children and families in the primary care setting. *Pediatrics.* 2017;139(1):e20151175. doi:10.1542/peds.2015-1175
123. Guzman L, Chen Y. Latino child poverty rose during the COVID-19 pandemic, especially among children in immigrant families. Hispanic Research Center. August 3, 2021. Accessed April 18, 2025. https://www.hispanicresearchcenter.org/research-resources/latino-child-poverty-rose-during-the-covid-19-pandemic-especially-among-children-in-immigrant-families
124. Guerrero AD, Zhou X, Chung PJ. How well is the medical home working for Latino and Black children? *Matern Child Health J.* 2018;22(2):175–183. doi:10.1007/s10995-017-2389-6
125. Rangel Gómez MG, López Jaramillo AM, Svarch A, et al. Together for Health: An initiative to access health services for the Hispanic/Mexican population living in the United States. *Front Public Health.* 2019;7:273. doi:10.3389/fpubh.2019.00273
126. Maalouf M, Fearon M, Lipa MC, Chow-Johnson H, Tayeh L, Lipa D. Neurologic complications of poverty: The associations between poverty as a social determinant of health and adverse neurologic outcomes. *Curr Neurol Neurosci Rep.* 2021;21(7):29. doi:10.1007/s11910-021-01116-z
127. National Institute for Health Care Management. The state of children's health in the United States. April 17, 2023. Accessed April 18, 2025. https://nihcm.org/publications/the-state-of-childrens-health-in-the-united-states
128. Llabre MM, Schneiderman N, Gallo LC, et al. Childhood trauma and adult risk factors and disease in Hispanics/Latinos in the US: Results from the Hispanic Community Health Study/Study of Latinos (HCHS/SOL) Sociocultural Ancillary Study. *Psychosom Med.* 2017;79(2):172–180. doi:10.1097/PSY.0000000000000394
129. Burke Harris N. *The Deepest Well: Healing the Long-Term Effects of Childhood Adversity.* Houghton Mifflin Harcourt; 2018.
130. Escobar-Galvez I, Yanouri L, Herrera CN, Callahan JL, Ruggero CJ, Cicero D. Intergenerational differences in barriers that impede mental health service use among Latinos. *Pract Innov (Wash DC).* 2023;8(2):116–130. doi:10.1037/pri0000204
131. Flanagan BE, Gregory EW, Hallisey EJ, Heitgerd JL, Lewis B. A social vulnerability index for disaster management. *J Homel Secur Emerg Manag.* 2011;8(1):3. doi:10.2202/1547-7355.1792
132. Barr RG, Avilés-Santa L, Davis SM, et al. Pulmonary disease and age at immigration among Hispanics. Results from the Hispanic Community Health Study/Study of Latinos. *Am J Respir Crit Care Med.* 2016;193(4):386–395. doi:10.1164/rccm.201506-1211OC
133. Bukstein DA, Friedman A, Gonzalez Reyes E, Hart M, Jones BL, Winders T. Impact of social determinants on the burden of asthma and eczema: Results from a US patient survey. *Adv Ther.* 2022;39(3):1341–1358. doi:10.1007/s12325-021-02021-0
134. Javed Z, Valero-Elizondo J, Cainzos-Achirica M, et al. Race, social determinants of health, and risk of all-cause and cardiovascular mortality in the United States. *J Racial Ethn Health Disparities.* 2024;11(2):853–864. doi:10.1007/s40615-023-01567-9
135. Bowser BP. Social-economic backgrounds to US county-based COVID-19 deaths: PLS-SEM analysis. *J Racial Ethn Health Disparities.* 2024;11(4):2304–2317. doi:10.1007/s40615-023-01698-z
136. Curtin SC, Tejada-Vera B, Bastian BA. Deaths: Leading causes for 2021. *Natl Vital Stat Rep.* 2024;73(4). doi:10.15620/cdc/147882

137. Rodriguez F, Hastings KG, Boothroyd DB, et al. Disaggregation of cause-specific cardiovascular disease mortality among Hispanic subgroups. *JAMA Cardiol.* 2017;2(3):240–247. doi:10.1001/jamacardio.2016.4653
138. Manjunath L, Hu J, Palaniappan L, Rodriguez F. Years of potential life lost from cardiovascular disease among Hispanics. *Ethn Dis.* 2019;29(3):477–484. doi:10.18865/ed.29.3.477
139. Whitley JC, Peralta CA, Haan M, et al. The association of parental and offspring educational attainment with systolic blood pressure, fasting blood glucose and waist circumference in Latino adults. *Obes Sci Pract.* 2018;4(6):582–590. doi:10.1002/osp4.307
140. Komulainen K, Mittleman MA, Jokela M, et al. Socioeconomic position and intergenerational associations of ideal health behaviors. *Eur J Prev Cardiol.* 2019;26(15):1605–1612. doi:10.1177/2047487319850959
141. Jain V, Al Rifai M, Khan SU, et al. Association between social vulnerability index and cardiovascular disease: A Behavioral Risk Factor Surveillance System study. *J Am Heart Assoc.* 2022;11(15):e024414. doi:10.1161/JAHA.121.024414
142. Hassel BC, Ayscue E, Dean S, Brooks-Uy V. Closing achievement gaps in diverse and low-poverty schools: An action guide for district leaders. Public Impact; Oak Foundation. 2018. Accessed April 18, 2025. https://files.eric.ed.gov/fulltext/ED589275.pdf
143. O'Day JA, Smith MS. *Opportunity for All: A Framework for Quality and Equality in Education.* Harvard Education Press; 2019.
144. Taylor J, Lindsay R, Ibrahim M, Kye P, Tegeler P. The persistence of school segregation in the United States, its effects on racial disparities in school funding, achievement, and discipline, and the failure of the US government to sufficiently address the problem. Report to the UN Committee on the Elimination of Racial Discrimination. Poverty & Race Research Action Council. July 2022. Accessed April 18, 2025. https://www.prrac.org/pdf/cerd-education-shadow-report-july2022.pdf
145. Madeux E. Educational funding inequality in southern US high schools. Ballard Brief. Brigham Young University. February 2024. Accessed April 18, 2025. https://ballardbrief.byu.edu/issue-briefs/educational-funding-inequality-in-southern-us-high-schools
146. Campbell KM, Rodríguez JE. Addressing the minority tax: Perspectives from two diversity leaders on building minority faculty success in academic medicine. *Acad Med.* 2019;94(12):1854–1857. doi:10.1097/ACM.0000000000002839
147. Rodríguez JE, Bliss C, Hawes KB, et al. Introspection to improve pipelines and graduate programs at University of Utah Health. *Fam Med.* 2021;53(8):730. doi:10.22454/FamMed.2021.377645
148. Zambrana RE, Carvajal D, Townsend J. Institutional penalty: Mentoring, service, perceived discrimination and its impacts on the health and academic careers of Latino faculty. *Ethn Racial Stud.* 2023;46(6):1132–1157. doi:10.1080/01419870.2022.2160651
149. Pololi L, Rodríguez J, Campbell K. Addressing disparities in academic medicine: What of the minority tax? *BMC Med Educ.* 2015;15(1):1–5. doi:10.1186/s12909-015-0290-9
150. Mendoza FS. How to increase Hispanics in medicine through the four Ps: Increase the pool, create effective pathways, support professional development, and change the politics. *J Natl Hisp Med Assoc.* 2025;3(1):3–20. Accessed August 15, 2025. https://jnhma.scholasticahq.com/article/136825-how-to-increase-hispanics-in-medicine-through-the-four-ps-increase-the-pool-create-effective-pathways-support-professional-development-and-change

151. Tyris J, Keller S, Parikh K. Social risk interventions and health care utilization for pediatric asthma: A systematic review and meta-analysis. *JAMA Pediatr.* 2022;176(2):e215103. doi:10.1001/jamapediatrics.2021.5103
152. Simoneau T, Gaffin JM. Socioeconomic determinants of asthma health. *Curr Opin Pediatr.* 2023;35(3):337–343. doi:10.1097/MOP.0000000000001235
153. Gao C, Sanchez KM, Lovinsky-Desir S. Structural and social determinants of inequitable environmental exposures in the United States. *Clin Chest Med.* 2023;44(3):451–467. doi:10.1016/j.ccm.2023.03.002
154. Malik R, Hamm K, Lee WF, Davis EE, Sojourner A. The coronavirus will make childcare deserts worse and exacerbate inequality. Center for American Progress. June 22, 2020. Accessed April 18, 2025. https://www.americanprogress.org/article/coronavirus-will-make-child-care-deserts-worse-exacerbate-inequality
155. Remor I, Raza R. Stabilizing childcare supply through a new funding mechanism. The Urban Institute. October 2021. Accessed April 18, 2025. https://www.urban.org/sites/default/files/publication/104929/stabilizing-child-care-supply-through-a-new-funding-mechanism_1.pdf
156. Zarate ME, Burciaga R. Latinos and college access: Trends and future directions. *J Coll Admiss.* 2010;209:24–29. Accessed April 18, 2025. https://files.eric.ed.gov/fulltext/EJ906627.pdf
157. Stern GM. Tuition-free college in New Mexico. *Hispanic Outlook on Education Magazine.* June 2022. Accessed April 18, 2025. https://www.hispanicoutlook.com/articles/tuition-free-college-new-mexico
158. National Center for Education Statistics. Loans for undergraduate students and debt for bachelor's degree recipients. US Dept of Education. Updated May 2023. Accessed April 18, 2025. https://nces.ed.gov/programs/coe/indicator/cub
159. Progress Report. Latinos are among the most burdened in student loan debt. Here's how advocates say that can be alleviated. UnidosUS. August 17, 2022. Accessed April 18, 2025. https://unidosus.org/progress-report/latinos-bear-the-brunt-of-the-countrys-1-7-trillion-in-student-loan-debt-heres-how-advocates-say-that-can-be-alleviated
160. Bartel AP, Kim S, Nam J, Rossin-Slater M, Ruhm CJ, Waldfogel J. Racial and ethnic disparities in access to and use of paid family and medical leave: Evidence from four nationally representative datasets. *Monthly Labor Review.* US Bureau of Labor Statistics. January 2019. doi:10.21916/mlr.2019.2
161. Glynn SJ, Farrell J. Latinos least likely to have paid leave or workplace flexibility. Center for American Progress. November 20, 2012. Accessed April 18, 2025. https://www.americanprogress.org/article/latinos-least-likely-to-have-paid-leave-or-workplace-flexibility
162. Economic Policy Institute. The impact of raising the minimum wage to $15 by 2025, by congressional district: Mapping the impact of the Raise the Wage Act of 2021 on workers. January 28, 2021. Accessed April 18, 2025. https://www.epi.org/publication/minimum-wage-to-15-by-2025-by-congressional-district
163. Economic Policy Institute. Why the US needs a $15 minimum wage: How the Raise the Wage Act would benefit US workers and their families. January 26, 2021. Accessed April 18, 2025. https://www.epi.org/publication/why-america-needs-a-15-minimum-wage
164. Shiro AG, Reeves RV. Latinos often lack access to healthcare and have poor health outcomes. Here's how we can change that. Brookings Institute. September 25, 2020. Accessed April 18,

2025. https://www.brookings.edu/articles/latinos-often-lack-access-to-healthcare-and-have-poor-health-outcomes-heres-how-we-can-change-that
165. Sanders B. News: Sanders introduces Medicare for all with 14 colleagues in the Senate. May 12, 2022. Accessed April 18, 2025. https://www.sanders.senate.gov/press-releases/news-sanders-introduces-medicare-for-all-with-14-colleagues-in-the-senate
166. Sharac J, Stolyar L, Corallo B, Tolbert J, Shin P, Robinson S. How community health centers are serving low-income communities during the COVID-19 pandemic amid new and continuing challenges. Kaiser Family Foundation. June 3, 2022. Accessed April 18, 2025. https://www.kff.org/medicaid/issue-brief/how-community-health-centers-are-serving-low-income-communities-during-the-covid-19-pandemic-amid-new-and-continuing-challenges
167. Vargas Bustamante A, Martinez LE, Balderas-Medina Anaya Y. California's physician shortage: White paper. UCLA Latino Policy & Politics Institute. 2020. Accessed April 18, 2025. https://latino.ucla.edu/wp-content/uploads/2021/08/LPPI-CPS-White-Paper-Design-Layout-reduced.pdf
168. Kreuter MW, Thompson T, McQueen A, Garg R. Addressing social needs in health care settings: Evidence, challenges, and opportunities for public health. *Annu Rev Public Health*. 2021;42: 329–344. doi:10.1146/annurev-publhealth-090419-102204
169. Jaffe S. NYC guarantees health care to all. *Lancet*. 2019;393(10169)e3–e4. doi:10.1016/S0140-6736(19)30157-6
170. Lopez Mercado D, Rivera-González AC, Stimpson JP, et al. Undocumented Latino immigrants and the Latino health paradox. *Am J Prev Med*. 2023;65(2):296–306. doi:10.1016/j.amepre.2023.02.010
171. Beard Morgan L, Rodriquez EJ, Juarez, JJ, Perez-Stable EJ. Black race matters in the Latino population. *Am J Public Health*. 2024;114(3):270–275. doi:10.2105/AJPH.2023.307452
172. Zambrana RE, Williams DR. The intellectual roots of current knowledge on racism and health: Relevance to policy and the national equity discourse. *Health Aff (Millwood)*. 2022;41(2): 163–170. doi:10.1377/hlthaff.2021.01439

Appendix 4A

Table 4A-1. Definition of Terms

Term	Definitions
Foreign-born Immigrants/ migrants/ unauthorized migrants	The *foreign-born* population consists of anyone living in the US who was not a citizen at birth, including naturalized US citizens, lawful permanent residents (immigrants), temporary migrants such as foreign students, humanitarian migrants (refugees and asylees), and unauthorized migrants.[1] In the US Immigration and Nationality Act, an *immigrant* is an individual seeking to become a Lawful Permanent Resident in the United States.[2]
US born	US citizenship is acquired by birth when a child is born in the territory of the United States. This includes US states, DC, Guam, Puerto Rico, the Northern Mariana Islands, and the US Virgin Islands.[3]
Generational status: Parental educational status First generation Second generation	*First-generation college student* means (a) an individual, both of whose parents did not complete a BA degree, or (b) in the case of any individual who regularly resided with and received support from only one parent, an individual whose only such parent did not complete a BA degree according to an amendment to the Higher Education Act of 1965 (1988).[4] This is used to determine eligibility for federal TRIO programs and Pell Grants.[5] *Second-generation college student* is used to refer to students whose parents or guardians earned at least one BA degree. *First generation* is often used in the immigration literature to refer to those who were born in the US and whose parents were born outside the US.
Settler colonialism/ colonization/ colonialism	*Settler colonialism* is "colonization in which colonizing powers create permanent or long-term settlements on land owned and/or occupied by other peoples, often by force."[7(p23)] By contrast, in other kinds of colonialism, colonizers may only focus on extracting resources back to their countries of origin. Settler colonialism usually includes oppressive governance, the dismantling of Indigenous cultural practices and lifeways, and the enforcement of codes of superiority, such as white supremacy.[7]
Racialized/ racialization/ colorism	*Racialization* is the process of manufacturing and utilizing the notion of race in any capacity; groups are designated as being part of a particular race and subjected to differential and/ or unequal treatment.[8] In countries other than the US, which has historically employed a Black-white binary, *colorism* or *racialization* have been named to acknowledge a mixture of different races.[9] As noted by Garcia, "the formation and expression of racial identity and identities is a function of socialization, experiences, and historical legacies."[10(p74),11]
Multiracial/Mixed-race ancestry	The US Census uses *multiracial* for people of 2 or more races.[6] Several terms are used to describe multiple races by US Census and others, including *mixed race* or "some other race" (Other race).[12-14] For example, Puerto Ricans have 66% European, 18% Indigenous, and 16% African ancestry while Mexicans have 45% European, 52% Indigenous, and 3% African ancestry. However, Mexican-origin populations were historically classified as white, and a majority of the Puerto Rican population has reported some other race (now called mixed race/multiracial).[15]
Mestizo	*Mestizo* is a term used throughout Latin America to characterize individuals with a mixed ancestry of white European and Indigenous.[16,17]

(Continued)

Table 4A-1. (Continued)

Term	Definitions
Indigenous Mexican	Communities that trace their roots back to populations and communities that existed prior to the arrival of Europeans. In the 2020 census, 19.41% of Mexicans identified as Indigenous. Mexican states with the highest percentages of persons who self-identified as being of Indigenous origin include Yucatan (65%), Oaxaca (69%), Chiapas (37%), Hidalgo (37%), and Campeche (47%).[18] Includes Pueblo peoples (Ancestral Pueblo, Anasazi), Hohokam, and Mogollon peoples who descended from those in the current US states of Colorado, Arizona, New Mexico, Utah, and Nevada, and Mexican states of Sonora and Chihuahua.[19]
Afro-Latino	Individuals of African descent who identify as *Afro-Latino* may share a racial identity with Black non-Latino persons and experience racism in everyday activities. However, most Afro-Latino persons share some amount of common ethnic, cultural, and linguistic characteristics with white and other Latino individuals in the US. The life experiences of Afro-Latinos are shaped by race, skin tone, and other factors in ways that differ from other Hispanics.[20,21] In 2020, ~6 million US adults identified as Afro-Latino, 2% of the US adult population and 12% of the adult Latino population. Puerto Ricans have 16% African ancestry compared with 3% for Mexicans.[22]
Traditionally and historically underrepresented	Groups that share involuntary historical incorporation into the US (via slavery, colonization, and land takeover), such as African Americans, Mexican Americans, AI/ANs, and Puerto Ricans. Mexican-origin people, Mexican Americans/Chicanos, and Puerto Ricans are predominantly historic citizen groups who were denied access to education, economic and social opportunity, and/or suffered past intergenerational, institutional discrimination in the US. There is much contemporary debate and controversy on the varying definitions of historically underrepresented, marginalized, and oppressed. NSF reports that Blacks, AI/ANs, Hispanics/Latinos, and NH/PIs are nationally underrepresented at many career stages in health-related sciences.[23] Individuals from these groups are also underrepresented when compared with their age cohorts in the biomedical and science workforce overall.
Structural racism	The historical and contemporary policies, practices, and norms that create and maintain white supremacy. Structural racism continues to disproportionately segregate communities of color from access to opportunity and upward mobility by making it more difficult for people of color to secure quality education, jobs, housing, health care, and equal treatment in the criminal legal system.[24]
SDOH	Conditions in the environments where people are born, live, learn, work, play, worship, and age that affect a wide range of health, functioning, and quality-of-life outcomes and risks. SDOH can be grouped into 5 categories: economic stability; education access and quality; health care access and quality, neighborhood and built environment; and social and community context.[25]
Political determinants	Involve the systematic process of structuring relationships, distributing resources, and administering power, operating simultaneously in ways that mutually reinforce or influence one another to shape opportunities that either advance health equity or exacerbate health inequities.[26]
Educationally disadvantaged	The denial of access to educational opportunities, the tendency to leave education at the first opportunity, and the hindrance of achievement by social and environmental factors.[27]
Economically disadvantaged	Socially disadvantaged individuals whose ability to compete in the free enterprise system has been impaired due to diminished capital and opportunities throughout their life course as compared with others in the same area who are not socially disadvantaged.[28]

Note: AI/AN = American Indian or Alaska Native; DC = District of Columbia; NH/PI = Native Hawaiian or Pacific Islander; NSF = National Science Foundation; SDOH = social determinants of health.

Table 4A-2. Timeline of Major Treaties, Laws, and Court Cases

Event	Description & Impact
Treaty of Guadalupe Hidalgo (1848)	Ended the Mexican–American war; México ceded 55% of its territory, relinquished all claims to Texas, and recognized the Rio Grande as its northern boundary with the US.
Gadsden Purchase (1854)	An agreement between the US and Mexico in which the US agreed to pay México $10 million for a 29,670 mi^2 portion of México that later became part of Arizona and New Mexico.
Treaty of Paris (1898)	Commissioners from the US and Spain met in Paris to produce a treaty to end the Spanish–American war. The islands of PR and Guam were placed under American control, and Spain relinquished its claim to Cuba.
California Sterilization Law (1909)	Authorized reproductive surgery on ~20,000 patients committed to California state homes or hospitals who were judged to be "mentally defective" and "unfit to reproduce."[29(p50)] The program did not designate specific racial/ethnic groups for sterilization, but existing racial hierarchies constructed Latinos/Mexicans/Mexican Americans as "immigrants of an undesirable type" that were inferior to whites; Latinas were 59% more likely to be sterilized than non-Latinas.[30(p611)]
Jones-Shafroth Act (1917)	Puerto Ricans were given statutory US citizenship. This act separated PR's government into executive, judicial, and legislative branches, and endowed Puerto Ricans with a bill of rights. Citizenship resulted in mass migration (~42,000 Puerto Ricans) to the US mainland in the subsequent decade due to WWI recruitment and labor opportunities. The majority settled in NYC. PR does not have voting representation in Congress, and Puerto Ricans with residency on the island are not eligible to vote in general elections, only in primaries. Only Puerto Ricans living on the US mainland can register to vote in their respective states.[31]
Immigration Act (Johnson Reed Act; 1924)	Limited the number of immigrants allowed entry into the US through a national origins quota. The quota provided immigration visas to 2% of the total number of people of each nationality in the US as of the 1890 Census. It completely excluded immigrants from Asia. Latin America was not included in the quota.[32,33]
Mexican Repatriation Program (1929-1939)	Scholars estimate that government authorities forcibly expelled 500,000 persons of Mexican origin from the US in the 1930s, with the majority of those removed being US citizens. Census data estimates indicate substantially lower numbers, limited governmental involvement, fewer citizens, and mainly voluntary departure. Voluntary decisions fit the repatriation strategy that had been common among young Mexican immigrants in the 1920s. Yet, the 1940s Bracero Program, designed by México and the US to replicate the 1920s pattern of circular migration, contributed to massive illegal immigration and unprecedented levels of deportation.[34]
Female sterilization in PR (1930-1965)	By 1953, an estimated 16% of Puerto Rican women aged 20-49 were sterilized, which increased to >34% by 1965. Informed consent procedures for sterilization were absent in hospitals as they had been for medical experiments. US policy in the 20th century, as a means to control overpopulation, justified sterilization as a way to introduce modern health care as an opportunity to bring Puerto Ricans out of poverty and into modernity.[35]
Population Control Law 116 (1937)	The institutionalization of the population control program was developed by the Eugenics Board. Funded by the US government and private contributions, it was designed to respond to Depression-era unemployment by catalyzing economic growth.[36]
Bracero Agreement (1942)	A bilateral agreement between the US and México in effect until 1964. It permitted Mexican nationals to serve as temporary agricultural workers during WWII labor shortages and required employers to pay a wage equal to that paid to US-born farmworkers and provide transportation and living expenses.[37]

(Continued)

Table 4A-2. (Continued)

Event	Description & Impact
Mendez v Westminster (1946)	Court case on racial segregation in the California public school system. The 9th Circuit Court of Appeals ruled that it was unconstitutional and unlawful to forcibly segregate Mexican American students by focusing on Mexican ancestry, skin color, and the Spanish language. This case upheld the Equal Protection Clause of the 14th Amendment and strengthened the landmark Supreme Court ruling in Brown v Board of Education (1954).[38]
Birth control experimentation in PR (mid-1950s)	The first large-scale human trial of the birth control pill was launched in a public housing project among 1,500 less-educated women in PR to conduct large-scale tests without informed consent.[39]
Operation Wetback (1954)	800 US Border Patrol officers performed a series of raids, roadblocks, and mass deportations, intentionally targeting undocumented Mexicans as a method of mass deportation to regulate Mexican migration. By the end of 1954, the campaign contributed to the deportation of >1 million people, mostly Mexican nationals.[40]
Cuban Refugee Program (1960-1970)	Provided daily necessities, employment opportunities, supplemental funds for resettlement, essential health services, federal assistance for local public school operating costs, training and educational opportunities, financial aid for the care and protection of unaccompanied children, and food distribution to Cuban refugees.[41]
Civil Rights Act (1964)	A landmark rights and US labor law in the US that outlawed discrimination based on race, color, religion, sex, or national origin. It prohibited unequal application of voter registration requirements and racial segregation in schools, employment, and public accommodations.[42]
Hart-Cellar Act (1965)	This act abolished the quota system that directed nearly 70% of immigration slots to northern Europeans. It loosened considerably the rules for immigration by prioritizing family reunification. It helped to shift the demographics of the US population by stimulating rapid growth of immigration numbers. In effect, when immigrants had naturalized, they were able to sponsor relatives in an ever-lengthening migratory process called chain migration.[43]
Cuban Adjustment Act (1966)	Granted work authorization permits and lawful permanent residency (green card status) to any Cuban native or citizen who settled in the US for at least 1 year. As thousands of Cuban exiles sought asylum, the Cuban population in the US grew from 79,000 to 439,000 in 1960-1970.[44]
Affirmative Action (1973)	Affirmative action policies were developed in the 1970s to expand opportunity for groups who have historically faced discrimination to address the effects of past policies. These groups included Blacks, AI/ANs, Mexicans, and Puerto Ricans. Their purpose was to ensure equal employment opportunities for applicants and employees. Affirmative action requirements intended to ensure that applicants and employees of federal contractors had equal opportunity for recruitment, selection, advancement, and every other term and privilege associated with employment, without regard to their race, color, religion, sex, sexual orientation, gender identity, national origin, disability, or status as a protected veteran. Under Executive Order 11246 (1965) and Section 503 (1973), affirmative action must actively engage in outreach initiatives that prioritize "women or minorities [that] are underutilized."[45]

(Continued)

Table 4A-2. (Continued)

Event	Description & Impact
Madrigal v Quilligan (1978)	Civil rights class action lawsuit filed by 10 Mexican American women against the LA County-USC Medical Center for involuntary or forced sterilization. The plaintiffs were residents of East LA, a predominantly Latino area with inadequate medical and educational resources. Unauthorized sterilizations among Mexican women with minimal English proficiency rose at the County Medical Center during the 1970s.[46]
OMB Statistical Policy Directive 15 (1977)	First US Census to publicly add Hispanic groups and make data available. The directive defined Hispanic groups as "a person of Mexican, Puerto Rican, Cuban, Central or South American or other Spanish culture or origin, regardless of race."[47(p37)] For more than 20 years, the current standards have provided a common language to promote uniformity and comparability for data on race and ethnicity for the population groups specified in the directive. However, the US Census expressed concern about 75% of Puerto Ricans claiming mixed race or another race.[15,48]
Refugee Act (1980)	Amended the earlier Immigration and Nationality Act and the Migration and Refugee Assistance Act. It raised the annual ceiling for refugees from 17,400 to 50,000, created a process for reviewing and adjusting the refugee ceiling to meet emergencies, and required annual consultation between Congress and the President. The act updated the definition of refugee to a person with a well-founded fear of persecution. Characterizing Salvadorans and Guatemalans as "economic migrants," the Reagan administration denied that the Salvadoran and Guatemalan governments had violated human rights and plummeted approval rates for Salvadoran and Guatemalan asylum cases to <3% in 1984. In the same year, the approval rate for Iranians was 60%, 40% for Afghans fleeing the Soviet invasion, and 32% for Poles. The act also created the Federal Refugee Resettlement Program to provide effective resettlement of refugees and assist them in achieving economic self-sufficiency as quickly as possible after arrival in the US.[49]
Immigration Reform and Control Act (1986)	Introduced civil and criminal penalties to employers who knowingly hired undocumented immigrants or individuals unauthorized to work in the US. However, the act also offered legalization, which led to lawful permanent residence and prospective naturalization to undocumented migrants who entered the country before 1982.[50]
Temporary Protection Act (1990–2000)	Allowed the Secretary of Homeland Security to designate a foreign country for temporary protection status due to conditions there that temporarily prevent the country's nationals from returning safely, or if the country is unable to adequately handle the return of its nationals due to ongoing armed conflict (e.g., civil war), environmental disaster (e.g., earthquake, hurricane), an epidemic, or other extraordinary and temporary conditions.[51]
The Personal Responsibility and Work Opportunity Act (1996)	Showcased a comprehensive bipartisan welfare reform plan to change the nation's welfare system into one that requires work in exchange for time-limited assistance. The act contained strong work requirements, a performance bonus to reward states for moving welfare recipients into jobs, state maintenance of effort requirements, comprehensive child support enforcement, and supports for families moving from welfare to work—including increased funding for childcare and guaranteed medical coverage.[52]

(Continued)

Table 4A-2. (Continued)

Event	Description & Impact
Nicaraguan Adjustment and Central American Relief Act (1997)	Provided immigration benefits and relief from deportation to a significant number of immigrants from Central America, Cuba, and former Soviet bloc countries who had applied for asylum.[53]
Secure Communities Program (2008-2017)	Utilized all law enforcement data systems and Criminal Alien Program resources to identify and take enforcement actions against criminal and other priority "aliens" while they were in the custody of another law enforcement or correctional agency.[24] Its active efforts in mass deportation resulted in the removal of >363,400 "criminal aliens" from the US.[54]
DACA (2012)	Allowed young adults (aged 15-30) who were brought to the US illegally as children to apply for temporary deportation relief and a 2-year work permit. As of March 31, 2025, there are 525,210 active DACA recipients.[37,55]
Act 20: The Export Services Incentives Act (2012)	Contributed to the transformation of PR into a tax haven by granting corporations and individuals (1) 4% maximum income tax on companies that export their goods or services outside of PR; (2) 100% exemption on income tax on dividends distributions; (3) 60% exemption of municipal license taxes; (4) 90% exemption of real and property taxes; and (5) 20-year tax decree, renewable for an additional 10-year period.[56]
Act 22: The Individual Investor Act (2012)	Incentivizes individuals to move to PR. The incentives are only available to individuals who were not a Puerto Rican resident within the last 15 years and meet the residency requirements. The act exempts all passive income obtained from investments from Puerto Rican taxes.[57]
Executive Order 13767 (2017)	Aimed to prevent undocumented immigration into the US through the construction of a physical wall on the border, "monitored and supported by adequate personnel so as to prevent illegal immigration, drug and human trafficking, and acts of terrorism."[58]
Student for Fair Admissions v President & Fellows of Harvard College (2023)	Petitioner SFFA sued Harvard College over its admissions process, alleging that the process violated Title VI of the Civil Rights Act of 1964 by discriminating against Asian American applicants in favor of white applicants. Harvard admitted that it used race as one of many factors in its admissions process but argued that its process adheres to the requirements for race-based admissions outlined in the Supreme Court's decision in Grutter v Bollinger. In June 2023, the Supreme Court ruled in favor of SFFA and held that affirmative action in college admissions is unconstitutional.[59]

Note: AI/AN = American Indian or Alaska Native; DACA = Deferred Action for Childhood Arrivals; LA = Los Angeles, California; NYC = New York City, New York; OMB = US Office of Management and Budget; PR = Puerto Rico; SFFA = Students for Fair Admissions; USC = University of Southern California; WWI = World War I; WWII = World War II.

REFERENCES

1. Azari SS, Jenkins V, Hahn J, Medina L. The foreign-born population in the United States: 2022. American Community Survey Briefs. US Census Bureau. April 2024. https://www2.census.gov/library/publications/2024/demo/acsbr-019.pdf
2. US Immigration. Immigrant definition. US Immigration Glossary. Accessed April 7, 2025. https://www.usimmigration.org/glossary/immigrant

3. US Immigration. US citizen definition. US Immigration Glossary. Accessed April 7, 2025. https://www.usimmigration.org/glossary/us-citizen
4. Higher Education Amendments of 1998, Federal TRIO Programs, Pub L No. 105-224, 112 Stat 1581, §402a (1998).
5. Clauss-Ehlers CS, Wibrowski CR. Building educational resilience and social support: The effects of the educational opportunity fund program among first- and second-generation college students. *J Coll Stud Dev*. 2007;48(5):574–584. doi:10.1353/csd.2007.0051
6. Jensen E, Jones N, Orozco K, et al. Measuring racial and ethnic diversity for the 2020 Census. US Census Bureau. August 4, 2021. Accessed April 7, 2025. https://www.census.gov/newsroom/blogs/random-samplings/2021/08/measuring-racial-ethnic-diversity-2020-census.html
7. MP Associates. Racial equity tools glossary. International City/County Management Association. May 25, 2022. Accessed April 7, 2025. https://icma.org/documents/racial-equity-tools-glossary
8. Dalal F. *Race, Colour and the Process of Racialization: New Perspectives from Group Analysis, Psychoanalysis and Sociology*. Brunner-Routledge; 2002.
9. Amaro H, Zambrana RE. Criollo, mestizo, mulato, LatiNegro, Indígena, White, or Black? The US Hispanic/Latino population and multiple responses in the 2000 census. *Am J Public Health*. 2000;90(11):1724–1727. doi:10.2105/ajph.90.11.1724
10. Garcia JA. A holistic alternative to current survey research approaches to race. In: Gómez LE, López N, eds. *Mapping Race: Critical Approaches to Health Disparities Research*. Rutgers University Press; 2013:83–104.
11. Javadi D, Murchland AR, Rushovich T, et al. Systematic review of how racialized health inequities are addressed in *Epidemiologic Reviews* articles (1979–2021): a critical conceptual and empirical content analysis and recommendations for best practices. *Epidemiol Rev*. 2023;45(1):1–14. doi:10.1093/epirev/mxad008
12. Parker K, Horowitz JM, Morin R, Lopez MH. Race and multiracial Americans in the US Census. Pew Research Center. June 11, 2015. Accessed April 21, 2025. https://www.pewresearch.org/social-trends/2015/06/11/chapter-1-race-and-multiracial-americans-in-the-u-s-census
13. Donella L. *Code Switch*. All mixed up: What do we call people of multiple backgrounds? NPR. August 16, 2016. Accessed April 21, 2025. https://www.npr.org/sections/codeswitch/2016/08/25/455470334/all-mixed-up-what-do-we-call-people-of-multiple-backgrounds
14. Horowitz JM, Budiman A. Key findings about multiracial identity in the US as Harris becomes vice presidential nominee. Pew Research Center. August 19, 2020. Accessed April 21, 2025. https://www.pewresearch.org/short-reads/2020/08/18/key-findings-about-multiracial-identity-in-the-u-s-as-harris-becomes-vice-presidential-nominee
15. Rodriguez C. *Changing Race: Latinos, the Census and the History of Ethnicity in the United States*. New York University Press; 2000.
16. Gonzalez-Barrera A. 'Mestizo' and 'mulatto': Mixed-race identities among US Hispanics. Pew Research Center. July 10, 2015. Accessed April 21, 2025. https://www.pewresearch.org/short-reads/2015/07/10/mestizo-and-mulatto-mixed-race-identities-unique-to-hispanics
17. Lugo-Lugo CR. "So you are a mestiza": Exploring the consequences of ethnic and racial clumping in the US Academy. *Ethn Racial Stud*. 2008;31(3):611–628. doi:10.1080/01419870701568882

18. Schmal JP. Indigenous Mexico in the 2020 Census: A state-by-state analysis. Indigenous Mexico. July 30, 2022. Accessed April 21, 2025. https://www.indigenousmexico.org/articles/indigenous-mexico-in-the-2020-census-a-state-by-state-analysis
19. Grandstaff J. Indian Tribes of the American Southwest. History How It Happened. December 2, 2019. Accessed April 21, 2025. https://historyhowithappened.com/indian-tribes-of-the-pre-columbian-american-southwest
20. Vera A, Pineda A. Blackness and Latinidad are not mutually exclusive. Here's what it means to be Afro-Latino in America. *CNN*. September 26, 2021. Accessed April 21, 2025. https://www.cnn.com/2021/09/26/us/black-latinos-afro-latinos-experience/index.html
21. Beard Morgan L, Rodriquez EJ, Juarez, JJ, Perez-Stable EJ. Black race matters in the Latino population. *Am J Public Health*. 2024;114(3):270–275. doi:10.2105/AJPH.2023.307452
22. Gonzalez-Barrera A. About 6 million US adults identify as Afro-Latino. Pew Research Center. May 2, 2022. Accessed April 21, 2025. https://www.pewresearch.org/short-reads/2022/05/02/about-6-million-u-s-adults-identify-as-afro-latino
23. Hamrick K. *Women, Minorities, and Persons with Disabilities in Science and Engineering*. National Science Foundation, National Center for Science and Engineering Statistics; 2019. Accessed April 21, 2025. https://ncses.nsf.gov/pubs/nsf19304
24. Urban Institute. Structural racism in America. October 5, 2021. Accessed April 21, 2025. https://www.urban.org/structural-racism-america
25. Office of Disease Prevention and Health Promotion. Social determinants of health. US Dept of Health and Human Services. Accessed April 21, 2025. https://health.gov/healthypeople/priority-areas/social-determinants-health
26. Dawes DE. *The Political Determinants of Health*. Johns Hopkins University Press; 2022.
27. Mortimore J, Blackstone T. *Disadvantage and Education*. Heinemann Educational Books; 1982.
28. Who is economically disadvantaged?, 13 CFR §124.104 (2013).
29. Stern AM, Novak NL, Lira N, O'Connor K, Harlow S, Kardia S. California's sterilization survivors: An estimate and call for redress. *Am J Public Health*. 2017;107(1):50–54. doi:10.2105/AJPH.2016.303489
30. Novak NL, Lira N, O'Connor KE, Harlow SD, Kardia SLR, Stern AM. Disproportionate sterilization of Latinos under California's eugenic sterilization program, 1920–1945. *Am J Public Health*. 2018;108(5):611–613. doi:10.2105/AJPH.2018.304369
31. Chavez HL, Partida MG. 1917: Jones-Shafroth Act. Library of Congress. August 17, 2020. Updated December 14, 2023. Accessed April 18, 2025. https://guides.loc.gov/latinx-civil-rights/jones-shafroth-act
32. Office of the Historian. The Immigration Act of 1924 (The Johnson-Reed Act). US Dept of State. Accessed April 18, 2025. https://history.state.gov/milestones/1921-1936/immigration-act
33. Massey DS, Pren KA. Unintended consequences of US immigration policy: Explaining the post-1965 surge from Latin America. *Popul Dev Rev*. 2012;38(1):1–29. doi:10.1111/j.1728-4457.2012.00470.x
34. Gratton B, Merchant E. Immigration, repatriation, and deportation: The Mexican-origin population in the United States, 1920–1950. *Int Migr Rev*. 2013;47(4):944–975. doi:10.1111/imre.12054

35. Gutiérrez ER, Fuentes L. Population control by sterilization: The cases of Puerto Rican and Mexican-origin women in the United States. *Latino(a) Res Rev.* 2010;7(3):85–100.
36. Krase K. Sterilization abuse: The policies behind the practice. National Women's Health Network. January 5, 1996. Accessed April 21, 2025. https://web.archive.org/web/20210918163517/https://nwhn.org/sterilization-abuse-the-policies-behind-the-practice
37. Cohn D. How US immigration laws and rules have changed through history. Pew Research Center. September 30, 2015. Accessed April 21, 2025. https://www.pewresearch.org/fact-tank/2015/09/30/how-u-s-immigration-laws-and-rules-have-changed-through-history
38. Chavez HL, Partida MG. 1946: Mendez v. Westminster. Library of Congress. August 17, 2020. Updated December 14, 2023. Accessed April 18, 2025. https://guides.loc.gov/latinx-civil-rights/mendez-v-westminster
39. Pendergrass DC, Raji MY. The bitter pill: Harvard and the dark history of birth. *The Harvard Crimson.* September 28, 2017. Accessed April 21, 2025. https://www.thecrimson.com/article/2017/9/28/the-bitter-pill
40. Hernandez KL. The crimes and consequences of illegal immigration: A cross-border examination of Operation Wetback, 1943 to 1954. *West Hist Q.* 2006;37(4):421–444. doi:10.2307/25443415
41. Mitchell WL. The Cuban Refugee Program. *Soc Secur Bull.* 1962;25(3):3–8. Accessed April 21, 2025. https://www.ssa.gov/policy/docs/ssb/v25n3/v25n3p3.pdf
42. US Dept of Labor. Legal highlight: The Civil Rights Act of 1964. Accessed April 21, 2025. https://web.archive.org/web/20210425123447/https://www.dol.gov/agencies/oasam/civil-rights-center/statutes/civil-rights-act-of-1964
43. Kammer J. The Hart-Celler Immigration Act of 1965. Center for Immigration Studies. September 30, 2015. Accessed April 21, 2025. https://cis.org/Report/HartCeller-Immigration-Act-1965
44. Chavez HL, Partida MG. 1966: The Cuban Adjustment Act of 1966. Library of Congress. August 17, 2020. Updated December 14, 2023. Accessed April 18, 2025. https://guides.loc.gov/latinx-civil-rights/cuban-adjustment-act
45. US Dept of Labor. Affirmative action frequently asked questions. Accessed April 21, 2025. https://web.archive.org/web/20240119025535/https://www.dol.gov/agencies/ofccp/faqs/AAFAQs
46. Chavez HL, Partida MG. 1978: Madrigal v. Quilligan. Library of Congress. August 17, 2020. Updated December 14, 2023. Accessed April 18, 2025. https://guides.loc.gov/latinx-civil-rights/madrigal-v-quilligan
47. US Office of Management and Budget. Directive no. 15: Race and ethnic standards for federal statistics and administrative reporting. 1978. Accessed April 10, 2025. https://spd15revision.gov/content/spd15revision/en/history/1977-standards.html
48. Gravlee CC, Dressler WW, Bernard HR. Skin color, social classification, and blood pressure in southeastern Puerto Rico. *Am J Public Health.* 2005;95(12):2191–2197. doi:10.2105/AJPH.2005.065615
49. Office of Refugee Settlement. The Refugee Act. US Dept of Health and Human Services. August 29, 2012. Accessed April 21, 2025. https://www.acf.hhs.gov/orr/policy-guidance/refugee-act
50. Chavez HL, Partida MG. 1986: Immigration Reform and Control Act of 1986. Library of Congress. August 17, 2020. Updated December 14, 2023. Accessed April 18, 2025. https://guides.loc.gov/latinx-civil-rights/irca

51. US Citizenship and Immigration Services. Temporary Protected Status. Updated April 7, 2025. Accessed April 21, 2025. https://www.uscis.gov/humanitarian/temporary-protected-status
52. Office of the Assistant Secretary for Planning and Evaluation. The Personal Responsibility and Work Opportunity Reconciliation Act of 1996. August 31, 1996. Accessed April 21, 2025. https://aspe.hhs.gov/reports/personal-responsibility-work-opportunity-reconciliation-act-1996
53. Rodriguez LA. Understanding the Nicaraguan Adjustment and Central American Relief Act. *ILSA J Int Comp Law*. 1996;5(2):28. Accessed April 21, 2025. https://nsuworks.nova.edu/ilsajournal/vol5/iss2/28
54. US Immigration and Customs Enforcement. Secure Communities. February 9, 2021. Accessed April 21, 2025. https://www.ice.gov/secure-communities
55. Immigration Forum. Current status of DACA: Explainer. August 11, 2025. Accessed August 15, 2025. https://immigrationforum.org/article/current-status-of-daca-explainer
56. Atiles J. The paradise performs: Blockchain, cryptocurrencies, and the Puerto Rican tax haven. *S Atlantic Q*. 2022;121(3):612–627. doi:10.1215/00382876-9826032
57. Sampas J. Puerto Rico: America's tax haven or vacation paradise. *Law Bus Rev Am*. 2015;21(1):49–83. Accessed April 21, 2025. https://core.ac.uk/download/pdf/147641481.pdf
58. Trump DJ. Executive order: Border security and immigration enforcement improvements. The White House. January 25, 2017. Accessed April 21, 2025. https://trumpwhitehouse.archives.gov/presidential-actions/executive-order-border-security-immigration-enforcement-improvements
59. *Students for Fair Admissions v President and Fellows of Harvard College*, 600 US 181 (2023).

5

Structural Inequities and Middle Eastern and North African American Health

Kristine J. Ajrouch, PhD, Nadia N. Abuelezam, ScD, Niaz Kasravi, PhD, Jen'nan G. Read, PhD, and Muniba Saleem, PhD

INTRODUCTION

The *Middle Eastern and North African* (*MENA*) category refers to persons who trace their ancestry to multiple countries and ethnicities throughout the Arab and non-Arab worlds, including parts of western Asia. MENA is sometimes also referred to as *South West Asia and North Africa* (*SWANA*). As a term, MENA emerged in the United States in the early 2000s after decades of lobbying for an official classification schema that would identify persons of Arab, Middle Eastern, and North African descent separately from other racial and ethnic groups and from their federal and Census classification as "white."[1] Today, MENA Americans continue to be counted as white in all federally collected data, including the US Census and national health surveys. Yet there is mounting evidence that a separate MENA category is needed to better identify and address health and other disparities within an increasingly diverse population.[2-4] The call to identify MENA populations builds from a long-standing and growing recognition that those who come from the MENA region have experiences that do not mirror those of white individuals.[5,6] There is a long history of MENA differential treatment including being overpoliced, charged, and easily deported.[7] Further, there is the immense diversity that exists within MENA, none of which is adequately captured in the aggregate white category.

In March 2024, the US Census announced that the Office of Management and Budget (OMB) updated their standards for maintaining, collecting, and presenting race/ethnicity data across federal agencies by including the MENA category.[8] As such, the category is now recognized as separate from the white category, though implementation of this new standard is yet to occur. The *MENA* category defines *Arab heritage* in a narrower way than previous definitions, limiting inclusion to those who trace their ancestry to one of 17 Arab League states: Algeria, Bahrain, Egypt, Iraq, Jordan, Kuwait, Lebanon, Libya, Morocco, Oman, Palestine, Qatar, Saudi Arabia, Syria, Tunisia, United Arab Emirates, and Yemen. It excludes some African countries which, nevertheless, are members of the

Arab League (Comoros, Djibouti, Mauritania, Somalia, and Sudan). *MENA* also includes those with ancestries to the non-Arab countries of Iran and Israel. This pan-ethnic categorization consists of people from multiple religions including those of various Christian, Jewish, Muslim, Baha'i, Zoroastrian, and other faiths, as well as an array of ethnicities that have long lived in Arabic-speaking countries, such as Amazigh, Assyrian, Chaldean, Copt, and Kurd. Further, those of MENA origins vary in terms of phenotype, ranging from lighter to darker skin, hair, and eyes.[9] This newly recognized racial/ethnic category promises to usher in a new era of research on MENA populations, particularly for Arab and Iranian Americans, making identification of this population more accessible. However, the plans to implement the collection of data that includes MENA are still not finalized and will require careful thought to ensure results yield meaningful and useful information.

Although the MENA term is relatively recent, MENA Americans have been part of the American mosaic dating back to the mid- to late-1800s and have a rich history that predates their arrival to the United States.[10] MENA societies are widely recognized for scientific discovery and influential developments in mathematics, astronomy, agriculture, literacy, and medicine.[11-13] Individuals with MENA ancestry have arrived in the United States for varied reasons, ranging from the desire to seek better economic and educational opportunities, family reunification, and most recently, refuge from political instability and wars.[14] MENA populations in the United States have made and continue to make meaningful contributions to the economy across an array of skilled professions, including the fields of medicine, arts, and business.[15] Establishing a MENA category is highly important for identifying health inequities. Though the literature on MENA health—primarily on those with Arab and Iranian ancestries—in the United States has expanded in the last decade, it still lags behind other ethnic and minority groups, largely due to an inability to identify MENA in large databases.[4,16,17] We first present the limited evidence available on MENA health.

Following the discussion of existing research on MENA health, this chapter provides an in-depth review of key barriers to achieving health equity for the MENA population. Specifically, we identify the ways in which structures of power have shaped the MENA experience in the United States. First, attention to US foreign policy illustrates how the Arab/MENA case is uniquely tied to global political developments[18] that can alter the profile and selectivity of MENA immigrants in different eras as well as silence and suppress the ability to fight for equal treatment. Second, and relatedly, US involvement in global conflicts has exacerbated prevailing antagonisms toward Muslims and the religion of Islam, both of which are conflated with being, or even looking, Arab or Middle Eastern.[19,20] Finally, the invisibility of MENA populations in federal statistics poses unique challenges, as there is limited ability to accumulate and track changes in data on key measures associated with health disparities. As such, economic, political, and social policies aimed at reducing racial/ethnic health inequities in the United States largely exclude

MENA individuals. In what follows, we elaborate on each of these barriers to illustrate how the current and historical contexts of structural racism evident in US foreign policy, the rise of Islamophobia, and MENA invisibility in data perpetuate oppression through unequal power relationships. Then, we discuss select systems of marginalization that help perpetuate health inequities: (1) immigration policy, (2) media, and (3) the criminal legal/national security system. Three actionable opportunities are proposed to begin to dismantle structural racism and improve health outcomes: (1) improving the presence of MENA individuals behind and in front of screens to improve media representation; (2) modifying policies that govern profiling in criminal legal systems and eliminate national security loopholes; and (3) advocating for a local MENA identifier wherever race and ethnicity data are collected. We then consider areas for further research, policy, and programming. The chapter concludes with a discussion that summarizes the key issues identified and action plans proposed.

EVIDENCE ON MIDDLE EASTERN AND NORTH AFRICAN HEALTH

The lack of a MENA marker in many large databases has required scholars interested in studying the health of the MENA population to capitalize on sources that include questions on respondents' nativity, place of birth, and/or ancestry. Such information is scarce in most nationally representative data sources. The National Health and Interview Survey (NHIS) and American Community Survey (collected by the US Census) are exceptions. However, each data source has its own shortcomings. NHIS, for example, only releases information on region of birth, rather than country, and after the 2019 survey redesign, they eliminated the question altogether. As such, the latest year that data are available on the MENA population is 2018, and the data only permit examination of foreign-born MENA without identifiers for the second and later generations. The American Community Survey permits examination of both foreign- and US-born individuals and contains information on country of birth and ancestry, but it has limited questions on health that focus only on disability. Disability is an important health indicator but tends to concentrate in older populations, thereby underestimating health disparities beyond disability, especially for foreign-born populations who tend to be younger.

Despite shortcomings, scholars have been innovative in using these national data sources to make inroads into knowledge on various aspects of MENA health.[14,21-24] Others have relied on convenience samples in areas of high MENA concentration, such as Arab/Middle Eastern American communities in Dearborn and Detroit, Michigan[25-28] or state-level data, such as the California Health Interview Survey,[29] or name algorithms[30,31] to examine the health of MENA populations. While not all areas of health have been well documented for MENA Americans, a few areas are well researched to identify health profiles and/or illustrate worse health than their white counterparts. Areas researched include diabetes and cardiovascular disease,[27,29,30,32] cancer,[33-36] and mental,[17,26,37,38] functional,[14,22,25,39] cognitive,[2,21,23,24] and maternal and infant health.[40-44]

General findings in the literature contradict research on immigrant health, finding nonexistent health advantages or worse health for immigrants from the Middle East and North Africa. Put differently, the oft noted and controversial *healthy immigrant effect*, whereby immigrants arrive in better health than their native-born counterparts, is less likely to be found among the MENA population living in the United States. This is true across consequential measures of functional,[14,22] self-rated,[45,46] and cognitive health.[21,24] Taken together, there is ample evidence to suggest significant health disparities among the MENA population. While it is true that the MENA population is largely hidden and hard to extricate from the white population, scholars have been innovative in doing so and in establishing patterns of poorer health that deserve further attention.

CURRENT AND HISTORICAL CONTEXT OF STRUCTURAL RACISM

There are three key sources of structural racism in the United States that are particularly relevant for the MENA population: US foreign policy, Islamophobia, and data invisibility. These serve as key foundations for the structural racism that is then perpetuated in the systems examined in this chapter, namely immigration, media, and the criminal legal/national security systems.

US Foreign Policy

Empire and *imperialism* are two words that are rarely used within the United States to describe US foreign policy, yet the expansion of American political, economic, cultural, media, and military influence beyond the boundaries of the United States has made the country ubiquitous.[47,48] From the proliferation of military bases worldwide[49] to cultural narratives,[50] US power has shaped the ways in which groups resist. Indeed, US foreign policy in the MENA region has been identified as key to the rise of an Arab/MENA identity. For instance, Abraham[51] argues that those of Arab ancestry may have all but melted into mainstream white America (notwithstanding that Arabs, both Christians and Muslims, especially those with darker complexions, always had unique challenges[52,53]) were it not for US foreign policy. US foreign policy drew attention to the MENA region following World War II, catapulting the group into a negative spotlight to which those with ancestral ties reacted by rediscovering or privileging their Arab identity. The Council on Foreign Relations states that there were three main US interests following World War II: ensuring the free flow of oil from the Persian Gulf, guaranteeing the survival and security of Israel, and limiting the influence of the former Soviet Union.[54] A general aversion toward Arabs specifically is thought to be borne out of a discomfort, if not outright opposition, to Arab and Arab American criticism of Israel through their advocacy and support for Palestinians.[55] In recent times, US foreign policy in the MENA region expanded to include countering terrorism and nuclear proliferation.[54] Such foreign policy foci influence US immigration policies, media portrayals, and domestic crime and legal policies involving MENA populations.

MENA integration experiences, particularly those of lighter-skinned Arab Americans, mirrored that of Southern Europeans in the early part of the 20th century. Yet, social distance increased for MENA populations over time, "created and reproduced by institutions of power ... and is manifested in government policies, mainstream cultural representations, public perceptions and attitudes, discriminatory behaviors, physical insecurity, and social and political exclusion."[18(p243)] While European immigrants overcame negative racialization processes to ultimately become white, in part by embracing domestic policies supporting racism toward non-whites (e.g., Irish Americans[56]), Arab and MENA ancestry populations separated from the European integration experience over time. In particular, the rise of the United States as a global superpower after World War II and its related foreign (not domestic) policy interests initiated the racialization of those in the Arab and MENA diaspora as non-white.[18] This distance intensified in the late 1960s due to political events in the MENA region, namely, the one-sided support evident in US foreign policy concerning the Arab–Israeli conflict,[57] which brought with it a barrage of negative stereotypes and selective policy enforcement toward Arab and MENA Americans.[58,59] US foreign policy efforts reflected a *clash of civilizations* mindset, ultimately driving US perceptions of Arabs as backward, threatening, and a danger to US values.[60,61] Relatedly, Arab and Middle Eastern diasporas faced backlash as a result of political instability and war and military violence in the MENA region, as well as white supremacy, Islamophobia, the criminalization of immigrants, and detentions in the diaspora as part of the same imperial process.[62] Such structures contribute to the importance of having racial and ethnic identities officially recognized in the United States as a means to gain voice and overcome silencing forces.

Researchers have historically faced substantial hurdles within academia to make Arab/MENA communities visible in scholarly work; the absence of a recognized racial/ethnic category justified marginalization of the population[63] and prevented any credible attempt to give voice to the Arab/MENA experience in the United States, especially when US foreign policy in the MENA region was openly criticized.[64] Whereas ethnic integration in the United States generally considers domestic arrangements and the legacy of colonialism, the integration of Arab/MENA populations is tied to global political developments.[18,55,65] Notably, the issues reviewed in this chapter draw from the inclusive MENA definition, but exclude those with ancestry to Israel. This is not an indication of the lack of importance of issues faced by those of Israeli ancestry. Modern anti-Semitism inflicted on those of the Jewish faith undeniably occurs and requires continued attention,[66] yet it has different origins and is qualitatively distinct from what Arabs, other

Middle Easterners, and those who are perceived as such experience in daily life.[67] A recent case in point illustrating these divergent experiences is the war in Gaza, particularly the killing of tens of thousands of civilians, including children. Human rights organizations are now calling these actions a genocide. Protests against the US support for the war resulted in accusations of anti-Semitism across various contexts, which included shutting down university student protests against investments supporting Israeli aggression. This was accompanied by police reprimanding and jailing protestors, universities preventing involved students from graduating, and talk by political candidates to deport those who protested.[68] Opposition to US support for the war also led to the House of Representatives to censure a representative (Rashida Tlaib) for speaking out against the US government's decision to financially aid Israel's fierce offensive on Gaza.[69] US efforts to extend its influence in the MENA region through foreign policy often results in the silencing of those aiming to identify injustices directed toward Arab/MENA groups (distinct from the Israeli situation) and also contributes to the rise of Islamophobia, or the fear of those who are from the region.

Islamophobia

Though the MENA population encompasses a vast diversity of religions, Islam or being Muslim are often conflated with being Arab or Middle Eastern. Hence, anyone who is perceived to be Muslim can be targeted by Islamophobic acts and policies. *Islamophobia* is defined by the United Nations as

> a fear, prejudice and hatred of Muslims that leads to provocation, hostility and intolerance by means of threatening, harassment, abuse, incitement and intimidation of Muslims and non-Muslims ... Motivated by institutional, political and religious hostility that transcends into structural and cultural racism, it targets the symbols and markers of being Muslim.[70]

In discussing Islamophobia, particularly in the context of MENA populations, it can be helpful to use the framework of *anti-Muslim racism*,[71] which emphasizes the perception of Muslims as a threat to the United States and often justifies treating them as enemies.[19] This framework can place Muslims, or those perceived as being Muslim, in a broader context of current and historical racism in the United States, furthering the potential to join the larger social justice movement in this country.[71] It is also important to remember that Islam is a religion and not a race, hence the experiences of Muslims from the MENA region and those of Black Muslims or other people of color can be vastly different. This framing, however, can more clearly reveal the shared racialized experiences of Muslims and other people of color in the United States and across the globe and incentivize solidarity for a more coordinated fight against white supremacy that is at the root of systemic othering and racism experienced by all communities of color.

Islamophobia in the United States is indeed largely rooted in US foreign policy, but also reflects many of this nation's historical foundations, such as the enslavement of African people, the genocide of Indigenous communities, and Jim Crow policies—all stemming from a belief in the superiority of the white race. The racialization of MENA populations is not only impacted by the legacy of white supremacy, but also via the three key areas where Islamophobia is most apparent today: on an individual level, through media portrayals, and by state-sanctioned policies.[71]

Individual acts of hate as well as anti-Muslim policies often (though not always) escalate at specific historical moments. The perception of Muslims as a threat to the United States often justifies treating them as enemies and leads to an increase in targeted violence.[19] Recent individual acts of hate following the War in Gaza include the murder of 6-year-old Wadea Al-Fayoume, who was stabbed 26 times in Plainfield, Illinois by his family's landlord on October 14, 2023,[72] and the shooting of three 20 year-old Palestinian American students in Burlington, Vermont on November 25, 2023.[73] Both acts of hate were linked to unfolding events in the Middle East. Studies also showed a devastating and vast rise in hate crimes following the attacks of September 11, 2001 (9/11) involving acts of vandalism, murder, harassment, and destruction of property—including places of worship.[74] According to the Federal Bureau of Investigation, anti-Muslim hate crimes saw a 17-fold increase from the year 2000 to 2001.[74] In 2016, following anti-immigrant rhetoric pushed by Donald Trump during his presidential campaign and consequent efforts to restrict immigrants from certain Muslim countries, a white man in Kansas walked into a restaurant in Kansas City, pulled a gun on two Indian nationals and said, "get out of my country." He then shot them, killing one and wounding the other, along with another man who tried to intervene. It was later revealed that the assailant believed the two men he targeted were Iranian, one of the countries included in Trump's anti-immigrant rhetoric.[75]

The ongoing refugee crises, driven in large part by foreign policy decisions of America and other Western nations—such as the displacement of millions of Iraqis after the US invasion of Iraq in 2003 and the subsequent military force used to fight the Islamic State of Iraq and Syria (ISIS)—and the promotion of anti-Muslim messaging by political leaders and the media are other policy and cultural factors that contribute to escalation. Yet, the people toward whom Islamophobia is directed are not always Muslim. Despite the religious, racial, cultural, and ethnic diversity of the region, US media has created a homogenizing Arab or MENA look, and those who fit that profile are potential targets of Islamophobic acts, whether they are from the MENA population or not.[76] An example of this is the tragic 2012 mass shooting by a white supremacist of a Sikh temple in Oak Creek, Wisconsin, ultimately leaving seven people dead.[77] Abboud et al.,[4] as well as others,[7,20,63] argue that Arabs and those from the MENA region are uniformly portrayed as Muslim, and Islam is portrayed as an uncivilized and violent religion, used to racialize anyone perceived as Muslim as inferior to white Americans.

In sum, Islamophobia often translates into structural racism and repression, taking the form of policies that discriminate against MENA populations on the individual, cultural, and societal levels.[19] Islamophobia can negatively influence health through experiences of identity stress at the individual, interpersonal, and institutional levels,[78] as well as shape perceptions of health care providers and availability of culturally appropriate services.[79,80] In other words, Islamophobia includes stigma and discrimination, both known to induce negative effects across physical, mental, and cognitive health dimensions.[81,82] Though the Council on American–Islamic Relations collects data on the prevalence and incidence of Islamophobia, the ability to systematically track and study the effects of such discrimination is stymied by MENA data invisibility.

Data Invisibility

MENA Americans are invisible in national statistics because they are considered white by OMB. Though this invisibility is now recognized as problematic by OMB's recent update to Policy Directive 15 to include MENA as a category requiring reporting across federal agencies,[8] MENA populations nevertheless have historically lacked and currently lack identification in data across political, social, and health landscapes. As a result, there has been an inability to properly identify MENA population size, demographics, and community needs. Hence, the ways in which MENA Americans are impacted by structural racism are difficult to document and challenging to address at scale across the United States. Data are known to be important to both combating structural inequities and perpetuating them in political, social, and health systems.[83] Further, data and documentation lead to opportunities for funding and dedicated resources to help address needs in known communities.[84] The collection of race and ethnicity data has been controversial in the United States since its beginnings in the late 1700s, and the identification of legally recognized racial and ethnic categories has shifted over time, often due to political motivations. Political motivations behind the collection of racial and ethnic data range from wanting to ensure white supremacy to remedying inequalities.[17,85,86] Accurate and robust collection of ethnicity and race data is the first critical step needed to identify and address disparities.

Health disparity statistics often exclude MENA populations because data is either not being collected on this population or this population is not disaggregated from the white race category. Invisibility and a lack of resources to address needs in this population begets a vicious cycle in addressing health disparities.[4] Without a dedicated identifier, it is difficult to collect data to understand population size, disease prevalence, and needs. Notably, the difficulty in identifying the MENA population in large, nationally representative datasets leads to a focus on ethnic enclaves, making it difficult to capture the diversity of the MENA population, or for that matter, generalize to the population level. For example, numerous health studies draw data from the largest, most visible population of MENA Americans in Wayne County, Michigan, due to the relative ease in seeing, and therefore identifying, this population. Yet, the socioeconomic profile of this enclave is much poorer than is observed among MENA Americans living in adjacent counties.[87] Further, identifying the social determinants of health disparities such as lack of knowledge, access to care and culturally sensitive providers, socioeconomic status, unfair treatment, and discrimination become challenging.[4]

An important aspect of ensuring health systems are equipped to meet the needs of the MENA American population is to overcome barriers to full participation in US society. Full participation includes being counted, and visibility would open avenues for developing culturally informed approaches to promoting good health. Yet, without estimates for MENA population size and needs, it is difficult to motivate dedicated funding towards addressing disparities experienced by this population. Further, without dedicated funding to address needs among MENA populations, fewer resources are available to support well-being, success, and support. This cycle (lack of identification → lack of funding → lack of identification) perpetuates disparities for MENA Americans in health, social services, and other sectors.

WAYS THAT MARGINALIZATION FLOWS THROUGH SYSTEMS TO PERPETUATE INEQUITIES

Examples of how marginalization of the MENA population flows through systems to perpetuate inequities can be seen through three key systems: immigration policy, media, and the criminal legal/national security systems. As noted previously, MENA populations are legally considered white along with those of European ancestry, yet MENA immigration patterns vary from European ancestry groups. Though both came in large numbers in the early 20th century, MENA immigration continued in large numbers after 1965 while European immigration considerably slowed by comparison. Racial and ethnic group membership has historically been tied to patterns of immigration and related policies, and that link continues today.[53] Laws permitting entry into the United States, as well as citizenship eligibility, have varied depending on national origins.[88,89] Second, media images, portrayals, and narratives have significant influence as sources of information regarding racial and ethnic groups, greatly shaping perceptions when direct interactions with members of these groups are limited or inaccessible.[90] The absence of representation, coupled with predominantly unfavorable media portrayals, is widely acknowledged to contribute to the cultivation of hostile attitudes, behaviors, and support for discriminatory policies towards the groups being depicted.[91] This phenomenon has been consistently observed in the case of media depictions of MENA individuals.[92,93] Finally, criminal legal systems dictate what is lawful or not, and often carry out their charge through profiling. Racial profiling at every level of the criminal legal system is a well-documented reality.[94] In fact, policies that racially profile—especially based on alleged national security concerns—are at the root of how many from the MENA population become involved in the US criminal legal system. In what follows, each system is discussed and illustrated.

Immigration and the Racialized Origins of the Middle Eastern/North African Category

US immigration policies have played a key role in shaping the composition of US racial and ethnic groups and have been particularly consequential for immigrants from the MENA region. Restrictive and discriminatory practices in the 18th, 19th, and early 20th centuries excluded or severely limited the entry of immigrants from the eastern hemisphere and reserved naturalization and citizenship to white persons who had resided in the United States for two or more years.[88,89] The 1882 Chinese Exclusion Act was the first to explicitly deny entry along racial lines, and it laid the foundation for the 1917 Immigration Act that created an "Asiatic Zone" that barred immigrants from most of the Asian continent. Four decades of progressively racist policies culminated in the 1924 National Origins Quota Act, which effectively made whiteness not only a prerequisite for citizenship, but also for entry into the United States.

Immigrants from the Middle East and North Africa were in a quandary regarding their racial classification; the majority were arriving from Syria and Lebanon but were neither African nor Asian. In order to gain the right to naturalization, they fought to prove Caucasian heritage and thus be counted as "white."[95] In 1915, the US Court of Appeals set an important precedent by ruling in favor of George Dow and extending the right of US citizenship to those from the Middle Eastern and North African regions.[96] Specifically, the ruling recognized them to be of Caucasian heritage, in large part due to their Christian affiliation and convincing argument that they migrated from the birthplace of the father of Christianity—Jesus Christ.[97] The fact that the majority of immigrants at the time were Christians played an important role in the pivotal court decision and reflected deeply entrenched preferences in the United States for a distinct type of white citizen, one that was lighter-skinned, Christian, and non-Asian. The conflation of race, region, phenotype, and religion worked in favor of MENA immigrants in the early part of the 20th century but would later hinder the migration and integration of darker-skinned and non-Christian MENA immigrants. In 1942, for example, Ahmad Hassan—a native of Yemen residing in Detroit—petitioned for US citizenship and was denied on the basis of his dark skin and the judge's determination that persons of the "Mohammedan world" could not be assimilated into "our civilization."[98]

Major waves of emigration from the Middle East began in earnest after the passage of the 1965 Immigration and Nationality Act. The act abolished national origin quotas and opened the door to migration from diverse world regions other than Western Europe. Lebanese, Syrian, Iranian, Palestinian, Assyrian, and Turkish immigrants made up the lion's share of Middle Eastern arrivals in the United States during the 1970s and 80s. The migration of these groups prior to the 1965 act meant that there were established communities in the United States that could provide economic and social support and ease the integration of newer immigrant arrivals. Importantly, though some immigrants arriving from these countries were darker in complexion, they were typically lighter-skinned and more phenotypically similar to US whites than later cohorts of MENA immigrants. This period of migration coincided with the end of the Civil Rights Movement and new federal standards on racial and ethnic classification. Federal agencies were tasked with enforcing Civil Rights laws and needed consistent and comparable data on race and ethnicity. In 1977, OMB issued Policy Directive 15, which established five broad racial/ethnic categories that guided the collection and reporting of all federal data: white, Black, Hispanic, Asian or Pacific Islander, and American Indian or Alaska Native.[99] The directive defined white as "a person having origins in any of the original peoples of Europe, North Africa, or the Middle East," and MENA fell squarely into that definition.[99(p37)] The standards further stipulated that Hispanic ethnicity be collected separately from the race question when possible, yielding the oft-used *non-Hispanic white* category as a reference group for measuring inequality. Several watershed events in the late 1980s and early 1990s altered the composition of immigration from the Middle East and North Africa. Political, economic, and civil unrest due to the ongoing Israeli–Palestinian conflict (1948–present), the Lebanese Civil War (1975–1990), the Iranian Revolution (1979), and the Iran–Iraq War (1980–1989) had a spillover effect, creating general instability in the region. The United States' involvement in the Gulf War (1990–1991) further destabilized the region, despite its success in liberating Kuwait. The Iraqi uprisings (1991), Yemeni Civil War (1994), and growing Islamic extremism were among the many factors motivating emigration from the Middle East during this time. In recognition of shifting trends in immigration, the 1980 US Census was the first to include a question on ancestry and also included Iran, Iraq, Saudi Arabia, Kuwait, and Yemen as response categories in the question on country of birth.[100] The 1990 and 2000 decennial censuses continued the practice, and results from the counts demonstrated rapid growth in the number of immigrants arriving from war-torn countries such as Iraq, Iran, Syria, and Yemen. Unlike their predecessors, a growing number were arriving as refugees rather than voluntary migrants.[101]

The diversity of newer arrivals from MENA compared with earlier waves of migration from the region cannot be overstated. Not only were the contexts in the sending regions more volatile but also the context of reception in the United States was less welcoming.[102,103] Civil unrest throughout the MENA region stagnated economic development and resulted in immigrants arriving with fewer socioeconomic resources, greater exposure to war-related trauma, and more accumulated stressors than earlier migrants.[104,105] In the aftermath of the terrorist attacks on 9/11, US attitudes and behaviors toward MENA immigrants became steadily more hostile, especially toward those who looked or sounded different from Western European whites.[38,106] Critical to the challenges around characterizing MENA people as white is the fact that the definition of white fails to capture the phenotypic, linguistic, and religious diversity that characterize later waves of immigrants from the MENA region. Most importantly, MENA Americans are less likely to share the white experience.[7,63] Renewed immigration from the MENA region following 1965 was a key element in shaping MENA Americans' experiences in the United States.[103] Immigration and the racialized origins of the MENA category therefore constitute a key structural system that has marginalized the MENA population to perpetuate inequities.

Media Representation and Depiction of Middle Eastern/North African and Muslim Individuals

The widespread conflation of the MENA population with the religion of Islam has been previously highlighted.[20] This issue is particularly prominent in media depictions, where MENA individuals are conspicuously absent behind the screens, as highlighted by the University of California, Los Angeles (UCLA) Hollywood Diversity Report.[107] Consequently, inaccurate, narrow, and one-dimensional portrayals of MENA characters prevail on screen.[92,108,109] This section critically examines the representation of MENA and Muslim individuals in US media, exploring the impact of these portrayals on both the depicted and non-depicted groups. Given that the majority of Americans have limited to no personal interactions with MENA and Muslim individuals in their everyday lives,[110] media sources become one of the primary and influential channels of information about these groups.[90,111] Understanding how MENA and Muslim individuals are portrayed across various media platforms becomes crucial in this context, as media exposure plays a significant role in shaping attitudes when direct experiences with members of the depicted group are scarce.[90,112,113]

MENA and Muslim individuals have historically faced underrepresentation and negative portrayals in the Western media landscape.[108,114,115] The aftermath of 9/11 witnessed a significant surge in media representations involving MENA and Muslim individuals, as documented in scholarly works.[117-119] Although there were some "good" depictions of MENA and Muslim characters as patriotic Americans working against the "bad" terrorists from these groups, much of the content remained overwhelmingly negative.[120] Numerous content analyses across newspapers, cable news, TV shows, movies, children's books, video games, and social media platforms have consistently demonstrated the underrepresentation and negative representation of MENA and Muslim individuals.[92,121-125] These portrayals often encompass themes of terrorism, violence, brutality, intolerance, exoticism, anti-Western norms, and gender inequality.[108,114,115] Ignoring the diversity of racial, ethnic, and religious identities encompassing MENA individuals, MENA characters in Hollywood are visually characterized with traits and tropes that have historically been used to marginalize other groups that are devalued by US society.[58] The characterizations often signal backwardness, violence, and gender oppression (e.g., dark skin and features, a distinctive hooked nose, veiled clothing), and characters are frequently represented as Muslims with extremist views.[115] The issue is not solely the presence of negative images; rather, it is the fact that they overwhelmingly dominate the narrative.

It is important to describe the *extent* to which media coverage involving MENA and Muslim individuals is negative. In an examination of 48,283 newspaper articles drawn from over a dozen American sources across a 20-year period, Bleich and van der Veen provided three important insights: (1) the average article mentioning Muslims or Islam in the United States is more negative than 84% of articles examined in this study; (2) news reports of other religious groups are much more balanced and nuanced, suggesting a specific bias among news reports referencing Muslims and Islam; and (3) these bias patterns are not specific to the United States but also found among newspapers published in the United Kingdom, Canada, and Australia.[126] Similarly, a content analysis of 320 television shows between 1996 and 2014 revealed that out of the 153 Middle Eastern characters represented in these shows, 70 (45.8%) were in the context of terrorism.[127] Interestingly, not only are references to terrorism in news articles five times more likely when the crime involves a Muslim versus a non-Muslim perpetrator,[127] such stories also receive greater attention and coverage within media.[128,129] Consequently, due to the strong association between terrorism and MENA and Muslim individuals portrayed in the media, people are more inclined to label crimes involving Muslim and Arab perpetrators as acts of terrorism.[130-132]

Exposure to these media images is influential in affecting the way outgroup members perceive MENA and Muslim individuals. Research consistently finds a positive relationship between exposure to negative media representations of MENA and Muslim individuals and unfavorable attitudes towards members of these groups.[92,133-136] These attitudes in turn are known to influence support for restrictive public policies targeting MENA and Muslim people domestically and internationally.[19,135,137,138] In addition, exposure to media depictions of Arabs as terrorists can increase perceptions that "a typical Arab person" is aggressive and angry, increasing the likelihood of hostile and violent actions against members of this group.[93] These research findings have been observed in short-term experimental and long-term survey research paradigms.[93,118,135,137,138] An important qualifier is whether or not individuals personally know someone from these groups. For example, research finds that Americans who personally know someone who is Muslim and rely on direct contact for information about Muslims tend to have more favorable impressions of them.[110,135]

MENA and Muslim individuals often report their dissatisfaction and frustration with the way in which media represents members of their groups and in turn its potential for influencing outgroup members' attitudes towards them.[139,140] Indeed, exposure to such media images is known to lead to detrimental outcomes for MENA and Muslim individuals. Pervasive stereotypes of racial/ethnic minorities in the media contribute to systemic racism, and frequent and repeated exposure to such images can lead to adverse psychological, social, and political consequences for the depicted group members.[19,38,141-145] For instance, Muslim immigrants who are exposed to negative media depictions of their religious ingroup are less likely to identify with their national communities,[146,147] more likely to avoid majority members,[148] and less likely to trust in their national governments.[147]

Interestingly, at times collective injustices and disadvantages can inspire minority communities to work together to improve the image and status of their group in the larger society.[149] Indeed, exposure to negative media images of Muslims was found to influence collective action among young Muslim Americans due to an increased sense of collective efficacy, a belief that Muslims can work together to improve their disadvantaged status in American society.[150] In sum, media representations become powerful sources that shape attitudes and perceptions, often becoming a major contributor to how people and cultures are understood. Related to the prevalence of negative images is the role of profiling and criminalization of MENA individuals in the criminal legal system.

Criminal Legal System

Profiling and criminalization in the name of national security encompasses the major structural role that the criminal legal system plays in the lives of MENA Americans. Many of those from MENA populations (though not all) who come in contact with the criminal legal system do so as a result of policies that are implemented in the name of "national security." Once groups are labeled as potential threats to the security of the nation and such labels are repeatedly portrayed in the media (as previously discussed), it becomes easier to sidestep equal protections and discriminate against people based on characteristics that are constitutionally protected.[151]

MENA populations in America's criminal legal apparatus are part of a larger problem of unequal treatment and profiling of people of color in this nation, and anti-terror policies are and must be seen as racial profiling initiatives.[152] *Racial profiling* is not the use of race *alone* as a reason for police and law enforcement to target individuals and groups.* Such policies, as well as increased incidents of individual discrimination and hate crimes against MENA populations, are most prevalent after incidents involving people or countries from the MENA region. Several examples in recent history highlight this fact. Following the 1979 Hostage Crisis, where Iranian students stormed the US embassy in Tehran, Iran and took American diplomats hostage, many people of Iranian descent living in the United States experienced heightened anti-Iranian sentiment, an experience that some say is common in their daily lives even today.[154] After the attacks of 9/11, policies and practices targeting people from the MENA region were also implemented. One such policy was the National Security Entry-Exit Registration System (NSEERS), which targeted people from 25 countries based on national origin, ethnicity, and religion.† Under this policy, certain nonimmigrant visa holders from the specified countries

---

*Other characteristics can also be used, including actual or perceived race, color, ethnicity, religion, nationality, sex, gender, gender identity or expression, sexual orientation, immigration or citizenship status, language, disability—including HIV status—housing status, occupation, or socioeconomic status.[153]
†These included Iran, Iraq, Libya, Sudan, Syria, Afghanistan, Algeria, Bahrain, Eritrea, Lebanon, Morocco, North Korea, Oman, Qatar, Somalia, Tunisia, United Arab Emirates, Yemen, Pakistan, Saudi Arabia, Bangladesh, Egypt, Indonesia, Jordan, and Kuwait.

were subjected to being fingerprinted, photographed, and interrogated upon entrance to the United States. Males older than the age of 16 who stayed in the country for more than one month were required to regularly report to government agencies and prove their residence, employment, or enrollment in educational institutions. While in effect, the NSEERS program registered roughly 90,000 Muslims, and thousands more were interrogated, detained, and/or deported for failure to comply.[155] In 2011, the Department of Homeland Security unlisted the countries covered by the NSEERS program but kept its infrastructure intact until 2016, when some provisions were dismantled.[156]

In addition to nationally implemented policies, some jurisdictions across the country engaged in other forms of surveillance and profiling of MENA populations, with little effectiveness and damaging long-term impact. Two such examples occurred in New York City, New York. From 2001 to 2014, the New York Police Department (NYPD) engaged in a surveillance and mapping program where a specialized demographics unit was created to infiltrate mosques, Muslim student groups, and Muslim-owned businesses in order to gather information. The program never led to any actionable information for law enforcement, faced multiple legal challenges, and only served to create further anxiety and mistrust of law enforcement in communities.[157] Further, in the weeks following 9/11 in New York City, local law enforcement engaged in large-scale sweeps across the city, casting a wide net in the name of the "War on Terror," leading to the arrest of more than 1,000 people as "special interest" detainees. Yet, most—often having been detained for long periods of time without being charged—were eventually only charged with overstaying their visas; some were detained for several months and ultimately deported back to their countries of origin, and many were forced to sign a special registry and live with the confusion and anxiety of what the future might hold for them. Neither NSEERS nor the local roundup programs proved effective in identifying any acts of terrorism,[151] but one real result was the terrorizing and tearing apart of countless families and communities by national and local government-sanctioned policies.[155,158]

Another policy targeting MENA populations was the USA PATRIOT Act, a hastened revision of US surveillance laws by Congress following 9/11. These revisions expanded the government's powers to spy on its own citizens in unprecedented ways while reducing necessary checks and balances such as judicial oversight, accountability, and people's ability to legally challenge those powers.[159] The expanded surveillance included monitoring phone calls and emails, collecting bank and credit reports, and tracking innocent people's online activity. Though many believed this policy was meant to apprehend terrorists, in reality it turned ordinary residents into suspects.[159] Key provisions of the USA PATRIOT Act were allowed to sunset in 2020.[160] The government's claims that the policy helped convict hundreds of people remains in serious doubt, and there is evidence of numerous incidents of government abuse of its expanded powers.[161] Although no court ever ruled it as unconstitutional, certain provisions of the act stand in stark contrast to the First and Fourth

Amendments of the US Constitution, which protect the right to free speech and offer protection from unreasonable searches and seizures, respectively.[159]

Anti-Muslim and anti-immigrant propaganda, along with discriminatory laws that target MENA populations, have tragic direct and collateral consequences. It is difficult to know the exact level of impact of criminal legal system involvement among MENA populations due to the challenges in identifying MENA populations (e.g., many are legally recognized as white). The negative health impacts of encountering law enforcement and being involved in the criminal legal system are well documented and include being more prone to physical and mental health issues. Those who encounter structural racism through the criminal legal system are more likely to have high blood pressure, cancer, asthma, and a plethora of infectious diseases.[162,163] Additionally, interactions with law enforcement can lead to the tragic occurrence of death at the hands of police; merely being a victim of or witnessing aggressive law enforcement increases the likelihood of suffering from a variety of posttraumatic issues, such as anxiety, lack of or lower-quality sleep, rapid heart rate, sweaty palms, and other similar trauma-induced symptoms.[164] Finally, children and families of individuals involved in the criminal legal system also suffer these consequences. Often referred to as *hidden victims*, children whose parents are involved in the system are more likely to suffer a myriad of issues, including economic hardships, anxiety, antisocial behavior, stress, and suspension or expulsion from school.[165] Studies focusing on the impact of 9/11 and the War on Terror on Muslim children and families also show an increase in symptoms of mental illness.[166]

In sum, due to sociopolitical realities and agendas, as well as anti-Muslim and racist policies that stem from them, people of the MENA region are often swept up in the criminal legal system by virtue of their origin. Data collection on this population is problematic, as police and others in the criminal legal system must decide how to categorize those of MENA descent.[152] Policies that target MENA and Muslim populations are often difficult to challenge because they are justified as national security concerns, and addressing hate crimes against those from the MENA region becomes challenging as this group is not considered a legal minority. The complexity around definitions of MENA and the wide discretion given to police and others in the criminal legal system to define the various situations in which MENA are targeted or implicated must be acknowledged.

DISMANTLING STRUCTURAL RACISM FOR IMPROVED HEALTH OUTCOMES

Three key areas for immediate intervention to dismantle structural racism are discussed: balanced media coverage, banning racial profiling, and using the MENA identifier at local levels.

Media Coverage

Media plays a significant role in shaping public perceptions, attitudes, and stereotypes. It has been observed that MENA and Muslim individuals have historically been subjected to negative and distorted portrayals in the media, perpetuating stereotypes and reinforcing biases. Part of the reason for the unidimensional and overwhelmingly negative representation of MENA and Muslim characters in American media is the absence of these groups behind the screen.[107] Accordingly, there is a critical need to support, invest in, and mentor MENA and Muslim content creators so they can create authentic, accurate, and diverse media. Some organizations have created databases to identify and locate MENA and Muslim talent to assist with these efforts (e.g., Pillars Fund, MENA Arts Advocacy Coalition, Arab American Screenwriters). Other efforts have urged media makers to be cognizant in their depictions of MENA and Muslim individuals in order to avoid the perpetuation of existing stereotypes and improve the quality of how these groups are represented in media (e.g., Riz Test, Obeidi-Alsultany Test, Muslim Women's Test).

Efforts to provide more balanced and positive media portrayals are critical, as research suggests that negative information (relative to positive information) receives more processing and exerts a greater influence on final impressions.[167,168] Some research has examined how more positive and balanced media depictions of MENA and Muslim individuals influence attitudes towards members of these groups.[118,137,138,169] For instance, a study comparing different media interventions' effectiveness for improving attitudes towards Muslims found that media messages highlighting the hypocrisy of blaming all Muslims, but not all Christians, for extremism were especially influential in reducing anti-Muslim attitudes.[170] Similarly, messages emphasizing media bias against MENA and Muslim groups are effective in reducing hostile attitudes towards members of these groups.[171] Counter-stereotypical representations in entertainment media, exemplified by shows like *Little Mosque on the Prairie*, have shown promise in mitigating prejudicial attitudes by fostering identification with MENA and Muslim characters.[169] This positive development aligns with recent endeavors to create television programs featuring MENA and Muslim protagonists that go beyond the confines of terrorism, such as *Ramy* and *Mo*. It is crucial to emphasize that media depictions do not need to be overwhelmingly positive to yield favorable outcomes. Even brief exposure to neutral and non-negative portrayals of MENA and Muslim individuals can lead to reduced hostility towards this group in both the short and long term.[138,171] These research findings underscore the importance of recognizing that the medium of media itself is not inherently problematic; rather, it is the content within it that determines whether positive or negative outcomes are likely in terms of attitudes towards different groups.

Ban Racial Profiling

A key solution available to policymakers interested in dismantling structural racism and helping end discriminatory policies that target people based on their race, ethnicity, religion, nationality, gender, and other inherent characteristics is to pass effective laws that ban and punish racial profiling. To specifically address much of the profiling targeted at MENA populations, it is important that such laws eliminate all national security loopholes (i.e., allowing for profiling if a group or individual is labeled a national security threat) in the absence of credible evidence linking such person(s) to a criminal activity or scheme.

Though many laws exist across different states, most do not have all the components necessary for an effective and enforceable law. A good policy must begin with a full and complete definition of *racial profiling*:

> discriminatory policing practices which target groups or individuals based on actual or perceived race, color, ethnicity, religion, nationality, sex, gender, gender identity or expression, sexual orientation, immigration or citizenship status, language, disability (including HIV status), housing status, occupation, or socioeconomic status in initiating law enforcement action against that individual, rather than an individual's behavior or other trustworthy information or circumstances, relevant to the locality and timeframe, that links a person [of a particular race, ethnicity, religion, national origin, etc.] to suspected unlawful activity.[153]

In addition to a comprehensive definition, these laws, which are needed on both state and federal levels, must have specific components in order to be effective (not only for MENA populations, but for all communities of color), including (1) banning *pretextual stops*—the use of alleged minor infractions by officers to inquire about other potentially illegal activity—of motorists and pedestrians; (2) prohibiting violations of the law and specifying penalties for officers and departments that are found to engage in the practice; (3) requiring mandatory data collection for all stops and searches of motorists and pedestrians; (4) requiring regular analysis and publication of the collected data on racial profiling; (5) creating an independent committee to review and respond to racial profiling complaints; and (6) allowing those who have been targets of racial profiling legal relief through the courts to stop officers and departments from engaging in the practice.[153]

Though effective anti-profiling laws on the federal and state level are key in helping end the systematic targeting of MENA populations in the criminal legal and national security apparatus, additional changes to policy and practice must also simultaneously occur in order to achieve meaningful systems transformation. These should include banning the use of paid informants and agent provocateurs that have been planted within MENA communities to essentially entrap individuals in alleged terror plots. Also, better classification of terror-related cases identified by law enforcement is needed, as current numbers are often unreliable and inflated due to wrongfully labeling many incidents of any alleged criminal activity by a person of MENA origin as potential terror threats and failing to reclassify criminal activity that was later proven to not be related to a terror plot.[152]

Those who support racial profiling often cite it as an effective tool for law enforcement. Yet racial profiling has always proven to be an ineffective and costly tactic.[152,153] Countless examples of its futility exist throughout American history, not the least of which are the ineffectiveness of the NSEERS program or the post-9/11 roundups in identifying and stopping potential terrorist acts. Data have in fact shown that racial profiling is an ineffective public safety tool in any context, such as in the so-called War on Drugs.[172] What most of these policies that rely on profiling and discrimination ultimately do is cast a wide net, waste limited law enforcement attention and resources, and fill the nation's prisons and jails disproportionately with people of color. They also create mistrust between communities and the law enforcement who are sworn to protect and serve them. Using reliable information instead of depending on general categories of race, ethnicity, nationality, religion, gender, or other characteristics will not only save time and resources but also achieve greater public safety more effectively. Additionally, it will help decrease the negative and often lifelong consequences experienced by those who come into contact with the criminal legal system.

Middle Eastern/North African Identifier at Local Levels

Underpinning all actionable opportunities to improve MENA health in a US context is the need for identification of MENA individuals in data across political, social, and health landscapes. Without a racial and ethnic identifier for MENA individuals in standard data collection methods, these individuals remain invisible and voiceless. Thus, action on the part of all organizations that collect racial/ethnic data to include a MENA identifier at the local levels will provide an important step towards making the MENA population visible. Structural interventions require appropriate and thorough data collection on MENA individuals to succeed. While President Biden recently signed the OMB Directive 15 incorporating a MENA checkbox in the 2030 Census, widespread use of a MENA category at the grassroots level is achievable in the short term. Health care, research, and other organizations and institutions that collect racial and ethnic data could begin to incorporate the MENA checkbox immediately (see Awad et al.[3] for guidance). Extensive and immediate use of the MENA checkbox at local levels will provide knowledge about the actual size of these communities as well as provide the data needed to begin to systematically address inequalities, given that a federally initiated and supported MENA identifier is not yet available. Further, extensive adoption of the checkbox will improve the chances that the additional structural interventions proposed earlier will succeed.

AREAS FOR FURTHER RESEARCH, POLICY, AND PROGRAMMING

The most pressing future direction is to include a MENA identifier in all data collection forms, with guidelines for use, data documentation, and analysis. Making a MENA identifier available will increase the ability to address disparities and inequalities. Accurate data permits opportunities to tackle educational and employment disparities to inform targeted interventions and policies that promote educational equity and support academic achievement as well as guide the development of initiatives that address barriers to employment, reduce occupational segregation, and promote economic integration. Socioeconomic status is a key determinant of health disparities and inequalities. Relatedly, making a MENA identifier available will facilitate the effective allocation of resources. Accurate data informs the need for community services and program funding. Specifically, it enables policymakers to identify areas with significant MENA populations to ensure adequate funding for social services, health care, language assistance programs, and cultural organizations. Further, it promotes the ability to tailor public infrastructure planning and improvement, such as schools, health care facilities, community centers, and transportation systems.

The additional benefits of including a MENA category within the US Census and other forms are extensive. First, a MENA identifier will allow for enhanced data accuracy and representation; enabling individuals with MENA heritage to self-identify accurately provides opportunities for more comprehensive and reliable data. Further, offering subcategories within the MENA category, such as Arab, Iranian, and Kurdish, will acknowledge the heterogeneity within the MENA population and enhance the granularity of data collection. The complexity of the MENA category suggests the need to specify groups under study.[173] There are political, historical, and current tensions that affect many of these groups, which adds to the complexity of creating a way in which we can talk about, understand, and therefore address the needs of these populations in a clear and inclusive way. For example, political tensions refer to explicit Islamophobia and racism by political candidates, including rhetoric against Arab or Muslim Senators or Representatives. Historical tensions include the surveillance and monitoring of MENA Americans as a result of events happening in the MENA region or due to political activity or protesting. Current tensions are illustrated in the war on Gaza and the American response, including the silencing of protestors, which likely impacts education and employment experiences. These data would then more accurately inform policy and programs to support and enhance the health of all. This will permit a more nuanced understanding of ethnic identities and socioeconomic dynamics to address critical intersections that produce systems of stratification.

Developing targeted policies and programs promotes cultural competency and inclusion. In particular, accurate data on the MENA population can inform the development of policies promoting cultural competency training for service providers, educators, health care professionals, and those working with refugee resettlement and law enforcement agencies. Culturally sensitive approaches foster inclusion, reduce biases, and improve service provision. Notably, such approaches support community engagement and empowerment by aiding in the identification of community leaders, organizations, and resources within the MENA population to facilitate targeted outreach, civic engagement, and capacity-building initiatives.

In sum, the identification of MENA people and disaggregation from the white category advances the ability to not only identify and address disparities between MENA and other groups but also improve the ability to detect disparities generally.[17] Future research, in particular, would benefit from prospective and longitudinal data collection alongside a focused engagement with the resiliency factors related to differences in migrant health patterns in MENA populations when compared with other migrant groups.[16,24] Identifying vulnerable populations will allow for eradicating disparities, noting commonalities across groups, and understanding what is unique to each group. A commitment to identify disparities across groups will be of interest to all.

CONCLUSION

The MENA population is complex, including individuals who come from a wide swath of nations in the Middle East (West Asia) and North Africa. Though the population is diverse, mounting evidence makes clear that an identifier is urgently needed to make this group visible in a uniform way. In particular, official recognition would provide reliable information that could balance the consistently negative images that arise when the media invokes the population during times of crisis, both in the United States and abroad. As discussed previously, the formation of negative attitudes, behaviors, and policies toward the MENA population has resulted largely from US foreign policies rather than domestic ones,[18,64] making MENA people somewhat unique from other minoritized groups. Yet, the ways that systems facilitate oppression of this group are addressable and begin with the ability to identify this group separately from other racial and ethnic populations in federally funded and collected data. The benefits of having a MENA identifier include being able to identify inequalities and health disparities. Identification is a critical first step to addressing challenges that will ultimately promote a healthy society for all.

REFERENCES

1. Mathews K, Phelan J, Jones NA, et al. 2015 National content test: Race and ethnicity analysis report. US Census Bureau. February 28, 2017. Accessed August 11, 2025. https://www.census.gov/programs-surveys/decennial-census/decade/2020/planning-management/plan/final-analysis/2015nct-race-ethnicity-analysis.html

2. Ajrouch KJ, Zahodne LB, Antonucci TC. Arab American cognitive aging: Opportunities for advancing research on Alzheimer's disease disparities. *Innov Aging.* 2018;1(3). doi:10.1093/geroni/igx034
3. Awad G, Ikizler A, Abdel-Salam L, Kia-Keating M, Amini B, El-Ghoroury N. Foundations for an Arab/MENA psychology. *J Hum Psychol.* 2022;62(4):591–613. doi:10.1177/00221678211060974
4. Abboud S, Chebli P, Rabelais E. The contested whiteness of Arab identity in the United States: Implications for health disparities research. *Am J Public Health.* 2019;109(11):1580–1583. doi:10.2105/AJPH.2019.305285
5. Maghbouleh N, Schachter A, Flores RD. Middle Eastern and North African Americans may not be perceived, nor perceive themselves, to be White. *Proc Natl Acad Sci USA.* 2022;119(7):e2117940119. doi:10.1073/pnas.2117940119
6. Suleiman M. *Arabs in America: Building a New Future.* Temple University Press; 1999.
7. Cainkar LA. *Homeland Insecurity: The Arab American and Muslim American Experience After 9/11.* Russell Sage Foundation; 2009.
8. Marks K, Jones N, Battle K. What updates to OMB's race/ethnicity standards mean for the Census Bureau. April 8, 2024. Accessed April 10, 2025. https://www.census.gov/newsroom/blogs/random-samplings/2024/04/updates-race-ethnicity-standards.html
9. Ajrouch KJ, Jamal A. Assimilating to a White identity: The case of Arab Americans. *Int Migration Rev.* 2007;41(4):860–879. doi:10.1111/j.1747-7379.2007.00103.x
10. Abdelhady D. The sociopolitical history of Arabs in the United States: Assimilation, ethnicity, and global citizenship. In: Nassar-McMillan SC, Ajrouch KJ, Hakim-Larson J, eds. *Biopsychosocial Perspectives on Arab Americans: Culture, Development, and Health.* Springer; 2014:17–43.
11. Chamsi-Pasha M, Chamsi-Pasha H. The contribution of Islamic culture to the development of medical sciences. *J Br Islamic Med Assoc.* 2020;6(2). Accessed April 10, 2025. https://www.jbima.com/article/the-contribution-of-islamic-culture-to-the-development-of-medical-sciences
12. Toomer GJ. *Eastern Wisedome and Learning: The Study of Arabic in Seventeenth-Century England.* Oxford University Press; 1996.
13. Modanlou HD. A tribute to Zakariya Razi (865–925 AD), an Iranian pioneer scholar. *Arch Iran Med.* 2008;11(6):673–677.
14. Read JG, Ajrouch KJ, West JS. Disparities in functional disability among Arab Americans by nativity, immigrant arrival cohort, and country of birth *SSM Popul Health.* 2018;7:100325. doi:10.1016/j.ssmph.2018.100325
15. New American Economy Research Fund. *Power of the Purse: Middle-Easterners and North Africans in America.* January 2019. Accessed April 10, 2025. https://research.newamericaneconomy.org/report/power-of-the-purse-middle-easterners-and-north-africans-in-america
16. Abuelezam NN, El-Sayed AM, Galea S. Relevance of the "immigrant health paradox" for the health of Arab Americans in California. *Am J Public Health.* 2019;109(12):1733–1738. doi:10.2105/AJPH.2019.305308
17. Awad GH. Lack of Arab or Middle Eastern and North African health data undermines assessment of health disparities. *Am J Public Health.* 2022;112(2):209–212. doi:10.2105/AJPH.2021.306590
18. Cainkar L. The social construction of difference and the Arab American experience. *J Am Ethn Hist.* 2006;25(2-3):243–278. doi:10.2307/27501698

19. Lajevardi N, Oskooii K, Saleem M, Docherty M. In the shadow of September 11: The roots and ramifications of anti-Muslim attitudes in the United States. *Adv Polit Psychol*. 2024;45(suppl 1): 87–118. doi:10.1111/pops.12943
20. Love E. *Islamophobia and Racism in America*. New York University Press. 2017
21. Al-Rousan T, Kamalyan L, Bernstein Sideman A, et al. Migration and cognitive health disparities: The Arab American and refugee case. *J Gerontol B Psychol Sci Soc Sci*. 2023;78(1):111–123. doi:10.1093/geronb/gbac129
22. Dallo FJ, Al Snih S, Ajrouch KJ. Prevalence of disability among US- and foreign-born Arab Americans: results from the 2000 US Census. *Gerontology*. 2009;55(2):153–161. doi:10.1159/000151538
23. Dallo FJ, Kindratt TB, Zahodne L. Prevalence of self-reported cognitive impairment among Arab American immigrants in the United States. *Innov Aging*. 2020;5(1). doi:10.1093/geroni/igaa058
24. Kindratt TB, Dallo FJ, Zahodne LB. Cognitive disability among Arab Americans by nativity status and arrival year: Lack of evidence for the healthy migrant effect. *J Racial Ethn Health Disparities*. 2022;9(5):2056–2062. doi:10.1007/s40615-021-01144-y
25. Ajrouch KJ. Health disparities and Arab-American elders: Does intergenerational support buffer the inequality–health link? *J Soc Issues*. 2007;63(4):745–758. doi:10.1111/j.1540-4560.2007.00534.x
26. Ajrouch KJ, Antonucci TC. Social relations and health: Comparing "invisible" Arab Americans to Blacks and Whites. *Soc Ment Health*. 2018;8(1):84–92. doi:10.1177/2156869317718234
27. Jaber LA, Brown MB, Hammad A, et al. Epidemiology of diabetes among Arab Americans. *Diabetes Care*. 2003;26(2):308–313. doi:10.2337/diacare.26.2.308
28. Patel MR, Green M, Tariq M, et al. A snapshot of social risk factors and associations with health outcomes in a community sample of Middle Eastern and North African (MENA) people in the US. *J Immigr Minor Health*. 2022;24(2):376–384. doi:10.1007/s10903-021-01176-w
29. Abuelezam NN, El-Sayed AM, Galea S, Gordon NP. Health risks and chronic health conditions among Arab American and White adults in Northern California. *Ethn Dis*. 2021;31(2):235–242. doi:10.18865/ed.31.2.235
30. Dallo FJ, Ruterbusch JJ, Kirma JD, Schwartz K, Fakhouri M. A health profile of Arab Americans in Michigan: A novel approach to using a hospital administrative database. *J Immigr Minor Health*. 2016;18(6):1449–1454. doi:10.1007/s10903-015-0296-8
31. Dallo FJ, Kindratt TB, Seaton R, Ruterbusch JJ. The disproportionate burden of COVID-19 cases among Arab Americans. *J Racial Ethn Health Disparities*. 2023;10(3):1108–1114. doi:10.1007/s40615-022-01298-3
32. Fritz H, DiZazzo-Miller R, Bertran EA, et al. Diabetes self-management among Arab Americans: patient and provider perspectives. *BMC Int Health Hum Rights*. 2016;16(1):22. doi:10.1186/s12914-016-0097-8
33. Bergmans R, Soliman AS, Ruterbusch J, et al. Cancer incidence among Arab Americans in California, Detroit, and New Jersey SEER registries. *Am J Public Health*. 2014;104(6):83–91. doi:10.2105/AJPH.2014.301954
34. Dallo FJ, Kindratt TB. Disparities in vaccinations and cancer screening among US- and foreign-born Arab and European American non-Hispanic white women. *Womens Health Issues*. 2015;25(1):56–62. doi:10.1016/j.whi.2014.10.002

35. Ayyash M, Ayyash M, Bahroloomi S, et al. Knowledge assessment and screening barriers for breast cancer in an Arab American community in Dearborn, Michigan. *J Community Health.* 2019;44(5):988–997. doi:10.1007/s10900-019-00671-4
36. Saad F, Ayyash M, Ayyash M, et al. Assessing knowledge, physician interactions and patient-reported barriers to colorectal cancer screening among Arab Americans in Dearborn, Michigan. *J Community Health.* 2020;45(5):900-909. doi:10.1007/s10900-020-00807-x
37. Amer M. *Arab American Mental Health in the Post September 11 Era: Acculturation, Stress, and Coping.* Dissertation. University of Toledo; 2005.
38. Awad GH, Kia-Keating M, Amer MM. A model of cumulative racial-ethnic trauma among Americans of Middle Eastern and North African (MENA) descent. *Am Psychol.* 2019;74(1): 76–87. doi:10.1037/amp0000344
39. Dallo FJ, Booza J, Nguyen ND. Functional limitations and nativity status among older Arab, Asian, Black, Hispanic, and White Americans. *J Immigr Minor Health.* 2015;17(2):535–542. doi:10.1007/s10903-013-9943-0
40. Lauderdale DS. Birth outcomes for Arabic-named women in California before and after September 11. *Demography.* 2006;43(1):185–201. doi:10.1353/dem.2006.0008
41. El-Sayed AM, Galea S. The health of Arab-Americans living in the United States: A systematic review of the literature. *BMC Public Health.* 2009;9(1):272. doi:10.1186/1471-2458-9-272
42. Abuelezam NN, Cuevas AG, Galea S, Hawkins SS. Maternal health behaviors and infant health outcomes among Arab American and non-Hispanic white mothers in Massachusetts, 2012–2016. *Public Health Rep.* 2020;135(5):658–667. doi:10.1177/0033354920941146
43. Samari G, Catalano R, Alcalá HE, Gemmill A. The Muslim Ban and preterm birth: Analysis of US vital statistics data from 2009 to 2018. *Soc Sci Med.* 2020;265:113544. doi:10.1016/j.socscimed.2020.113544
44. Hyder A, Barnett KS. Low birth weight and preterm birth among Arab-American women in Ohio. *Matern Child Health J.* 2021;25(4):574–583. doi:10.1007/s10995-020-03095-y
45. Abdulrahim S, Baker W. Differences in self-rated health by immigrant status and language preference among Arab Americans in the Detroit Metropolitan Area. *Soc Sci Med.* 2009;68(12): 2097–2103. doi:10.1016/j.socscimed.2009.04.017
46. Read JN, Amick B, Donato KM. Arab immigrants: A new case for ethnicity and health? *Soc Sci Med.* 2005;61(1):77–82. doi:10.1016/j.socscimed.2004.11.054
47. Boggs C. *Origins of the Warfare State: World War II and the Transformation of American Politics.* Routledge; 2016.
48. Said EW. *Orientalism.* Pantheon Books; 1978.
49. Vine D. *Base Nation: How US Military Bases Abroad Harm America and the World.* Metropolitan Books; 2015.
50. Said EW. *Culture and Imperialism.* Vintage Books; 2012.
51. Abraham N. Anti-Arab racism and violence in the United States. In: McCarus E, ed. *The Development of Arab-American Identity.* University of Michigan Press; 1994:155–214.
52. Bayoumi M. Racing religion. *CR New Centennial Rev.* 2006;6(2):267–293. doi:10.1353/ncr.2007.0000
53. Gualtieri S. Becoming White: Race, religion and the foundations of Syrian/Lebanese ethnicity in the United States. *J Am Ethn Hist.* 2001;20(4):29–58. doi:10.2307/27502745

54. Council on Foreign Relations. Modern history and US foreign policy: Middle East and North Africa. Accessed August 11, 2025. https://education.cfr.org/learn/learning-journey/middle-east-and-north-africa-essentials/modern-history-and-us-foreign-policy-middle-east-and-north-africa
55. Pennock PE. *Rise of the Arab American Left: Activists, Allies, and Their Fight against Imperialism and Racism, 1960s–1980s*. University of North Carolina Press; 2017.
56. Ignatiev N. *How the Irish Became White*. Harvard University Press; 1994.
57. Abu-Laban B, Suleiman MW, eds. *Arab Americans: Continuity and Change*. Association of Arab-American University Graduates; 1989.
58. Stockton R. Ethnic archetypes and the Arab image. In: McCarus E, ed. *The Development of Arab-American Identity*. University of Michigan Press; 1994:119–153.
59. US Commission on Civil Rights. Civil rights issues facing Arab Americans in Michigan. Accessed April 10, 2025. https://www.usccr.gov/files/pubs/sac/mi0501/ch5.htm#_ftn3
60. Huntington S. *The Clash of Civilizations and the Remaking of World Order*. Touchstone; 1996.
61. Slade S. The image of the Arab in America: Analysis of a poll on American attitudes. *Middle East J*. 1981;35(2):143–162. Accessed April 10, 2025. https://www.jstor.org/stable/4326196
62. Naber NS. Imperial whiteness and the diasporas of empire. *Am Q*. 2014;66(4):1107–1115. doi:10.1353/aq.2014.0068
63. Naber N. Ambiguous insiders: An investigation of Arab American invisibility. *Ethn Racial Stud*. 2000;23(1):37–61. doi:10.1080/014198700329123
64. Cainkar LA. Palestine—and empire—are central to Arab American/SWANA studies. *J Palestine Stud*. 2021;50(2):4–21. doi:10.1080/0377919X.2021.1899513
65. Howell S, Shryock A. Cracking down on diaspora: Arab Detroit and America's "War on Terror." *Anthropological Q*. 2003;76(3):443–462. doi:10.1353/ANQ.2003.0040
66. Stanley T. Antisemitism and safety fears surge among US Jews, survey finds. *AP News*. February 13, 2024. Accessed April 10, 2025. https://apnews.com/article/jewish-muslim-antisemitism-islamophobia-hamas-israel-us-d4220df14c7a40403ba61781f3f87854
67. Marvasti A. Being Middle Eastern American: Identity negotiation in the context of the war on terror. *Symb Interact*. 2005;28(4):525–547. doi:10.1525/si.2005.28.4.525
68. Householder M, White E. Police break up pro-Palestinian camp at the University of Michigan. *AP News*. May 21, 2024. Accessed April 10, 2025. https://apnews.com/article/israel-palestinians-gaza-campus-protests-michigan-335904cf0ecb308a111eaa8bc86aeaf5
69. Amiri F. House votes to censure Rep. Rashida Tlaib over her Israel-Hamas rhetoric in a stunning rebuke. *AP News*. Updated November 8, 2023. Accessed April 10, 2025. https://apnews.com/article/congress-house-censure-resolution-tlaib-8085189047a4c40f2d44ada4604aa076
70. United Nations. International Day to Combat Islamophobia. Accessed August 11, 2025. https://www.un.org/en/observances/anti-islamophobia-day
71. Naber N, Junaid R. The 21st century problem of anti-Muslim racism. *Jadaliyya*. July 25, 2019. Accessed August 11, 2025. https://www.jadaliyya.com/Details/39730
72. Yan H, Parks B, Mascarenhas L, Langmaid V. 2023. A 6-year-old Palestinian-American was stabbed 26 times for being Muslim, police say. His mom couldn't go to his funeral because she was stabbed, too. *CNN*. October 16, 2023. Accessed April 10, 2025. https://www.cnn.com/2023/10/16/us/chicago-muslim-boy-stabbing-investigation/index.html

73. Llamas T, Alsharif M. Palestinian students shot in Vermont say the suspect waited for and targeted them. *NBC News*. January 17, 2024. Accessed April 10, 2025. https://www.nbcnews.com/news/us-news/palestinian-students-shot-burlington-vermont-interview-hospital-recovercna133822
74. Human Rights Watch. The September 11 backlash. In: *"We Are Not the Enemy": Hate Crimes Against Arabs, Muslims, and Those Perceived to be Arab or Muslim after September 11*. Human Rights Watch; 2002. Accessed April 11, 2025. https://www.hrw.org/reports/2002/usahate/usa1102-04.htm
75. CBS News. Kansas Man Charged with Hate Crime in Fatal Shooting of Indian Engineer. *CBS News*. June 9, 2017. Accessed April 10, 2025. https://www.cbsnews.com/news/adam-purinton-faces-hate-crime-charges-in-fatal-shooting-of-indian-engineer
76. Alsultany E. *Broken: The Failed Promise of Muslim Inclusion*. New York University Press; 2022.
77. Mentzer R. Wisconsin's Sikh community a decade after fatal temple shooting. *NPR*. July 28, 2022. Accessed August 11, 2025. https://www.npr.org/2022/07/28/1114335390/wisconsins-sikh-community-a-decade-after-fatal-temple-shooting
78. Samari G. Islamophobia and public health in the United States. *Am J Public Health*. 2016;106(11):1920–1925. doi:10.2105/AJPH.2016.303374
79. Ali S, Awaad R. Islamophobia and public mental health: Lessons learned from community engagement projects. In: Moffic H, Peteet J, Hankir A, Awaad R, eds. *Islamophobia and Psychiatry: Recognition, Prevention, and Treatment*. Springer; 2019: 375–390.
80. Laird LD, de Marrais J, Barnes LL. Portraying Islam and Muslims in MEDLINE: A content analysis. *Soc Sci Med*. 2007;65(12):2425–2439. doi:10.1016/j.socscimed.2007.07.029
81. Hatzenbuehler ML, Phelan JC, Link BG. Stigma as a fundamental cause of population health inequalities. *Am J Public Health*. 2013;103(5):813–821. doi:10.2105/AJPH.2012.301069
82. Williams DR, Mohammed SA. Discrimination and racial disparities in health: evidence and needed research. *J Behav Med*. 2009;32(1):20–47. doi:10.1007/s10865-008-9185-0
83. Prewitt K. The Census race classification: Is it doing its job? *Ann Am Acad Pol Soc Sci*. 2018;677(1):8–24. doi:10.1177/0002716218756629
84. Farley R, Haaga J, eds. *The American People: Census 2000*. Russell Sage Foundation; 2005.
85. Robbin A. Classifying racial and ethnic group data in the United States: The politics of negotiation and accommodation. *J Gov Inf*. 2000;27(2):129–156. doi:10.1016/S1352-0237(00)00131-3
86. Strmic-Pawl HV, Jackson BA, Garner S. Race counts: Racial and ethnic data on the US Census and the implications for tracking inequality. *Sociol Race Ethn*. 2018;4(1):1–13. doi:10.1177/2332649217742869
87. Read JG, Ajrouch KJ. US Census study. Submitted to the Arab Community Center for Economic and Social Services Arab American Research Initiative. 2023. Accessed August 11, 2025. https://www.arabnarratives.org/narrative/arab-americans-a-community-portrait
88. Budiman A, Tamir C, Mora L, Noe-Bustamante L. Facts on US immigrants, 2018. Pew Research Center. August 20, 2020. Accessed April 10, 2025. https://www.pewresearch.org/race-and-ethnicity/2020/08/20/facts-on-u-s-immigrants-current-data
89. Cohn D. How US immigration laws and rules have changed through history. Pew Research Center. September 30, 2015. Accessed August 11, 2025. https://www.pewresearch.org/short-reads/2015/09/30/how-u-s-immigration-laws-and-rules-have-changed-through-history

90. Blumer H. Race prejudice as a sense of group position. *Pac Sociol Rev.* 1958;1(1):3-7. doi:10.2307/1388607
91. Dixon T. Media stereotypes: Content, effects, and theory. In: Oliver MB, Raney A, Bryant J, eds. *Media effects: Advances in Theory and Research.* Routledge; 2019:243-257.
92. Hawkins I, Coles SM, Saleem M, Moorman JD, Aqel H. How reel Middle Easterners' portrayals cultivate stereotypical beliefs and policy support. *Mass Commun and Soc.* 2022;27(1):1-25. doi: 10.1080/15205436.2022.2062000
93. Saleem M, Anderson CA. Arabs as terrorists: Effects of stereotypes within violent contexts on attitudes, perceptions, and affect. *Psychol Violence.* 2013;3(1):84-99. doi:10.1037/a0030038
94. The Sentencing Project. Report to the United Nations on racial disparities in the US criminal justice system. April 19, 2018. Accessed April 10, 2025. https://www.sentencingproject.org/reports/report-to-the-united-nations-on-racial-disparities-in-the-u-s-criminal-justice-system
95. Naff A. *Becoming American: The Early Arab Immigrant Experience.* Southern Illinois University Press; 1993.
96. *Dow v United States,* 226 F 145 (1915).
97. Gualtieri SMA. *Between Arab and White: Race and Ethnicity in the Early Syrian American Diaspora.* University of California Press; 2009.
98. In Re Ahmed Hassan, 48 F Supp 843 (ED Mich 1942).
99. US Office of Management and Budget. 1977 race and ethnic standards for federal statistics and administrative reporting. 1978. Accessed April 10, 2025. https://spd15revision.gov/content/spd15revision/en/history/1977-standards.html
100. Farley PM. Local authorities' use of private law. *Adopt Foster.* 1991;15(2):41-44. doi:10.1177/030857599101500208
101. US Dept of Homeland Security. Yearbook of Immigration Statistics. Accessed September 24, 2023. https://www.dhs.gov/immigration-statistics/yearbook
102. European and North American Ewing Sarcoma Study Groups. EWING 2008 Results Summary. Accessed September 24, 2023. https://www.sarcoma.org.au/news/news/ewing-2008-results-summary
103. Jamal A, Naber N, eds. *Race and Arab Americans Before and After 9/11: From Invisible Citizens to Visible Subjects.* Syracuse University Press; 2008.
104. Haas SA, Ramirez D. Childhood exposure to war and adult onset of cardiometabolic disorders among older Europeans. *Soc Sci Med.* 2022;309:115274. doi:10.1016/j.socscimed.2022.115274
105. Reynolds MM, Chernenko A, Read JG. Region of origin diversity in immigrant health: Moving beyond the Mexican case. *Soc Sci Med.* 2016;166:102-109. doi:10.1016/j.socscimed.2016.07.018
106. Pew Research Center. Modern immigration wave brings 59 million to US, driving population growth and change through 2065. Chapter 1: The nation's immigration laws, 1920 to today. September 28, 2015. Accessed April 10, 2025. https://www.pewresearch.org/race-and-ethnicity/2015/09/28/chapter-1-the-nations-immigration-laws-1920-to-today
107. Ramón A-C, Tran M, Hunt D. UCLA Hollywood Diversity Report presents: Streaming Television in 2023. UCLA Entertainment and Media Research Initiative. December 2024. Accessed April 10, 2025. https://socialsciences.ucla.edu/hollywood-diversity-report-2024
108. Alsultany E. *Arabs and Muslims in the Media: Race and Representation after 9/11.* New York University Press; 2012.

109. Yuen NW, Chin C, Deo M, DuCros F, Lee JJ, Milman N. Terrorists and tyrants: Middle Eastern and North African (MENA) actors in prime time television. MENA Arts Advocacy Coalition. 2018. Accessed August 11, 2025. https://archive.thinkprogress.org/uploads/2018/09/MENATandT_Presentation_FullDoc_Final.pdf
110. Mohamed B. Muslims are a growing presence in US, but still face negative views from the public. Pew Research Center. September 1, 2021. Accessed April 10, 2025. https://www.pewresearch.org/short-reads/2021/09/01/muslims-are-a-growing-presence-in-u-s-but-still-face-negative-views-from-the-public
111. Pew Research Center. Benedict XVI viewed favorably but faulted on religious outreach: Public expresses missed views of Islam, Mormonism. September 25, 2007. Accessed August 11, 2025. https://assets.pewresearch.org/wp-content/uploads/sites/5/legacy-pdf/358.pdf
112. De Fleur ML, Ball-Rokeach SJ. *Theories of Mass Communication*. 5th ed. Longman; 1989.
113. Harwood AE, Smith GE, Cayton T, Broadbent E, Chetter IC. A systematic review of the uptake and adherence rates to supervised exercise programs in patients with intermittent claudication. *Ann Vasc Surg*. 2016;34:280–289. doi:10.1016/j.avsg.2016.02.009
114. Said EW. *Covering Islam: How the Media and the Experts Determine How We See the Rest of the World*. Vintage Books; 1997.
115. Shaheen JG. Reel bad Arabs: How Hollywood vilifies a people. *Ann Am Acad Pol Soc Sci*. 2003;588:171–193. Accessed April 10, 2025. https://www.jstor.org/stable/1049860
116. Abrahamian E. The US media, Huntington and September 11. *Third World Q*. 2003;24(3):529–544. doi:10.1080/01436590320000844556
117. Bail CA. The fringe effect: Civil society organizations and the evolution of media discourse about Islam since the September 11th attacks. *Am Sociol Rev*. 2012;77(6):855–879. doi:10.1177/0003122412465743
118. Lajevardi N. The media matters: Muslim American portrayals and the effects on mass attitudes. *J Polit*. 2021;83(3):1060–1079. doi:10.1086/711300
119. Martin P, Phelan S. Representing Islam in the wake of September 11: A comparison of US television and CNN online messageboard discourses. *Prometheus*. 2002;20(3). doi:10.1080/08109020210141371.
120. Alsultany E. Arabs, Muslims, and Arab Americans: Constructing an evil other. In: Campbell C, ed. *The Routledge Companion to Media and Race*. Routledge; 2016;241–249.
121. Ahmed S, Matthes J. Media representation of Muslims and Islam from 2000 to 2015: A meta-analysis. *Int Commun Gaz*. 2017;79(3):219–244. doi:10.1177/1748048516656305
122. Awan I. Islamophobia and Twitter: A typology of online hate against Muslims on social media. *Policy Internet*. 2014;6(2):133–150. doi:10.1002/1944-2866.POI364
123. Dill KE, Gentile DA, Richter WA, Dill JC. Violence, sex, race, and age in popular video games: A content analysis. In: Cole E, Daniel JH, eds. *Featuring Females: Feminist Analyses of the Media*. American Psychological Association; 2005:115–130.
124. Dixon TL, Williams CL. The changing misrepresentation of race and crime on network and cable news. *J Commun*. 2015;65(1):24–39. doi:10.1111/jcom.12133
125. Nacos BL, Torres-Reyna O. *Fueling Our Fears: Stereotyping, Media Coverage, and Public Opinion of Muslim Americans*. Bloomsbury; 2007.

126. Bleich E, van der Veen AM. *Covering Muslims: American Newspapers in Comparative Perspective*. Oxford University Press; 2021.
127. Betus AE, Kearns EM, Lemieux AF. How perpetrator identity (sometimes) influences media framing attacks as "terrorism" or "mental illness". *Commun Res*. 2020;48(8):1133–1156. doi:10.1177/0093650220971142
128. Kearns EM, Betus AE, & Lemieux AF. Why do some terrorist attacks receive more media attention than others? *Justice Q*. 2019;36(6):985–1022. doi:10.1080/07418825.2018.1524507
129. Mitnik SP, Freilich JD, Chermak SM. Post-9/11 coverage of terrorism in the New York Times. *Justice Q*. 2020;37(1):161–185. doi:10.1080/07418825.2018.1488985
130. D'Orazio V, Salehyan I. Who is a terrorist? Ethnicity, group affiliation, and understandings of political violence. *Int Interact*. 2018;44(6):1017–1039. doi:10.1080/03050629.2018.1500911
131. Huff C, Kertzer JD. How the public defines terrorism. *Am J Polit Sci*. 2018;62(1):55–71. doi:10.1111/ajps.12329
132. West K, Lloyd J. The role of labeling and bias in the portrayals of acts of "terrorism": Media representations of Muslims vs. non-Muslims. *J Muslim Minor Aff*. 2017;37(2):211–222. doi:10.1080/13602004.2017.1345103
133. Lajevardi N, Oskooii KAR, Walker HL, Westfall AL. The paradox between integration and perceived discrimination among American Muslims. *Polit Psychol*. 2020;41(3):587–606. doi:10.1111/pops.12640
134. Nisbet EK, Zelenski JM, Murphy SA. The nature relatedness scale: Linking individuals' connection with nature to environmental concern and behavior. *Environ Behav*. 2009;41(5):715–740. doi:10.1177/0013916508318748
135. Saleem M, Yang GS, Ramasubramanian S. Reliance on direct and mediated contact and public policies supporting outgroup harm. *J Commun*. 2016;66:604–624. doi:10.1111/jcom.12234
136. Shaver JH, Sibley CG, Osborne D, Bulbulia J. News exposure predicts anti-Muslim prejudice. *PloS one*. 2017;12(3):e0174606. doi:10.1371/journal.pone.0174606
137. Bruneau E, Kteily N. The enemy as animal: Symmetric dehumanization during asymmetric warfare. *PLoS ONE*. 2017;12(7):e0181422. doi:10.1371/journal.pone.0181422
138. Saleem M, Prot S, Anderson CA, Lemieux AF. Exposure to Muslims in media and support for public policies harming Muslims. *Commun Res*. 2017;44(6):841–869. doi:10.1177/0093650215619214
139. Sirin S, Fine M. *Muslim American Youth: Understanding Hyphenated Identities through Multiple Methods*. New York University Press; 2008.
140. Tsfati Y. Hostile media perceptions, presumed media influence, and minority alienation: The case of Arabs in Israel. *J Commun*. 2007;57(4):632–651. doi:10.1111/j.1460-2466.2007.00361.x
141. Cano-Gamez E, Trynka G. From GWAS to function: Using functional genomics to identify the mechanisms underlying complex diseases. *Front Genet*. 2020;11:424. doi:10.3389/fgene.2020.00424
142. Littlefield MB. The media as a system of racialization: Exploring images of African American women and the new racism. *Am Behav Sci*. 2008;51(5):675–685. doi:10.1177/0002764207307747

143. Obermaier M, Schmuck D, Saleem M. I'll be there for you? Effects of Islamophobic online hate speech and counter speech on Muslim in-group bystanders' intention to intervene. *New Media Soc.* 2021;25(9):2339-2358. doi:10.1177/14614448211017527
144. Quintero Johnson JM, Saleem M, Tang L, Ramasubramanian S, Riewestahl E. Media use during COVID-19: An investigation of negative effects on the mental health of Asian versus white Americans. *Front Commun.* 2021;6. doi:10.3389/fcomm.2021.638031
145. Ramasubramanian S, Doshi MJ, Saleem M. Mainstream versus ethnic media: How they shape ethnic pride and self-esteem among ethnic minority audiences. *Int J Commun.* 2017;11: 1879-1899. Accessed April 10, 2025. https://ijoc.org/index.php/ijoc/article/view/6430
146. Kunst JR, Tajamal H, Sam DL, Ulleberg P. Coping with Islamophobia: The effects of religious stigma on Muslim minorities' identity formation. *Int J Intercult Relat.* 2012;36(4):518-532. doi:10.1016/j.ijintrel.2011.12.014
147. Saleem M, Wojcieszak ME, Hawkins I, Li M, Ramasubramanian S. Social identity threats: How media and discrimination affect Muslim Americans' identification as Americans and trust in the US government. *J Commun.* 2019;69(2):214-236. doi:10.1093/joc/jqz001
148. Saleem M, Ramasubramanian S. Muslim Americans' responses to social identity threats: Effects of media representations and experiences of discrimination. *Media Psychol.* 2019;22(3): 373-393. doi:10.1080/15213269.2017.1302345
149. van Zomeren M, Postmes T, Spears R. Toward an integrative social identity model of collective action: A quantitative research synthesis of three socio-psychological perspectives. *Psychol Bull.* 2008;134(4):504-535. doi:10.1037/0033-2909.134.4.504
150. Saleem M, Hawkins I, Wojcieszak ME, Roden J. When and how negative news coverage empowers collective action in minorities. *Commun Res.* 2021;48(2):291-316. doi:10.1177/0093650219877094
151. Patel F. Ending the "national security" excuse for racial and religious profiling. Brennan Center for Justice. July 22, 2021. Accessed December 6, 2023. https://www.brennancenter.org/our-work/analysis-opinion/ending-national-security-excuse-racial-and-religious-profiling
152. Cainkar L. Racial control under the guise of terror threat: Policing of Muslim, Arab, and SWANA communities. *Crit Stud Terrorism* 2023;16(1):152-174. doi:10.1080/17539153.2023.2166194
153. Kasravi N. *Born Suspect: Stop-and-Frisk Abuses and the Continued Fight to End Racial Profiling in America*. National Association for the Advancement of Colored People; 2014. Appendix III. Accessed August 11, 2025. https://search.issuelab.org/resource/born-suspect-stop-and-frisk-abuses-and-the-continued-fight-to-end-racial-profiling-in-america.html
154. Asma-Sadeque S. Fears of increased 'Iranophobia' grip Iranian-American community. *Al Jazeera.* January 29, 2020. Accessed April 10, 2025. https://www.aljazeera.com/news/2020/1/29/fears-of-increased-iranophobia-grip-iranian-american-community
155. Center for Constitutional Rights. National Security Entry-Exit Registration System (NSEERS) Freedom of Information Act (FOIA) Request. 2017. Accessed August 11, 2025. https://ccrjustice.org/node/6205
156. American Civil Liberties Union. National Security Entry-Exit Registration System. Accessed August 11, 2025. https://www.aclu.org/issues/immigrants-rights/immigrants-rights-and-detention/national-security-entry-exit-registration

157. Bridge Initiative. Factsheet: The NYPD Muslim Surveillance and Mapping Program. Georgetown University. May 11, 2020. Accessed August 11, 2025. https://bridge.georgetown.edu/research/factsheet-the-nypd-muslim-surveillance-and-mapping-program
158. Fields G, Nasir N. Muslims recall questionable detentions that followed 9/11. *AP News*. October 4, 2021. Accessed August 11, 2025. https://apnews.com/article/immigration-africa-canada-religion-asia-bf725e0016e88eef2abc73bedd0c5718
159. American Civil Liberties Union. Surveillance ender the USA/PATRIOT Act. October 23, 2021. Accessed August 11, 2025. https://www.aclu.org/documents/surveillance-under-usapatriot-act
160. Electronic Privacy Information Center. PATRIOT Act. Accessed August 9, 2025. https://epic.org/issues/surveillance-oversight/patriot-act
161. American Civil Liberties Union. Myths and realities about the Patriot Act. June 22, 2005. Accessed August 11, 2025. http://www.aclu.org/documents/myths-and-realities-about-patriot-act
162. Binswanger IA, Krueger PM, Steiner JF. Prevalence of chronic medical conditions among jail and prison inmates in the USA compared with the general population. *J Epidemiol Community Health*. 2009;63(11):912–919. doi:10.1136/jech.2009.090662
163. Massoglia M, Pridemore WA. Incarceration and health. *Annu Rev Sociol*. 2015;41(1):291–310. doi:10.1146/annurev-soc-073014-112326
164. Laurencin CT, Walker JM. Racial profiling is a public health and health disparities issue. *J Racial Ethn Health Disparities*. 2020;7(3):393–397. doi:10.1007/s40615-020-00738-2
165. Martin E. Hidden consequences: The impact of incarceration on dependent children. *NIJ J*. 2017;278. Accessed August 11, 2025. https://nij.ojp.gov/topics/articles/hidden-consequences-impact-incarceration-dependent-children
166. Sirin SR, Choi E, Tugberk C. The impact of 9/11 and the War on Terror on Arab and Muslim children and families. *Curr Psychiatry Rep*. 2021;23(8):47. doi:10.1007/s11920-021-01264-6
167. Baumeister RF, Bratslavsky E, Finkenauer C, Vohs KD. Bad is stronger than good. *Rev Gen Psychol*. 2001;5(4):323–370. doi:10.1037/1089-2680.5.4.323
168. Soroka S, Fournier P, Nir L. Cross-national evidence of a negativity bias in psychophysiological reactions to news. *Proc Natl Acad Sci USA*. 2019;116(38):18888–18892. doi:10.1073/pnas.1908369116
169. Murrar S, Brauer M. Entertainment-education effectively reduces prejudice. *Group Processes Intergroup Relat*. 2018;21(7):1053–1077. doi:10.1177/1368430216682350
170. Bruneau E, Kteily N, Laustsen L. The unique effects of blatant dehumanization on attitudes and behavior towards Muslim refugees during the European 'refugee crisis' across four countries. *Eur J Soc Psychol*. 2018;48(5):645–662. doi:10.1002/ejsp.2357
171. Moore-Berg SL, Karpinski A. Race and social class as intersecting social categories. *Soc Psychol*. 2021;52(4):227–237. doi:10.1027/1864-9335/a000451
172. Mann B. After 50 years of the War On Drugs, "What good is it doing for us?" *NPR*. June 17, 2021. Accessed April 11, 2025. https://www.npr.org/2021/06/17/1006495476/after-50-years-of-the-war-on-drugs-what-good-is-it-doing-for-us
173. Abuelezam NN, El-Sayed A, Galea S, Gordon NP. Understanding differences within ethnic group designation: comparing risk factors and health indicators between Iranian and Arab Americans in Northern California. *BMC Public Health*. 2021;21(1):1074. doi:10.1186/s12889-021-11121-z

6

We Are the Ocean

Laufou Jacob Fitisemanu Jr., MPH, Maile Tauali'i, PhD, MPH,
Yvette C. Paulino, PhD, and Fuimaono Nia Aitaoto, PhD, MPH, MS

INTRODUCTION

'O le vasa le alofi—*The ocean is our convening space.*
Samoan: Assertion that the sea is a *connecting space* rather than *a separating void.*

The Pacific Ocean's 25,000 islands are home to Indigenous Pacific Islanders, stewards of one-third of the earth's surface area (see Figure 6-1 and Box 6-1).[1] The islands situated entirely within the Pacific Ocean have historically been described in western geopolitical terms as island groups known as Micronesia, Melanesia, and Polynesia.[2] North of the Equator and east of the Philippines are the islands of Micronesia, which form an arc that spans from Palau, Guam, and the Commonwealth of the Northern Mariana Islands (CNMI) in the west through the Federated States of Micronesia (FSM; formerly the Caroline Islands), Nauru, and the Marshall Islands to Kiribati in the east. In the eastern Pacific, largely enclosed within an invisible triangle formed by the Hawaiian Islands to the north, Aotearoa (New Zealand) to the southwest, and Rapa Nui (Easter Island) far to the east, are the many ("poly") islands of Polynesia. Other components of this widely scattered collection, from west to east, include Tuvalu, Uvea (Wallis), Futuna, Tokelau, Samoa (formerly Western Samoa), American Samoa, Tonga, Niue, the Cook Islands, and French Polynesia (including the Society, Tuamotu, and Marquesas Islands).[3] The great arc of islands located north and east of Australia and south of the Equator is called Melanesia, home to the peoples of New Guinea island, the Bismarck Archipelago, Solomon Islands, Vanuatu (the New Hebrides), New Caledonia, and Fiji. It is important to note that Melanesia is the only subregion in Oceania to be named according to the skin color of the people (from the Greek words *melas* [black] and *nēsos* [island]) and is seen as a negative representation of Melanesians, though there is a movement to "re-present" Melanesia through "Melanesianism" which "embraces the subregion's ethno-linguistic and cultural diversities."[4(p111)]

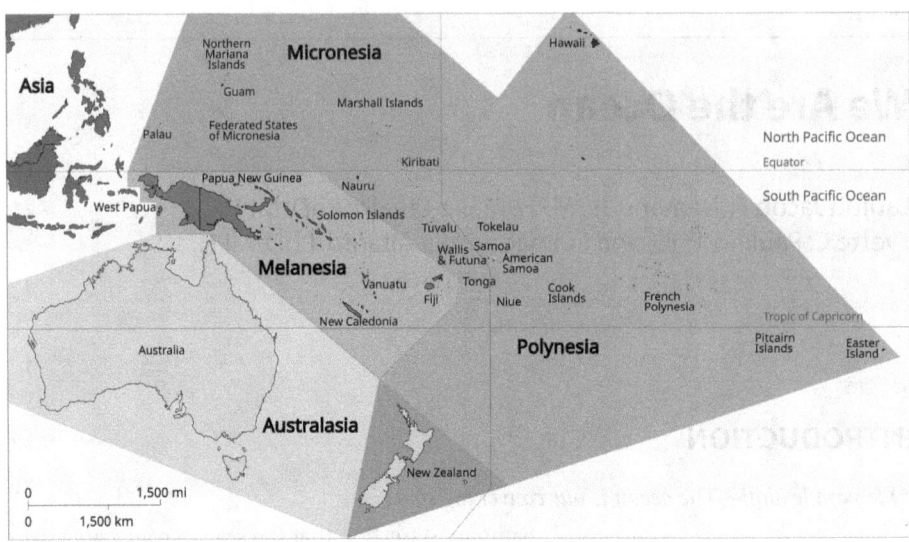

Source: Cruickshanks.[1] Reprinted under the terms of the CC-BY SA license (https://creativecommons.org/licenses/by-sa/3.0/deed.en).

Figure 6-1. We Are Oceania

Oceania is generally considered one of the most colonized, or least decolonized, regions in the world.[5] With the ending of the Trust Territory of the Pacific Islands, the Northern Mariana Islands became a "commonwealth" of the United States, and the new republics of FSM, the Marshall Islands, and Palau signed Compacts of Free Association with the United States. Guam remained an unincorporated territory of the United States and the only island in Micronesia that has yet to exercise political self-determination.[6] Britain's high commissioner in New Zealand continues to administer Pitcairn, and the other former British colonies remain members of the Commonwealth of Nations, recognizing the British King as their titular head of state and vesting certain residual powers in the British government or the King's representative in the islands. Australia did not cede control of the Torres Strait Islands, inhabited by a Melanesian population, or Lord Howe and Norfolk Island, whose residents are of European ancestry. New Zealand retains indirect governance over Niue and Tokelau and has kept close relations with another former possession, the Cook Islands, through a compact of free association. Chile rules Easter Island (Rapa Nui) and Ecuador rules the Galápagos Islands. The Aboriginal peoples of Australia, the Māori of Aotearoa (New Zealand) and the Kānaka Māoli of Hawai'i, despite movements demanding more cultural recognition, greater economic and political considerations, or even outright sovereignty, have remained minorities in countries where massive waves of migration have completely changed their societies.

In his 1994 essay "Our Sea of Islands," the visionary scholar Dr. Epeli Hau'ofa explained that this region can be considered from two perspectives. The external, foreign

Box 6-1. Oceania Facts

- Land area: 3.5 million mi²
- Water area: 63 million mi²
- 25,000 islands
- 1,000+ languages
- 26+ nations and territories
- 44,491,724 population

perspective tends to view Oceania as "islands in a far sea," where islands are tiny specks of land flung out in a vast, expansive sea.[7(p7)] This perspective is widespread in the western academic contexts, where the Pacific region is thought of as a vast but insignificant void between the formidable continents of Asia and the Americas. Another perspective is from those who relate to the region as their ancestral home and are at peace on their islands, as well as with the deep ocean that surrounds them. For these people, the region is Oceania and is known as home, to be a "sea of islands." Dr. Hauʻofa also wrote that "[t]he world of Oceania is not small; it is huge and growing bigger every day," because these islands are still being birthed and are continually growing, along with the knowledge of how to explore Oceania and live in harmony with it.[7(p6)]

Growing imperialism during the 19th century resulted in the occupation and military control of much of the Pacific by European powers, and later Japan and the United States. In 1874, the British took control of Fiji and only three major island groups remained independent in Polynesia: Tonga, Hawaiʻi, and Sāmoa. The Euro-American powers considered all three under their own spheres of interest with Americans taking a specific interest in Hawaiʻi, the British in Tonga, and the Germans, British, and Americans all claiming a right to determine the future of Sāmoa. Hawaiʻi's King Kalākaua understood that inaction would lead to a gradual erosion of Hawaiian independence, so he developed a plan, the Pacific Confederacy (also referred to as the Polynesian Confederacy), to unite the remaining independent Polynesian groups in an explicitly anti-colonial polity based upon their shared cultural and ethnic heritage. This alliance did not materialize. In 1898, the United States illegally annexed Hawaiʻi and in 1899 Germany occupied western Samoa (now the Independent State of Samoa) while the United States claimed eastern Samoa (now American Samoa) through cession treaties signed in 1900 (Tutuila) and 1904 (Manuʻa). Only the Kingdom of Tonga retained independence as the singular example of uninterrupted Indigenous governance in the Pacific. In the western Pacific, the United States gained control of Guam from Spain in 1898.[8] Germany possessed the Northern Mariana Islands, creating the division between Guam and the northern islands of the Mariana Islands, and acquired other islands in Micronesia through the German–Spanish Treaty of 1899. During World War I, Japan took the Northern Mariana Islands and the rest of the islands in Micronesia. Japan controlled most of the western region during the Pacific War (World War II); however, by the end of that war, Japan

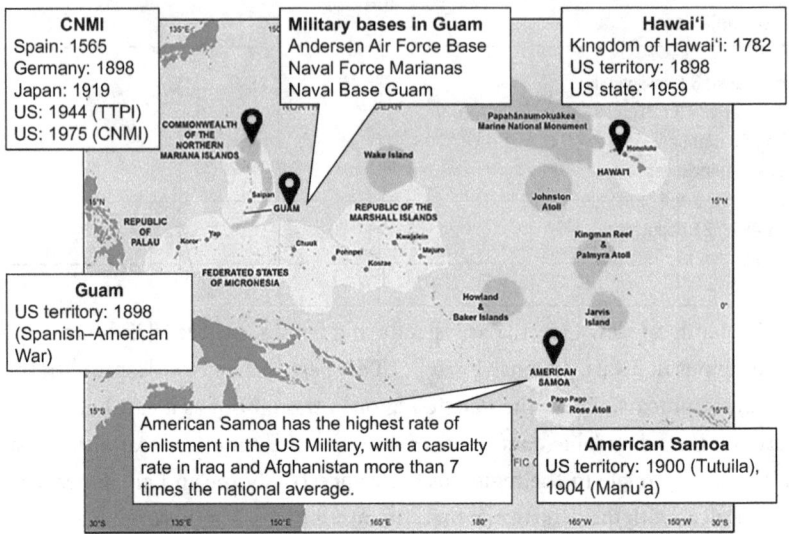

Source: Pacific Islander Center for Primary Care Excellence. Adapted with permission.
Note: CNMI = Commonwealth of the Northern Mariana Islands; TTPI = Trust Territory of the Pacific Islands.
Figure 6-2. US Political Relationships in the Pacific

was defeated and islands under its control came under the control of the United States.[9] The United Nations placed the islands, with the exception of Guam, under a trusteeship known as the Trust Territory of the Pacific Islands, administered by the United States.[10]

Though the Pacific Confederacy was not borne to fruition, it and similar events have reshaped the understanding of Pacific Islanders from "colonial encounter" to people who actively engaged and sought to shape regional and global networks by developing and engineering relationships between different island groups. This created a more complex, less colonially derived understanding of Pacific peoples and allows another dimension through which we can understand and rethink the field of world history itself. See Figure 6-2 for a map of US political relationships in the Pacific.

VISIBILITY AND REPRESENTATION IN DATA

Ko hai ho hingoa?—Who is your name?
                    Tongan: Emphasizing the semantic construct of names
                    as living entities rather than inanimate labels.

In the United States, *Native Hawaiian or Other Pacific Islander* was one of the six racial and ethnic groups created after the US Office of Management and Budget (OMB) issued a federal register notice, "Revisions to the Standards for the Classification of Federal Data on Race and Ethnicity," in 1997 that separated the Asian and *Native Hawaiian or Other*

Pacific Islander (*NHOPI*) racial categories. In 2024, "Other" was removed from the category, creating the term *Native Hawaiian or Pacific Islander* (*NH/PI*). The revised OMB directive defines *NH/PI* as people having origins in any of the original peoples of Hawai'i, Guam, Samoa, or other Pacific Islands. While disaggregation of the NH/PI and Asian categories is helpful, the definition created by the OMB directive does little to acknowledge the heterogeneity of the vastly diverse peoples, languages, cultures, worldviews, and demographics that are combined into the NH/PI category. It is therefore imperative that disaggregation of Oceanic cultural identities *within* the federal NH/PI designation be promoted along with disaggregation from the Asian category. Data gaps will continue to persist as long as OMB and Census categorizations fail to acknowledge the granular realities that are rendered statistically invisible when combined into a seemingly homogenous grouping. It should be a prioritized goal to revise and optimize the federal designation to promote accurate, granular data collection to better understand protective factors, disease prevalence, and lived experiences for each group. In order to account for multiracial NH/PIs, improved efforts are also needed to ensure that federal datasets reporting NH/PI "alone and in combination" are tabulated and made accessible for all datasets that are reported for NH/PI "alone." See Figure 6-3 for a current NH/PI population map of the United States.[11]

In addition to the difficulty of accurately characterizing NH/PI identities through existing demographic categories, the population data landscape is further complicated by the need to account for multiple legal residence statuses, some of which are unique to NH/PIs. Because of the turbulent histories of American imperialism, colonization, and militarization, the nation states of Oceania have come to affiliate with the United States through different mechanisms, and these geopolitical relationships have direct impacts on how NH/PIs interface (or don't interface) with US health systems. Depending on their place of origin/residence, NH/PIs can fall under various immigration statuses, including US citizens, immigrants, permanent residents, citizens of Compact of Free Association (COFA) nations, and US nationals. American Samoa has the singular standing as the only American territory where US citizenship is not extended at birth; rather, people born in American Samoa are considered US nationals, not US *citizens*, a distinction that some American Samoans believe gives them second-class status. Unlike American Samoa, FSM, the Republic of the Marshall Islands, and the Republic of Palau are not American territories, but autonomous sovereign nations with treaty relationships through COFA. This free association arrangement permits citizens of COFA signatory nations to lawfully reside in the United States but does not grant the same status as a *lawful permanent resident*. Until Congressional action restored Medicaid eligibility for COFA citizens in 2020,[12] thousands of legal nonimmigrants were barred from accessing Medicaid coverage for over 20 years.[13] The decades-long struggle to reinstate Medicaid eligibility for Micronesians from COFA signatory nations is just one example of how the immigration system privileges certain legal statuses over others, and how these distinctions directly contribute to inequitable access to health services.

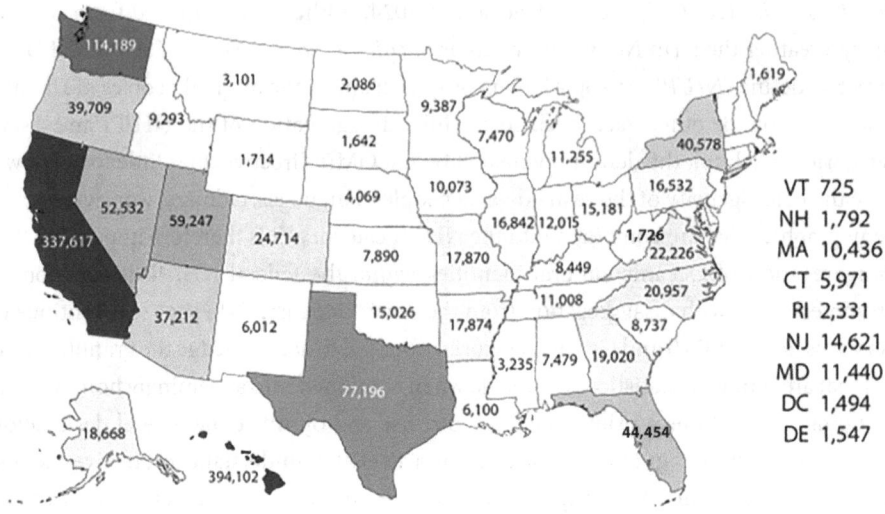

Source: Prior.[11] Reprinted with permission of Kem C. Gardner Policy Institute, University of Utah.

Note: NH/PI = Native Hawaiian or Pacific Islander. States with the highest number of NH/PIs include Hawai'i, California, Washington, Texas, and Utah (67% of US NH/PI population). The NH/PI population is among the fastest growing populations, with a 30% increase since the 2010 Census. The US NH/PI population is expected to double by 2050.

Figure 6-3. US NH/PI Population by State, 2020

HEALTH, WELLNESS, AND WISDOM ACROSS TIME AND SPACE

'A'ohe Pau ka 'Ike i ka Hālau Ho'okahi—Not all knowledge is taught in the same school.
Hawaiian: Encouraging knowledge seeking
and information sharing from diverse sources.

Prior to contact with the western world, the peoples of Moana Nui (a term with cognate analogs in many Polynesian languages referring to the Pacific Ocean) were reported to be strong, healthy, and statuesque. Demonstration of this health is evident in the human population expansion and growth as deep-sea voyagers navigated the largest ocean on the earth and established societies with populations numbering in the hundreds of thousands. See Box 6-2 for a list of select societal achievements. It is estimated that the average lifespan of Pacific Islanders in precolonial contexts was seemingly as high as 70 or 80 years. By contrast, the typical life expectancy of British contemporaries was closer to 40 or 50 years. Early documentation by western explorers describes the incredible health of Oceanic ancestors. During Captain James Cook's contact with the islands, he documents that "old men are often to be seen" and goes on to cite a specific story of "the oldest looking man that any of the party had ever seen, and they thought he could not be short of 100 years old."[14(p721)] Today, the life expectancy of NH/PIs in the United States is slightly higher than the US average (76 years) and comparable to the

Box 6-2. Notable Achievements of Oceania Peoples

- The ancestors of today's CHamoru were the first explorers to conduct transoceanic travel in the western Pacific region.
- 'Iolani Palace in Hawai'i had electricity before the White House.
- Tonga was the only Oceanian nation to maintain native sovereignty and avoid foreign colonization.
- Hawaiian-language newspapers were the first in the United States to use colored ink.
- Samoa's Mau a Pule independence movement espoused civil disobedience in the early 1900s, ahead of better-known nonviolent social movements in India and the United States.
- Within 13 years of the introduction of written language, Hawai'i had a 91% literacy rate—an achievement unparalleled in the world.
- The Māori of Aotearoa/New Zealand were the first to discover subantarctic islands including Maungahuka (Auckland Islands) and Tini Heke (Snares Islands).
- Ceremonial and commercial exchange networks spanning hundreds of miles (such as the Melanesian "Kula exchange") have operated for centuries throughout Oceania.
- King Kalakaua of Hawai'i was the first sovereign monarch to circumnavigate the earth.

United Kingdom (80 years).[15,16] Life expectancy, which varies across the Pacific from 64 years in Nauru to 77 years for Native Hawaiians in Hawai'i, is impacted by many determinants such as diet.

The traditional Oceanic diet was acclaimed as the source of the active vitality and robust physiques noted by nearly every foreign observer who encountered NH/PIs during the Age of (European) Exploration. Accounts of early colonial foodways almost universally describe the Indigenous diet as varied and nutritious, with the largest proportion of calories provided by plant foods. Indeed, Joseph Banks of the Cook Expedition asserted that the native diet was so "productive of sound health" that it rendered "physicians almost useless."[17(p347)] University of Hawai'i analyses suggest the nutritional composition of caloric intake at the time of European contact was roughly 78% carbohydrate, 10% fat, and 12% protein.[18] Another assessment revealed that a neotraditional Samoan diet was strongly associated with decreased abdominal circumference and healthier high-density lipoprotein cholesterol levels.[19] By comparison, the typical American diet today consists of 45% carbohydrates, 40% fat, and 15% protein.[20] Many of the ancestral foods cultivated throughout Oceania are touted for their healthy properties today, such as taro poi (probiotic and hypoallergenic starch),[21] breadfruit (gluten free, complete protein),[22] and coconut haustorium (nutrient rich, lactose free).[23]

The restoration and revitalization of traditional foods and foodways is prolific among NH/PI communities, both in the islands and where the diaspora has led them. Motivated by the high rates of metabolic illness, NH/PI researchers and health providers investigated the impact of returning to a traditional pre-contact diet. The late Dr. Noa Emmett Aluli is revered for his legacy of the protection and preservation of land, famous for living by the motto of "the health of the land, is the health of our people, is the health of our nation." But his work on the Moloka'i Heart Study and the Moloka'i Diet is what birthed

> **Box 6-3. Case Studies: Restoring Traditional Food and Lifestyle**
>
> **Hoʻoulu ʻĀina** is a 100-acre nature preserve nestled in the back of Kalihi valley on the island of Oʻahu, cared for by Kōkua Kalihi Valley Comprehensive Family Services, a nonprofit community health center and Federally Qualified Health Center. Through 4 interwoven program areas, Hoʻoulu ʻĀina seeks to provide people of their *ahupuaʻa* (land division) and beyond the freedom to make connections and build meaningful relationships with the *ʻāina* (land), each other, and themselves. Here, the community comes together around forest, food, knowledge, spirituality, and healthy activity.[26]
>
> **Paepae o Heʻeia** is a private nonprofit organization dedicated to caring for Heʻeia Fishpond – an ancient Hawaiian fishpond located in Heʻeia Uli, Koʻolaupoko, Oʻahu. Their vision is to perpetuate a foundation of cultural sustainability for communities (*ʻohana*) of Hawaiʻi through education. Their mission is to implement values and concepts from the model of a traditional fishpond to provide intellectual, physical, and spiritual sustenance for our community.[27]

the movement to cultivate and immerse Native Hawaiians in traditional food systems to reverse the impact of the Western/colonial diet.[24,25]

Today there are countless nonprofit organizations, health care systems, community groups, schools, and families who are actively working to restore NHs/PIs to traditional food and lifestyle, due to the overwhelming evidence that it restores the health of the people (see Box 6-3).[26,27] Both land and sea are food-cultivating systems used in the arsenal to fight the epidemic proportions of metabolic illnesses in the NH/PI community. Unfortunately, there are many barriers that inhibit and hinder this lifesaving work. Water restrictions, rising sea levels, climate change, the prioritization of tourism, lack of land availability, toxic chemicals, unexploded ordinances from military test bombing, and damage caused by military testing are just a few of the challenges that NH/PI communities face when working for traditional food restoration.

The restoration of traditional food systems and the revival of lifestyles that approach the level of physical activity of NH/PI ancestors will be instrumental in revitalizing wellness among NH/PIs living in Oceania and the continental United States.

Jede ak eō—Look up to the frigate bird.
> Marshallese: Advisement to learn from experienced, knowledgeable sources; frigate birds were used as navigational aids as their flight paths indicated the direction and proximity of land.

The peoples of Oceania have knowledge as profound as the ocean that surrounds them. Knowledge of sustainability and resourcefulness is the result of a thousand years of development on untouched land and ocean highways navigated by technical skill and empirical wisdom accumulated over generations of scientific exploration, observation, and experimentation. Concepts of conservation originate in islands where water is sacred, and land is family. Indeed, the CHamoru names of some of the villages in Guam originate from the body parts of Puntan, a deified ancestor whose body became the island. Ancient Indigenous practices of agriculture, land tenure, and aquaculture that have sustainably maintained entirely self-sufficient island societies for centuries have recently been "discovered" by modern science and acknowledged as best practices in natural conservation. Indigenous islander knowledge is also being tapped by modern science sectors, who are excited to understand the practical relevance of substances and practices that have been long understood in island communities. For example, promising research into the antiretroviral properties of prostratin—derived from the Samoan *mamala* folk remedy for treating hepatitis—may lead to advancements in the treatment of AIDS.[28]

The prostratin research and clinical trials are also a pioneering example of a research approach that acknowledges Indigenous knowledge holders as stakeholders and collaborators, rather than just subjects or informants; in this case, legal arrangements have been negotiated to protect the intellectual property of Samoa by ensuring that the people of Samoa will share in the proceeds of any commercial pharmaceutical products that may be derived from prostratin. A similar example is the recent "discovery" that traditional Oceanic architecture and house-building practices are more resistant to cyclones than some western housing structures, prompting modern architects to adapt some of the weather-resistant features of traditional homes (such as Vanuatuan *nakamal* and Samoan *fale*) into contemporary buildings.[29,30]

IMPACTS OF COLONIZATION, OCCUPATION, AND DISENFRANCHISEMENT

Keleun ieng soupeidi—Upright like a hibiscus tree in the wind.
            Pohnpeian: Praising those who maintain dignity
            in resistance to external forces.

Despite having thrived in Oceania for millennia, NH/PIs face continual and increasing pressures to abandon their island homes to join the growing diasporic communities on the US mainland. Hawai'i, for example, ranks fourth in the nation for percent population decline[31] with an average of over 11,500 net out-migrants leaving for the continental United States.[32] Some of these pressures, such as limited opportunities for social mobility and economic development, lead many NH/PIs from island territories to join the US military, with the prospect of professional skills training, higher education benefits, and steady income that often exceeds other employment options on-island. American Samoa (governed by the US Navy 1900–1951) and the Freely Associated States (under US governance 1947–1986; Palau until 1994) are recognized as having the highest military enlistment rates per capita, and soldiers from these areas have experienced some of the highest casualty rates in US conflicts in the Middle East.[33] Based on recruiting data from 2003, Pacific Islander Americans were 249% overrepresented in the military.[34] Beside disproportionately exposing NH/PI soldiers to the atrocities of war, the United States used several Pacific islands to test nuclear weapons and military occupation of island homelands like Hawai'i and Guam continues to prohibit customary utilization of natural resources, restrict access to culturally significant places and arable land, pollute potable water, destroy marine life, and interfere with traditional aquaculture—all of which have deleterious effects on individual and social wellness.[35] Between 1946 and 1958, the United States used the Marshall Islands as an atom bomb testing ground. During that time, 67 atomic bombs were dropped in the islands, on and around the atolls of Bikini, Enewetak, Rongelap, and Utrik.[36] As a result, these islands are unhabitable, and residents were forced to migrate to other islands and the United States. Furthermore, radioactive waste, soil, and ordnance remain scattered around the islands. On Runit Island, 3.1 million cubic meters of irradiated waste is precariously stored in a massive hole covered by concrete, an unsustainable solution which is not being urgently addressed, even as the makeshift receptacle leaks waste into the surrounding oceanic environment.

The widespread militarization of parts of Oceania—such as Guam, where the US military owns roughly one-third of the island's land area—has led to significant loss of customary land in order to build airfields, housing barracks, and military facilities. Military occupation not only displaces Indigenous residents but prevents the traditional utilization of arable land and prohibits wellness-promoting practices tied to ancestral spaces and sustainable agriculture and animal husbandry. The impacts of militarization on the public health of Oceania are serious and long reaching. Military activities in Hawai'i (where the US military controls >200,000 acres) include hundreds of toxic military sites that have destroyed landscapes and poisoned potable water sources.[37,38] In Guam, military activities on the northern half of the island have contributed to groundwater pollution, forcing the closure of several wells in the Northern Guam Lens Aquifer which supplies approximately 80% of the island's drinking water.[39] Atomic weapon detonation testing (and nuclear waste storage) in the Marshall Islands (by the US) and French Polynesia (by France) caused irreparably devastating impacts on the resident populations, including the exposure of over 100,000 Oceanian people to radioactive fallout. In 2023, Bill S.1751 was introduced in Congress to amend the Radiation Exposure Compensation Act to add Guam, thereby making radiation survivors from Guam eligible for compensation.[40] Although the bill was unsuccessful, residents of Guam, including Guam's representative to Congress and the Pacific Association for Radiation Survivors advocacy group, continue to fight for the amendment.

Cultural and linguistic genocide, combined with immigration and occupation, have created societies where Indigenous NH/PIs are minorities in their own homelands and/or where native languages are no longer the daily means of communication (e.g., Hawai'i, Aotearoa/New Zealand, Guam, French Polynesia, New Caledonia, Rapa Nui/Easter Island). These dynamics contribute to culture clashes, alienation, and imposter syndrome which impact individual and social wellness as people and communities strive to walk (often in isolation) in multiple realities with conflicting standards of excellence and indicators of success.[41] The pressure to preserve and embody ancestral values, language, and cultural traits while pursuing success and achievement as defined by colonially imposed cultural norms contributes to the allostatic load in ways that can negatively impact health.[42] The imposition of non-native economic systems that rely on cash transactions and introduced market goods/services have detrimentally contributed to the foodways of Oceania in ways that elevate the prestige and reliance on imported (often processed) foods that rely on foreign supply chains, while devaluing the nutrient-dense, natural foods that have been a source of nutrition and livelihood for millennia. People who would otherwise be able to assume a local trade and raise a family among their ancestral lands are subjected to the daily pressures of market competition and foreign measures of success, which frequently cause NH/PIs to seek higher education or corporate trajectories in stress-inducing contexts where many feel an expectation to sacrifice Indigenous language, culture, and worldview to achieve mainstream indicators of success.

THE UMBRELLA OF (IN)VISIBILITY: HOW MARGINALIZATION PERPETUATES INEQUITIES

Hiaʻ rā he ta ma hiaʻ la faʻ—Press on the branch until it breaks.
                    Rotuman: Expression of commitment to seeing
                    an objective through to completion.

In 1977, OMB created for the first time racial and ethnic categories for federal data collection and reporting; one of which was *Asian or Pacific Islander*, or *API*. This aggregated identifier brought multiple populations together in one category.[43] In 1997, in response to significant efforts by NH/PI advocates, OMB revised the standards for the classification of federal data on race and ethnicity. These revisions included splitting the racial category *Asian or Pacific Islander* into two categories, *Asian* and *Native Hawaiian or Other Pacific Islander*.[44] Major reasons for disaggregation included the following:

1. The need to identify health disparities and issues within Native Hawaiian and Pacific Islander populations apart from Asian populations within the United States.
2. The need to recognize and protect the unique relationship and political status that Native Hawaiians and certain other Pacific Islanders have with the United States.

OMB standards are intended to apply to all federally collected data and reporting in the following areas: education, the national census, medical research, disease statistics, zoning for Congressional districts, the Voting Rights Act, and compliance with federal law and statutory regulations. In addition, many private and nonprofit agencies, such as the Joint Commission, encourage the use, at a minimum, of the race and ethnicity categories from the OMB.

Table 6-1 lists the common acronyms, definitions, and sources used in policy and programs associated with NH/PIs.[43-52] While these acronyms are presented in the order they appear in legislation or official federal guidance, they are not preclusive or subsuming of

Table 6-1. Acronyms in Common Usage

Acronym/Label	Definition
native Hawaiian	≥50% blood quantum Native Hawaiian (lowercase "n" specifically used in the definition).[45]
AAPI	Asian American or Pacific Islander. The federal government defines the term *AAPI* to include "all people of Asian, Asian American, or Pacific Islander ancestry who trace their origins to the countries, states, jurisdictions and/or the diasporic communities of these geographic regions."[46] The pan-racial identity of *Asian American* was created in the 1960s. Chinese American, Filipino American, and Japanese American college students in the SF Bay Area were concerned with the living conditions in primarily Asian American residential areas and took inspiration from the advances made by the Black Civil Rights Movement.[47]
Native American	Defined by the Native American Programs Act of 1974 as "American Indians, Native Hawaiians, other Native American Pacific Islanders (including American Samoan Natives), and Alaska Natives." In that legislation the definitions include the following: "'Native Hawaiian' means any individual any of whose ancestors were natives of the area which consists of the Hawaiian Islands prior to 1778" and "'Native American Pacific Islanders' means an individual who is Indigenous to a [US] territory or possession located in the Pacific Ocean, and includes such individual while residing in the [US]."[48]
API	In 1977, OMB created racial and ethnic categories for federal data collection and reporting, one of which was *Asian or Pacific Islander*, or *API*.[43]
NHOPI	In 1997, OMB separated this API aggregation into two distinct groups: those of Asian descent (A) and those of *Native Hawaiian and Other Pacific Islander* descent (*NHOPI*).[44]
COFA	Agreements between the US and the Pacific Island sovereign states of FSM (Chuuk, Kosrae, Pohnpei, and Yap), the Republic of the Marshall Islands, and the Republic of Palau, collectively known as FAS. COFA allows FAS citizens to access federal programs and travel freely to and access opportunities in the US and its territories. In return, the US assumes responsibility for the defense of FAS and can utilize the land for military purposes. As per this agreement, the US provides economic assistance to FAS.[49,50] Since its first enactment, COFA has been amended or renewed a few times. In March 2024, Congress renewed the renegotiated COFA agreements for $7.1 billion in economic assistance over the next 20 years.[51]
NH/PI	As of March 2024, OMB announced revisions for race and ethnicity statistical standards. "Other" was removed from *Native Hawaiian or Other Pacific Islander*, creating the term *NH/PI*.[52]

Note: COFA = Compact of Free Association; FAS = Freely Associated States; FSM = Federated States of Micronesia; OMB = US Office of Management and Budget; SF = San Francisco, California.

preceding terms, nor are they representative terms. The racial category *NH/PI* is complex because it represents a people that collectively span the spectrum of both Indigenous to the United States and immigrants to this country, with all the complex relationships in policies those expansive definitions cover. And none of these acronyms are representative of how any NH/PI group refers to themselves. These are simply terms we have unfortunately been labeled with, usually inaccurately. Based on consultation with community organizations and advocates, *NH/PI* is the preferred acronym used in this chapter (while other acronyms are cited throughout).

Today, the implementation of this policy continues, sometimes with difficulty, both within the federal government and within private sector organizations and institutions which undertake and report on research involving populations within the United States. The former API category has continued to be used along with a newer *Asian American or Pacific Islander (AAPI)* identifier, yet neither category is recognized by OMB as an appropriate federal definer of a class of people or a racial grouping. The negative impacts of continued use of an API category are considerable both for Asian and for NH/PI populations.

When a small racial group is combined with another larger racial group, the status of the large group can skew the data and mask the status of the smaller group. An example of masking is seen in the age-adjusted death rate for Asians and/or Pacific Islanders, which is 350 per 100,000 (524/100,000 for the total US population), while the age-adjusted death rate for Native Hawaiians, a subset of the Pacific Island group, is 901 per 100,000. Even more alarming are the statistics for individuals who identify as Native Hawaiian alone (disaggregated from those who identify as Native Hawaiians and ≥1 other race), which is 2,200 per 100,000.[53] Justification for racial category aggregation is limited and weak. With technological advances, the ability to record, track, and report on smaller populations is not only possible but also essential for identifying and addressing identified health issues in the populations. The continued use of a combined API category has negative impacts on both Asian and NH/PI populations. A case study highlighting the issue of data disaggregation can be found in Box 6-4.[54]

One of the most egregious consequences of aggregating Asians and NH/PIs is the creation of an image in the public eye of a monolithic Asian Pacific Islander identity that inaccurately depicts Asians and NH/PIs as a single, homogenous community. Dozens of Asian-serving organizations exist across the United States that use nebulous terminology like *Asian Pacific, Asian Pacific Islander, Asian Pacific American*, and more to name their organizations and articulate their mission statements, but such entities (with very few exceptions) are overwhelmingly Asian in the composition of their leadership, membership, and service populations. The fact that the US Asian population is 15 times larger than the NH/PI population means that NH/PIs are always numerically disadvantaged and statistically underrepresented when aggregated with Asians, which makes acquisition of resources, requests for competitive grant funding, and political representation even harder to attain.[31] Policymakers and resource distributors need to be more informed of the implications of allocating funding for Asians *and* NH/PIs to entities that have little capacity or interest in serving NH/PIs.

So long as funders (including federal, state, and local governments) continue to disburse funding for combined Asian and NH/PI communities, guardrails should be

Box 6-4. Case Study: It's Not Just Data Disaggregation

An example of the harms that are experienced via a lack of data disaggregation is teen pregnancy and infant mortality rates which are conflated in *API* designations.

When the Utah Department of Health first disaggregated Asian and NH/PI birth outcomes data, drastic disparities were revealed that had long been rendered statistically invisible. In 2015, only 42% of NH/PI mothers in Utah had received prenatal care services in the first trimester of pregnancy (compared with 74.2% statewide) and the NH/PI infant mortality rate was 10.5 deaths per 1,000 live births (more than twice as high as the state average). The alarming rate of infant death and lack of prenatal care among NH/PI mothers prompted the first statewide BRFSS study conducted in English, Tongan, and Samoan. The larger sample sizes and improved self-response options of this study provided unprecedented data insights and statistical significance that had not been previously possible, even with data pooling of survey samples over multiple years.

These findings were used in close collaboration with NH/PI community partners and advisors to inform the development of an evidence-based intervention delivered through a culture-based framework called "It Takes a Village: Giving Our Babies the Best Chance." This program was piloted in 2015 and has since been recognized as a promising practice by AMCHP in 2018, and formal evaluation has demonstrated that It Takes a Village "effectively raised awareness, improved knowledge, and increased self-efficacy" for addressing maternal and infant health among NH/PIs. The project continues to be successfully implemented by NH/PI partner organizations.[54]

Note: AMCHP = Association of Maternal & Child Health Programs; API = Asian or Pacific Islander; BRFSS = Behavioral Risk Factor Surveillance System; NH/PI = Native Hawaiian or Pacific Islander.

instituted that require grantees to demonstrate meaningful (not just "equitable") engagement of NH/PIs and Asians. A case study discussing the impact of disaggregated data on health intervention is found in Box 6-5.[55] Funding allocation decisions should also take the relative gravity of health disparities into consideration and not just sheer population size. As an example, the Type 2 diabetes prevalence rate among NH/PIs is significantly higher than among Asians, but because the total Asian population is many times larger, there are more Asians diagnosed with diabetes than NH/PIs. When funders seek to address health disparities, it is critical that small populations with serious disparities, like NH/PIs with diabetes, not be dismissed in favor of large populations that are more numerous but may have less serious disparities.

"POVERTY" AND FINANCIAL SECURITY

Angang chok aramas—Success is achieved through collaboration.
            Chuukese: Admonition to work together to achieve mutual benefit for all.

Conventional definitions of poverty aren't always shared between and within communities, especially since the term itself is associated with stigmatized connotations and moral judgments. Ancestral notions of wealth and income in Oceania frequently

Box 6-5. Case Study: Visibility Enables Action

> Inconsistent data collection and reporting standards are a significant barrier to accurately understanding NH/PI health indicators, and therefore an impediment to informing intervention. The challenges encountered by the NHPI Data Policy Lab (coordinated by the UCLA Center for Health Policy Research) while compiling COVID-19 morbidity and mortality data illustrate the barriers posed by inconsistent data standards. Compilation and monitoring of data initially required lab members to manually locate and decipher all state-level COVID-19 websites. This required significant amounts of time and effort due to the frequent changes in state reporting sites and the data collection quality check process which required entries to be verified by separate lab members. According to Calvin Chang of the NHPI Data Policy Lab, "the presentation of data gaps, where states were not reporting a disaggregated NH/PI category, also posed unique challenges. Traditional data visualizations focus on only displaying data that exists and suppressing areas where data does not. Compiling this data required manually examining each state dashboard that did not report disaggregated NH/PI COVID-19 data to determine whether NH/PI data was being explicitly aggregated under an 'Asian Pacific Islander' or 'Other' category or if it could not be determined if any NH/PI data was being reported. These states had to be checked regularly, in addition to states that were already reporting disaggregated NH/PI data, to track changes in how NH/PI data was being reported" (email, May 21, 2023). These dynamics of changing parameters, data suppression/omission, and datasets with varying race categorizations all contribute to the difficulty of obtaining reliable data with which to inform interventions and policies to address determinants of health for NH/PIs.
>
> The efforts of the NHPI Data Policy Lab are also an example of the positive impact that accurate, disaggregated data can have on policy prioritization of NH/PIs and funding allocation to NH/PI communities. A study published by the lab in May 2021 highlighted that the COVID-19 death rate for NH/PIs in California (123/100,000) was higher than the overall state death rate (84/100,000) and the Asian category death rate (74/100,000).[55] Additionally, the study showed that 7 Asian groups exceeded the aggregate Asian and state averages, and that among NH/PIs, the death rate among Samoans was considerably higher than the aggregate NH/PI rate. None of these disparities would have been evident unless Asian and NH/PI data were disaggregated. In many states, NH/PI populations were not considered a priority population for COVID-19 vaccination and testing because NH/PI data were combined (and rendered invisible) within combined "Asian and Pacific Islander" categories. In states and counties where disaggregated data were collected, the dismal disparities in case rates, hospitalizations, and deaths were clear, allowing NH/PIs to advocate for heightened prioritization and increased access to resources to mitigate the disproportionate impacts of the pandemic on NH/PIs.

Note: NH/PI = Native Hawaiian or Pacific Islander; UCLA = University of California, Los Angeles.

applied to *communal* substance and mutual benefit, and were often measured in terms of generosity, redistribution, and shared surplus, rather than accumulation. Social functions like weddings and funerals served multiple roles of strengthening human relationships, exchanging goods and services, and redistributing surplus resources. If wealth was measured in terms of sharing and extensive social networks, then poverty could be defined as the lack of strong reciprocal relationships. Village/clan/family systems based on subsistence farming and communal network economies frequently clash with introduced "modern" financial systems based on profit maximization, cash economy, and commodification. The incongruence of these value systems has profound impacts on health, especially notions of mental health related to perceived self-worth and self-image. Some of the highest rates of suicide have been reported in Pacific island countries such as Kiribati (30.6/100,000 population), Micronesia (29/100,000), Vanuatu (21/100,000), Solomon Islands (17.4/100,000), Samoa (14.6/100,000), Australia (11.3/100,000), New Zealand (10.3/100,000), and Fiji (9.5/100,000), all of which were above the 2019 global age-standardized suicide rate of 9.0 per 100,000.[56] Pacific Islander youth are at high risk for suicide and suicide attempts.[57] Suicide rates reached epidemic proportions in Oceania in correlation with modernizing cultural changes that drastically changed social roles and expectation in ways that devalued Indigenous wealth and service and esteemed foreign concepts of economic success and worth.[58] The alarmingly high rates of suicide and suicide attempts among NH/PIs are indicative of the complex dynamics between individual wellness, community health, and cultural resilience, and emphasize the critical need for systems-level monitoring, prevention, and intervention efforts.

Conspicuous consumption based on the commodification of introduced foreign prestige goods has major impacts on financial wellness in ways that can perpetuate cycles of overspending and debt to fulfill social obligations. This is relevant to the NH/PI experience in the United States because of the strong correlation between food insecurity (and nutrition-related health status) and financial insecurity.[59] While ostentatious gift-giving and lavish social functions are rooted in values of generosity and reciprocity, the overextension of certain social practices can impact socioeconomic stability and (if viewed negatively by younger generations) can discourage the perpetuation of cultural practices that may be seen as overly burdensome. Tongan funerary customs typically include exchanges of money, food, woven mats, and other textiles between the extended families of the deceased. These ritual exchanges can sometimes become so extravagant as to become financially burdensome[60]; it is not unheard of for some families to accumulate significant debt or forgo mortgage or utility payments to meet family obligations. The existence of robust cultural safety nets provided by communal resource sharing practices can be a protective factor, but there are instances where such customs may negatively impact the ability to afford health insurance or needed health services.

INTERSECTING SYSTEMS OF OPPRESSION AND INEQUITY

Housing and Homelessness/Houselessness

Indigenous peoples are considered traditional stewards of the lands they inherit from prior generations. The perpetuation of this stewardship is at risk when Indigenous peoples are dispossessed of their ancestral lands. In 2018, the United Nations held its 17th session of the Permanent Forum on Indigenous Issues focused on Indigenous peoples' collective rights to lands, territories, and resources, which was fitting considering at the time an estimated 370 million around the world were being dispossessed of their ancestral lands.[61] The Reverend Joaquin Flores Sablan from Guam once stated, "Land ownership was the greatest security, particularly inherited property which they treated as a sacred trust from their parents. To part with the land was the same as committing suicide."[62(p142)] The displacement from ancestral lands, whether forced through militarization, rising cost in real estate, or natural hazards, poses significant challenges for NH/PIs (who may, and often do, retain Indigenous identities as immigrants or refugees residing away from their ancestral home islands).

While *homelessness* and *houselessness* are often used interchangeably, the term *houselessness* can highlight the distinction between a *house* (a physical structure) and a *home* (a place of belonging and community). *Houselessness* can also encompass individuals living in nontraditional shelters like vehicles, while *homelessness* is often associated with living on the streets or in emergency shelters. Ultimately, both terms describe a lack of stable housing. Homelessness, and more recently houselessness, in the United States has increased 6% since 2017, and NH/PIs experienced the highest rate (171/10,000) followed by American Indian, Alaska Native, or Indigenous (83/10,000); Black, African American, or African (59/10,000); Hispanic/Latino (29/10,000); white (15/10,000); multiracial (13/10,000); and Asian or Asian American (6/10,000).[63] This pattern of homelessness is seen across the native homelands of NH/PIs. In 2023, Hawaii was reported to have the 4th highest state homelessness rate in the United States.[64] The recent Maui fires have only further exacerbated homelessness in Hawai'i. Saipan in the Northern Mariana Islands experienced a record high of homelessness in 2018, a 637% increase from the previous year, after Super-typhoon Yutu.[65] Guam's annual point-in-time count revealed an increase from 790 homeless individuals before the COVID-19 pandemic in 2020 to 1,087 in 2022.[66]

Economics

The stewardship of land and natural resources has helped to balance and sustain the economies of Indigenous communities, but this balance was interrupted when communities shifted from a subsistence economy to a cash economy. In most of the Pacific Islands, subsistence was primarily based on farming and fishing. Indigenous NH/PI communities thrived on Indigenous economies such as trade networks among islands. For example, the Indigenous economic systems in Micronesia were based on kinship relations that involved the exchange of food, goods, and tributes between larger islands and smaller islands within an archipelago chain. Within the Micronesian island chain of Yap, the main island of Yap would receive tribute goods such as shells, mats, and coconut oil from the smaller outer lying islands of Ulithi and Namonuito who were also distantly related to each other. The main island of Yap would reciprocate in kind by providing bananas, taro, breadfruit, and other crops, which were usually harder to grow in the outer island areas.

> **Box 6-6. Case Study: Disproportionate Economic Burden of Basic Costs of Living**
>
> In the US-affiliated Pacific Islands, high shipping and import costs raise living expenses.[69] In FSM, 39%–54% of household budgets are devoted to food costs, significantly surpassing the 10%–15% average in the United States.[70] To cope with these expenses, many FSM households rely on remittances from relatives working abroad, including places like Guam or the mainland US. Economic aggregate data shows that each FSM household receives, on average, $840 in remittances each year.[70]

Note: FSM = Federated States of Micronesia.

This system stabilized interisland networks, food security, and resource management in the region.[67]

Wage-based labor was introduced as subsistence living was replaced with a cash economy. New costs such as land taxes forced people into employment for wages and away from farming. This also created an economic incentive to use land for other means besides farming. Similarly, subsistence fishing was transformed into a cash commodity. An unincorporated US territory such as Guam lacks sovereignty over much of its land and natural resources. For example, there is limited restriction on who can own land on Guam and the United States decides Guam's maritime boundaries and limits without the island's consultation.[6] Disparities also exist between NH/PIs living in Pacific territories and those residing in Hawai'i and the continental United States. According to the 2020 US Island Areas Censuses, the median household income in the territories ranged from $28,352 in American Samoa, $31,362 in CNMI, to $58,289 in Guam; the average household income for all NH/PIs residing in Hawai'i and the continental United States in 2019 was $66,695.[68] These disparities are exacerbated by the disproportionate economic burden that higher costs of living place on the residents of the US-affiliated Pacific Islands, as described in Box 6-6.[69,70]

Many NH/PIs migrate westward toward the mainland United States for economic opportunities. Economic growth is dependent on the development of a skilled labor force. According to the US Bureau of Labor Statistics, the employment–population ratio among NH/PIs aged 16 years and older was 63%. Similarly, 64% attained at least a high school degree while unemployment was 4%.[71] Even though many NH/PIs are gainfully employed, factors such barriers to higher education likely contribute to their annual median income of $74,000, which is lower than the median income of $80,000 among non-Hispanic whites.[72]

Health Care

Indigenous peoples are masters of the art of traditional healing. Prior to colonialism, Indigenous health systems relied largely on traditional healers such as the *kahunas* in Hawaii and the *yo'åmtes* in Guam and the Northern Mariana Islands. While the practice of traditional healing declined over decades as modern medicine transformed health care systems, there has been a renewed interest in revitalizing traditional healing practices among the current generation of NH/PIs.[73,74] Still, western health care models are largely used in NH/PI native communities. The Constitution of the World Health Organization refers to health as a fundamental human right and this human right includes "access to the health services they need, when and where they need them, without suffering financial hardship."[75] Despite this assertion, there is no consensus among American legislators on whether to treat health care as a human right. This impasse directly impacts the health of the most marginalized, including many NH/PIs. Access to allopathic health care services varies for NH/PIs depending on place of residence. Despite having health insurance, many NH/PIs do not access the health care system. Distrust of the health care system, competing priorities on time and resources, misalignment of values, race discordance between provider and patient, and lack of childcare or transportation are examples of access barriers that extend beyond health care. These barriers to health care may be amplified in states outside of the Pacific, as NH/PIs are a smaller percentage of the population and many health care systems focus their efforts on larger minority populations, resulting in health care systems that are misaligned with NH/PI communities. Examples include nutrition education that is not representative of foods from the Pacific or patient-focused care that excludes the family in education or support coordination. When a health care system is uneducated or unaware of the unique needs of a community, health care may not resonate or reach them. Although data on health care access for NH/PI communities are limited (due to data aggregation with Asian Americans) there are efforts to compile and further evaluate this kind of information. For example, the Association of Asian Pacific Community Health Organizations' report *The Health of Asian Americans, Native Hawaiians, and Pacific Islanders Served at Health Centers: An Analysis of the 2021 Uniform Data System* highlights the differences between AA- and NHPI-serving health centers in the United States.[76]

Collectively, there are close to two million people residing in NH/PI-serving US-affiliated jurisdictions, with Hawaiʻi making up the largest portion. Every jurisdiction has at least one public-serving hospital. Hawaii has the most hospitals, including the US-ranked Queen's Medical Center. All jurisdictions provide some form of health insurance coverage. US-supported coverage, including Medicaid, CHIP, and Medicare, are only available in the state of Hawaiʻi and territories of American Samoa, the Commonwealth of the Northern Mariana Islands, and Guam. Table 6-2 shows the distribution of health care and health care services across US-affiliated Pacific islands.[68,77–82]

Acceptance and collaboration were universal values in Oceania, where every individual had roles and contributions that were integral to the success of the community. While NH/PI cultural norms that honor aging/elderly populations and embrace gender diversity are supportive community determinants of health, these norms are sometimes at odds with modern health systems, western clinical practices, and systemic public policies. The advocacy group United Territories of Pacific Islanders Alliance Washington (UTOPIA-Washington) asserts that glaring disparities persist in the health status of NH/PI

Table 6-2. Health Care Access Among NH/PI Jurisdictions Affiliated With the United States

	American Samoa	CNMI	FAS	Guam	Hawai'i
Population[68,77]	49,710	47,329	105,987 (FSM) 54,446 (Marshall Islands) 17,976 (Palau)	153,836	1,455,271
Operating hospitals[78,79]	1	1	4 (FSM) 2 (Marshall Islands) 1 (Palau)	3[a]	28[a]
Insurance coverage[68,80]	39.8%	64.8%	47.6% (FSM) 58.9% (Marshall Islands) 64.7% (Palau)	81%	96.8%
Medicaid and CHIP[81,82]	Yes	Yes	FAS migrants to US: yes FAS migrants to territories: up to the territory	Yes	Yes
Medicare[81,82]	Yes	Yes	FAS migrants to US and territories: yes	Yes	Yes

Note: CHIP = State Children's Health Insurance Program; CNMI = Commonwealth of the Northern Mariana Islands; FAS = Freely Associated States; FSM = Federated States of Micronesia; NH/PI = Native Hawaiian or Pacific Islander. FSM includes the islands of Chuuk, Kosrae, Pohnpei, and Yap.
[a]Includes military hospitals.

lesbian, gay, bisexual, transgender, queer, and questioning (LGBTQ+) populations due to significant barriers to gender-affirming treatments, hormone therapy, gender confirmation surgeries, and mental health services for gender dysphoria. While NH/PI societal values may lend to more general acceptance of gender nonconformity, this accommodation is not seen consistently in health care systems or governments, and policy barriers still exist even in states where insurance coverage is approved for gender-affirming therapies. Furthermore, "gender-affirming care is not integrated into medical schools, contributing to a knowledge gap and provider shortage of specialists who are qualified to serve transgender and gender nonconforming populations" (T. Vaina, A. Suluai, T. Johnson, UTOPIA-Washington, email, June 15, 2023).

RESISTANCE, REFORMATION, RESTORATION

Minesngon para ginanña—Success through perseverance.
    CHamoru: Encouraging advancement and improvement despite challenging barriers.

If indeed, as the evidence supports, the people of Oceania enjoyed a state of optimal health prior to colonization, it follows logically that the way to return to wellness is to *decolonize* our communities by undoing the prejudicious practices and foreign systems that were imposed through colonization. However, the issue is not as straightforward as it might seem. While many aspects of colonization were forcibly implemented by European and American religious orders and government regimes, many foreign cultural traits were voluntarily adopted by ancestors and in many cases syncretized or otherwise integrated into what are now considered NH/PI cultures. Introduced food products such as turkey tails, mangoes, SPAM, lamb flaps, pineapples, salted meats, and tinned fish are now so prevalent in Oceania that many NH/PIs would be hard pressed to imagine traditional feasts that don't include these foods. A full return to a precolonial diet devoid of any introduced foods would be a major challenge for mosted NH/PIs, not just in terms of behavior change, but because many staple cultivars are no longer produced at sufficient scale to fulfill increased demand. The challenge is even more difficult for diasporic NH/PI populations living in the continental United States, where growing seasons and climate zones are less suited for growing tropical produce.

The overemphasis on health disparities and inequities is demoralizing and fails to uplift the incredible assets of Oceania peoples who continue to persist, innovate, and advance despite statistical invisibility, dismal health indicators, and disproportionate burden of disease. The same legacy of resilient perseverance, Indigenous ingenuity, and oneness of people/land that sustained NH/PI societies through military occupation, cultural genocide, and colonial imperialism are unique, untapped strengths that can bolster efforts to improve, change, and/or replace systemic structures that prevent NH/PIs from achieving optimal health, individually and collectively.

Even if a total return to precolonial foodways and societal dynamics may not be fully achievable, NH/PIs can make significant gains in health and wellness by resisting and replacing systems and policies that obstruct equitable access to the places, relationships, and resources that nurtured their ancestors and that are best suited to nurture their communities today. The brief discussions that follow are offered as select examples of policy barriers to optimal wellness and some possible policy solutions.

IMPACTS OF INJUSTICE AND POLICY BARRIERS

Nā Wai 'Ehā: The Four Waters

For over 160 years, massive diversion systems have drained nearly dry the famous four waterways of central Maui: the Waiheʻe River, and Waiehu, ʻĪao, and Waikapū Streams.[83] This injustice was initiated to support plantation agriculture, with a focus on sugarcane. This caused great harm to the natural environment and Native Hawaiian traditional farming that relied on the free-flowing streams. As a result, many cultural harms were inflicted, with many unresolved to this day. Although there are no longer sugar plantations on Maui, the Nā Wai 'Ehā legendary waters have not been returned and remain today "a mere trickle of their former selves."[83(p128)]

Climate Change Front Line

The Pacific Islands are one of the first regions to experience the devastating impacts of climate change. Due to the low-lying nature of many of the islands, they are threatened by flooding, coastal erosion, salinization, and storm surges. The Pacific's small island states contribute to only 0.03% of global greenhouse gas emissions, yet they are facing an unequal share of climate change threats. The current pace of sea level rise has not been seen for 5,000 years, and it is predicted that by the middle of this century, there will be an average sea level rise of between 25 cm and 58 cm along the coastlines of Pacific Island countries.[84] This rise would be devastating for islands that sit at or just above sea level. Furthermore, if global temperatures increase by 2°C (3.6°F) above pre-industrial levels, as is becoming increasingly likely, it is estimated that 90% of the coral reefs in much of the Pacific Island region could suffer severe degradation, which will have a devastating effect on the marine species that depend upon these ecosystems.[84] Climate change is affecting fisheries and many threatened marine species. Climate change impacts will become increasingly severe and widespread in the coming decades. Fortunately, climate change is a priority of the "Blue Continent" where leaders from key organizations such as the Pacific Islands Forum, the Micronesian Islands Forum, and the Pacific Island Health Officers' Association continue to incorporate the protection of the ocean and islands in high-level strategic planning and implementation efforts.

Invisibility Results in Disparities in Education

Compared with the general population, NH/PI students have significantly lower college attainment rates; between 2015 and 2019, only 17.8% had obtained a four-year degree. By contrast, approximately 32% of the total population held a four-year degree or higher in the same period.[85] A large percentage of Samoans (58.1%), Tongans (54.2%), Native Hawaiians (50.0%), and Guamanians or Chamorros (47.0%) who attend college leave without earning a degree.[86] The educational disparities begin early in the K–12 pathway. For example, disaggregation of Pacific Islanders from the Asian Pacific Islander group of third to fifth grade students in Hawaii public schools revealed that reading performance of Native Hawaiian students was overestimated by 14% to 16% and Pacific Islander students by 30% to 35% compared with white students.[87] Recently, the Center for American Progress acknowledged gaps in educational experiences of Pacific Islander children in the K–12 system and suggested the creation of a few policies including a policy to increase college readiness for Pacific Islanders and a policy to preserve Native Hawaiian and other Indigenous languages.[88]

Unfortunately, NH/PIs have been largely overlooked in policy considerations at the federal, state, and local levels, as well as in the development of school/campus services and programs. This is partly due to a lack of understanding of the needs, challenges, and experiences of NH/PI students, particularly in the various social and institutional contexts in which they pursue their educational goals.

IMPACTS OF REVITALIZATION AND RESTORATION

O Kāne-au-loli-ka-honua, honu neʻe pū ka ʻāina—Oh Kāne Who Transforms the World, like a sea turtle crawling, so the land changes.
                         Hawaiian: Supplication that acknowledges the transformational, dynamic nature of ecosystems.

The peoples of Oceania are from places and spaces that feed and heal. Their islands are among the newest lands on this planet, full of life and beauty. These islands have fed generations of people because their ancestors gifted the knowledge to live in balance with their environment. As decolonization takes shape and a return to traditional knowledge of how to farm, hunt, fish, and live takes root, the people of Oceania begin to see their health return to that of their ancestors. Language revitalization has allowed many to read and understand the knowledge of their ancestors. Traditional land and sea stewardship increases their longevity and ability to thrive just as their great grandparents did. Ancient healing practices and the revitalization of ceremonies begin to repair the deep sorrows and pains their people suffer from because of colonization and exploitation. Programs and efforts to support the peoples of Oceania will benefit the entire earth because their knowledge and experience will allow all people of this planet to live in ways that make the earth productive and fertile (*momona*).

ʻĒwekea Piʻi Moʻo Lāʻau Lapaʻau: A Healer in Every Home

An intensive course utilized an *ʻāina*-based (land-based; generally refers to initiatives that utilize the natural environment and traditional knowledge for learning, healing, or skill development) immersive teaching model that is rooted in spirituality, supported by lineal knowledge traditions, and developed through trained practices that were acquired by Kahuna Lāʻau Lapaʻau Levon Ohai, Kahu Keoki Kīkaha Pai Baclayon, and Kumu Leinaʻala Bright. Nā Kumu Lāʻau Lapaʻau, with the support of Sustain Hawaiʻi and the Administration for Native Americans, offered a unique opportunity to engage in this deep foundational course with the objective of helping interested students become cultural practitioners of *lāʻau lapaʻau* (curing medicine, often plant based) and perpetuate Hawaiʻi's tradition of health and healing (see https://www.ewekea.org).

Mana Academy: Embodying the Dreams and Aspiration of Our Ancestors

Mana Academy is an accredited public charter school that was founded in 2013 in response to academic achievement gaps observed among Pacific Islanders and other communities living in Salt Lake County, Utah. Armed with a mission and a mandate to close the achievement gap in their community, the founders of Mana Academy created a unique school model that taps into and leverages shared cultural values to create a space where scholars feel a sense of belonging, connectedness, and purpose. With this foundation in place, Mana Academy engages key partners—educators, parents, cultural practitioners, local colleges and universities, and experts in various professions—to create learning experiences that will develop lifelong learners equipped with real-world skills and the competence to excel in life (see https://www.themanaacademy.org).

Ke Kula 'o Samuel M. Kamakau Laboratory Public Charter School

Ke Kula 'o Samuel M. Kamakau Laboratory Public Charter School is a family-based Hawaiian language immersion school offering a comprehensive multilevel (Pre-K–8) educational program. The school was established in January 2000 in response to the expressed needs of Native Hawaiian families to increase student achievement through culturally based education, while addressing the educational needs of multiple generations of learners. Ke Kula 'o Kamakau contributes to the ongoing development of Hawaiian language education through research, teacher training, and resource development.

> 'O ko ke Kula 'o Samuel M. Kamakau ala nu'ukia, 'oia ho'i, ka mālama 'ana i honua mauli ola i waiwai i ka 'ike a me ka lawena aloha o nā kūpuna i mea e lei ai lākou i ka lei o ka lanakila.
>
> The mission of Ke Kula 'o Samuel M. Kamakau is to foster success for all members of their learning community by providing a culturally healthy and responsive learning environment . . .
>
> Ma o ka 'ōlelo Hawai'i e ola ai nā iwi o nā kupuna iā lākou. 'O ke Kumu Honua Mauli Ola ka pou hale o lākou. Lei 'ia nā 'ano a'o a pau i ka lanakila ma o ka 'ike kino. 'O nā 'ohana ke kula, ke kaiaulu nā kōko'okolu e kāko'o ai i ia hale.
>
> The Hawaiian language is the foundation that enables them to honor ancestors and perpetuate traditions. The principles of Kumu Honua Mauli Ola, the Hawaiian Educational philosophy, form the support structure of the school. All learning styles are supported so that the children will attain equitable success. Families, school and community are equal partners of their success.[89]

Hā'ena Community-Based Subsistence Fishing Area

The Hā'ena Community-Based Subsistence Fishing Area includes the waters and submerged lands from the shoreline to a distance of one mile off the northwestern coast of Kaua'i. The purpose of the Hā'ena Community-Based Subsistence Fishing Area is to (1) sustainably support the consumptive needs of the *Hāʻena ahupuaʻa* (the Hāʻena land division) through culturally rooted, community-based management; (2) ensure the sustainability of nearshore ocean resources in the area through effective management practices, including the establishment of limits on the harvest of aquatic life; (3) establish the *Makua Puʻuhonua* (Marine Refuge) for the preservation and protection of this nursery habitat for juvenile reef fishes; (4) recognize and protect customary and traditional Native Hawaiian fishing practices that are exercised for subsistence, cultural, and religious purposes in the area; and (5) facilitate the substantive involvement of the community in resource management decisions for the area through dialogue with community residents and resource users.[90]

Perpetuating Cultural Wisdom in Healing

Medicinal plants have been used in traditional healing and passed orally through generations for thousands of years in the Mariana Islands. The identification of approximately 70 medicinal plants[91] and Indigenous healing practices[73] have recently been documented. To perpetuate the knowledge and healing practices, the University of Guam is piloting a *Yoʼåmte* or traditional healer apprenticeship through its CHamoru Studies Program with guidance from community partners, especially CHamoru traditional healers.[92] The pilot program content includes Indigenous health and healing, CHamoru health care practices, and traditional healing practicum and field work. Leaders of the pilot program are interested in expanding apprenticeship rotations to other islands in the Marianas, enhancing community gardens to include medicinal plants, and collaborating with Western practitioners to complement healing, to name a few.

Revitalizing Indigenous Language in the School System

Chief Huråo Academy began in 2005 as an immersion program with a mission to promote and perpetuate the CHamoru language and culture. The curriculum emphasized nine cultural values of *aguaiya* (to love), *agofliʼe'* (to be non-judgmental), *aʼumitde* (to be humble; to be selfless), *afaʼmaolek* (to forgive; to reciprocate), *arespeta* (to respect), *amamåhlao* (to have shame; to have moral and ethical boundaries), *ageftao* (to be giving) *aʼadahi* (to care for others/surroundings), and *aʼagradesi* (to be grateful).[93] The academy now includes a *Neni* or preschool program that was launched in 2018 and the *Faneyåkan Sinipok* or a full CHamoru immersion cohort of kindergarten students that was launched in 2019 in one of Guam's public elementary schools.[94,95] Summer programs are open to all children and offer a variety of cultural exposure to oral traditions, song, dance, weaving, cooking, and living off the land. Teens who have participated in the summer programs often return as *Pineksai* volunteers to help teach and care for the younger children. The academy's main community focus is the *Eskuelan Mañaina*, a program that teaches parents to become fluent in order to use the language with their children at home.

CATALYSTS FOR CHANGE TO REDUCE DISPARITIES AND IMPROVE HEALTH EQUITY

- Disaggregate NH/PI from Asians in data; this is essential for identifying and addressing identified health issues in the NH/PI population. The continued use of a combined API category has negative impacts on both Asian and NH/PI populations.
- Recommend usage of "NH/PI" as the preferred acronym in printed references.
- The health care system must serve all communities and recognize that misaligned values between communities and health care will result in a failed health care system and continued health disparities. All communities should have access to culturally safe and respectful care.
- Remove/revise policies that prohibit customary usage and access to ancestral lands and waters by lineal descendants of traditional custodians and residents.
- Provide funding and resources to facilitate the universal teaching of Indigenous languages and decolonized history in public schools in the state of Hawai'i, the territories of Guam and American Samoa, CNMI, and the signatory nations of COFA.
- Increase funding for research opportunities and tertiary education scholarships for students of NH/PI ancestry.
- Increase funding opportunities for sustainable economic development and renewable energy infrastructure in all Oceania territories and freely associated states.
- Mandate that recipients of AAPI funding provide meaningful allocation of resources and services in benefit of NH/PI.
- Formally codify the White House Initiative on AAs and NH/PIs as a permanent entity with funded personnel and operational resources.
- Evaluate and review all federal agencies to review and revise policies and procedures that exclude and/or potentially harm NH/PIs (with inclusion of NH/PI evaluators in the process).

CONCLUSION: RECONNECTIONS

Whatungarongaro te tangata, toitū te whenua—As humankind disappears, the land remains.

> Māori: Assertion that the timelessness of ancestral places and the power of indigeneity transcend beyond individual lifetimes.

The nations of Oceania have existed for far longer than the United States of America and the social institutions, worldviews, and governance systems that emerged from this area were time-tested and optimized to ensure that their people not only survived, but thrived, on some of the most remote islands on the planet. The European explorers—who ventured into the Pacific centuries after these ancestors had already traversed the largest ocean on earth—were universally impressed by the robust health and vitality of the islanders they encountered. These foreigners encountered sophisticated societies that sustainably maintained healthy populations through the cultivation of nutrient-dense superfoods like breadfruit (which Europeans introduced to the Americas). The colonizers brought devastating diseases that decimated island populations, priming them for invasion, occupation, and annexation. The imposition of non-native governance, languages, religions, and economies forever altered the balance of relationships between and among people, land, and ocean; the disharmony and disruption were correlated with a decline in general health, signaled by the emergence of noncommunicable diseases like diabetes, metabolic syndrome, obesity, and cardiovascular disease. Modern science and medicine are now beginning to acknowledge that the so-called Stone Age ancestors, long dismissed as noble savages (but savages nonetheless), were custodians of cultures and worldviews that have immense relevance to humanity's search for optimal health in all its dimensions.

Just as antiretroviral therapies derived from Oceania's native healers are being recognized as lead candidates for new HIV treatment,[96] the world has much to gain by emulating ancient Oceanian practices that have long nurtured intrepid voyagers, whose descendants now number 1.5 million in the United States. These people have persisted and thrived in the face of pandemics and imperialism and their outsized influences on modern American society are clearly visible in words like *tattoo*, *wiki*, and *taboo* (derived from Polynesian languages), sports like surfing (an Oceanian invention)[97] and football (Samoans and Tongans are 28 times more likely to play in the National Football League than any other ethnic group),[98] and popular entertainment (NH/PI performers like Dwayne Johnson are among the highest paid and most recognizable in the world).[99] If the people of these sea of islands have been able to contribute so much to the world despite displacement and the overthrow of ancestral systems, how much more positive change can be brought about by validating Indigenous science to resist systemic inequities, restore healthful institutions and policies, and revitalize the individual and collective health of NH/PIs and all Americans?

ACKNOWLEDGMENTS

Meitaki ma'ata, tangkiu, vinaka vakalevu, ko rabwa, fakaaue, tubwa kōr, fakafetai, fa'afetai lava, mahalo piha, mālō 'aupito, si yu'os ma'åse.

This paper is the product of continuous community consultation, review, and collaboration with many NH/PIs whose expertise and lived experiences have contributed immeasurably to this effort, including Keith Camacho, Calvin Chang, Timaima Vakalala Clawson, Victoria-Lola Leon Guerrero, Taffy Johnson, Keawe'aimoku Kaholokula, Melisa Laelan, Adrianna Suluai, Sina Uipi, and Tepatasi Vaina.

REFERENCES

1. Cruickshanks. Oceania UN Geoscheme Regions. Wikimedia Commons. Accessed April 14, 2025. https://commons.wikimedia.org/wiki/File:Oceania_UN_Geoscheme_Regions.svg
2. Lal BV, Fortune K. *The Pacific Islands: An Encyclopedia*. University of Hawaii Press; 2000:63.
3. West FJ, Foster S. Pacific Islands. Encyclopedia Britannica. Accessed April 14, 2025. https://www.britannica.com/place/Pacific-Islands
4. Kabutaulaka T. Re-presenting Melanesia: Ignoble savages and Melanesian alter-Natives. *Contemp Pac*. 2015;27(1):110–145. doi:10.1353/cp.2015.0027
5. Aldrich R. *France and the South Pacific Since 1940*. University of Hawai'i Press: 1993.
6. Kuper KG, Bradley J. *Giha Mo'na: A Self-Determination Study for Guåhan*. University of Guam Press; 2021.
7. Hau'ofa E. Our sea of islands. *Contemp Pac*. 1994;6(1):148–161. doi:10.30687/LGSP/2785-2709/2023/02/002
8. Sater W. *Chile and the United States: Empires in Conflict*. University of Georgia Press, 1990.
9. Tewari N, Alvarez AN. *Asian American Psychology: Current Perspectives*. CRC Press; 2008.
10. UN SC Res 21 (Apr 2, 1947). Accessed August 6, 2025. https://digitallibrary.un.org/record/111988?v=pdf
11. Prior H. Exploring Utah's Pacific Islander groups: A detailed analysis. Kem C. Gardner Policy Institute, University of Utah. September 2024. Accessed August 11, 2025. https://d36oiwf74r1rap.cloudfront.net/wp-content/uploads/2024/09/Pacific-Islanders-FS-Sep2024.pdf
12. Consolidated Appropriations Act, 134 Stat 1182, Pub L 116-26 (2021).
13. Personal Responsibility and Work Opportunity Reconciliation Act, 110 Stat 2105, Pub L 104-193 (1996).
14. Cook J. *The Journals of Captain James Cook on His Voyages of Discovery*. Beaglehole JC, ed. Vol 3. Hakluyt Society at the University Press; 1967–1974.
15. Wu Y, Uchima O, Browne C, Braun K. Healthy life expectancy in 2010 for Native Hawaiian, White, Filipino, Japanese, and Chinese Americans living in Hawai'i. *Asia Pac J Public Health*. 2019;31(7):659–670. doi:10.1177/1010539519875614
16. Panapasa SV, Mau MK, Williams DR, McNally JW. Mortality patterns of Native Hawaiians across their lifespan: 1990-2000. *Am J Public Health*. 2010;100(11):2304–2310. doi:10.2105/AJPH.2009.183541
17. Banks J. *The Endeavor Journal of Joseph Banks, 1769–1771*. Vol 2. State Library of New South Wales. Accessed April 14, 2025. https://acms.sl.nsw.gov.au/_transcript/2015/D33961/a1193b.html
18. Fujita R, Braun K, Hughes C. The traditional Hawaiian diet: A review of the literature. *Pac Health Dialog*. 2004;11(2):250–259. Accessed August 11, 2025. http://pacifichealthdialog.nz/pre-2013-archive/Volume2011/no2/PHD1120220p2502025920Fujita20orig.pdf
19. DiBello JR, McGarvey ST, Kraft P, et al. Dietary patterns are associated with metabolic syndrome in adult Samoans. *J Nutr*. 2009;139(10):1933–1943. doi:10.3945/jn.109.107888
20. Kanahele GH. *Ku Kanaka Stand Tall: A Search for Hawaiian Values*. University of Hawai'i Press; 1986.
21. Brown AC, Valiere A. The medicinal uses of poi. *Nutr Clin Care*. 2004;7(2):69–74. Accessed April 14, 2025. https://pmc.ncbi.nlm.nih.gov/articles/PMC1482315

22. Liu Y, Brown PN, Ragone D, Gibson DL, Murch SJ. Breadfruit flour is a healthy option for modern foods and food security. *PLoS One*. 2020;15(7):e0236300. doi:10.1371/journal.pone.0236300
23. Manivannan A, Bhardwaj R, Padmanabhan S, Suneja P, Hebbar KB, Kanade SR. Biochemical and nutritional characterization of coconut (*Cocos nucifera* L.) haustorium. *Food Chem*. 2018;238:153–159. doi:10.1016/j.foodchem.2016.10.127
24. Aluli NE. Prevalence of obesity in a Native Hawaiian population. *Am J Clin Nutr*. 1991;53(suppl 6):1556S–1560S. doi:10.1093/ajcn/53.6.1556S
25. Shintani TT, Hughes CK, Beckham S, O'Connor HK. Obesity and cardiovascular risk intervention through the ad libitum feeding of traditional Hawaiian diet. *Am J Clin Nutr*. 1991;53(suppl 6):1647S–1651S. doi: 10.1093/ajcn/53.6.1647S
26. Kōkua Kalihi Valley Comprehensive Family Services. Hoʻoulu ʻĀina. Accessed April 11, 2025. https://hoouluaina.org
27. Paepae o Heʻeia. Accessed April 11, 2025. https://paepaeoheeia.org
28. Johnson HE, Banack SA, Cox PA. Variability in content of the anti-AIDS drug candidate prostratin in Samoan populations of *Homolanthus nutans*. *J Nat Prod*. 2008;71(12):2041–2044. doi:10.1021/np800295m
29. United Nations Educational, Scientific, and Cultural Organization. *Safeguarding Indigenous Architecture in Vanuatu*. 2017. Accessed April 14, 2025. https://unesdoc.unesco.org/ark:/48223/pf0000248144
30. Wilson C. Samoa's architects look to the past to boost climate resilience. *Thomas Reuters Foundation News*. October 2, 2014. Accessed April 14, 2025. https://news.trust.org/item/20141001140022-jt1y3
31. US Census Bureau. New vintage 2021 population estimates available for the nation, states and Puerto Rico. December 21, 2021. Accessed April 14, 2025. https://www.census.gov/newsroom/press-releases/2021/2021-population-estimates.html
32. Vila G. Vintage 2024 county population estimates for the state of Hawaii: July 1, 2020 through July 1, 2024. State of Hawaii, Research & Economic Analysis Division. Accessed May 22, 2025. https://files.hawaii.gov/dbedt/census/popestimate/2024/county-pop/2024_county-pop-est_highlights.pdf
33. US House of Representatives. American Samoa death rate in the Iraq War is highest among all States and US Territories. March 23, 2009. Accessed April 14, 2025. https://web.archive.org/web/20090809113322/http://www.house.gov/list/press/as00_faleomavaega/asdeathratehighestamongstates.html
34. Kane T. Who bears the burden? Demographic characteristics of US military recruits before and after 9/11. The Heritage Foundation. November 7, 2005. Accessed April 11, 2025. https://web.archive.org/web/20100326234926/http://www.heritage.org/Research/Reports/2005/11/Who-Bears-the-Burden-Demographic-Characteristics-of-US-Military-Recruits-Before-and-After-9-11
35. Davis S. Colonialism, militarization, tourism, and environment as nexus. In: Davis S, ed. *The Empires' Edge: Militarization, Resistance, and Transcending Hegemony in the Pacific*. University of Georgia Press; 2015:91–114.

36. Rose JJ. The remote Marshall Islands complicate US Pacific policy. *The Interpreter*. October 27, 2022. Accessed April 11, 2025. https://www.lowyinstitute.org/the-interpreter/the-remote-marshall-islands-complicate-us-pacific-policy
37. Niheu K, Turbin LM, Yamada S. The impact of the military presence in Hawai'i on the health of na Kanaka Maoli. *Pac Public Health*. 2006;13(2):172–179.
38. Sicard S. How much land does the military really own?. *Military Times*. August 13, 2022. Accessed August 6, 2025. https://www.militarytimes.com/off-duty/military-culture/2022/08/15/how-much-land-does-the-military-really-own
39. Bradley J. *An Analysis of the Economic Impact of Guam's Political Status Options*. June 12, 2000. Accessed April 14, 2025. https://decol.guam.gov/sites/default/files/Academic-Study-An-Analysis-of-the-Economic-Impact-of-Guams-Political-Status-Options-Bradley-Joseph-2000.pdf
40. Radiation Exposure Compensation Act Amendments of 2023, S. 1751, 118th Cong. (2023).
41. Mori WS. On the lack of Native Hawaiian and Pacific Islander individuals in the physician workforce. *JAMA Netw Open*. 2021;4(9):e2125399. doi:10.1001/jamanetworkopen.2021.25399
42. Guidi J, Lucente M, Sonino N, Fava GA. Allostatic load and its impact on health: A systematic review. *Psychother Psychosom*. 2021;90(1):11–27. doi:10.1159/000510696
43. US Office of Management and Budget. 1977 race and ethnic standards for federal statistics and administrative reporting. 1978. Accessed April 14, 2025. https://spd15revision.gov/content/spd15revision/en/history/1977-standards.html
44. US Office of Management and Budget. 1997 Standards for Maintaining, Collecting, and Presenting Federal Data on Race and Ethnicity. 1997. Accessed April 14, 2025. https://spd15revision.gov/content/spd15revision/en/history/1997-standards.html
45. Hawaiian Homes Commission Act (Act of July 9, 1921), 42 Stat 108, Pub L 85-733 (1920).
46. The White House. The White House Initiative on Asian Americans and Pacific Islanders: Final report to the President. January 25, 2025. Accessed April 14, 2025. https://bidenwhitehouse.archives.gov/wp-content/uploads/2025/01/WHIAANHPI-Report-to-the-President-Rising-Together-WH.pdf
47. Nittle NK. History of the Asian American Civil Rights Movement. *ThoughtCo*. March 3, 2021. Accessed April 14, 2025. https://www.thoughtco.com/asian-american-civil-rights-movement-history-2834596
48. Native American Programs Act of 1974, 42 USC §2991 (1974).
49. Compact Act of 1986, Pub L 99-239, 99 Stat 1770 (1986).
50. Palau Compact of Free Association Act, Pub L 99-658, 100 Stat 3672 (1986).
51. US Congress Joint Economic Committee. How the renewed Compacts of Free Association support US economic, national security, and climate goals. May 2024. Accessed August 9, 2025. https://www.jec.senate.gov/public/index.cfm/democrats/2024/5/how-the-renewed-compacts-of-free-association-support-u-s-economic-national-security-and-climate-goals
52. US Office of Management and Budget. Revisions to OMB's Statistical Policy Directive No. 15: Standards for maintaining, collecting, and presenting federal data on race and ethnicity. March 29, 2024. Accessed April 14, 2025. https://www.federalregister.gov/documents/2024/03/29/2024-06469/revisions-to-ombs-statistical-policy-directive-no-15-standards-for-maintaining-collecting-and

53. Ghosh C. Healthy People 2010 and Asian Americans/Pacific Islanders: Defining a baseline of information. *Am J Public Health*. 2003;93(12):2093–2098. doi:10.2105/ajph.93.12.2093
54. Utah Department of Health. Utah health status update: It Takes a Village: Addressing infant mortality disparities by giving Utah Pacific Islander babies the best chance. April 2018. Accessed August 11, 2025. https://ibis.utah.gov/ibisph-view/pdf/opha/publication/hsu/2018/1804_ItTakesAVillage.pdf
55. Ponce NA, Shimkhada R, Tulua A. Disaggregating California's COVID-19 data for Native Hawaiians & Pacific Islanders and Asians fact sheet. NHPI Data Policy Lab, University of California, Los Angeles. May 26, 2021. Accessed April 14, 2025. https://healthpolicy.ucla.edu/our-work/publications/disaggregating-californias-covid-19-data-native-hawaiians-and-pacific-islanders-and-asians
56. World Health Organization. Suicide worldwide in 2019: Global health estimates. 2021. Accessed April 14, 2025. https://www.who.int/publications/i/item/9789240026643
57. Mathieu S, de Leo D, Koo YW, Leske S, Goodfellow B, Kõlves K. Suicide and suicide attempts in the Pacific Islands: A systematic literature review. *Lancet Reg Health West Pac*. 2021;17:100283. doi:10.1016/j.lanwpc.2021.100283
58. Lowe ED. Epidemic suicide in the context of modernizing social change in Oceania: A critical review and assessment. *Contemp Pac*. 2019;31(1):105–138. doi:10.1353/cp.2019.0007
59. Rabbitt MP, Reed-Jones M, Hales LJ, Burke MP. Household food security in the United States. US Dept of Agriculture, Economic Research Service. September 2024. Accessed August 10, 2025. https://ers.usda.gov/sites/default/files/_laserfiche/publications/109896/ERR-337.pdf?v=28148
60. Kaʻili T. *Marking Indigeneity: The Tongan Art of Sociospatial Relations*. University of Arizona Press; 2017.
61. United Nations. Lands, natural resources represent life for Indigenous peoples, not mere commodities, speakers stress as permanent forum begins session. April 16, 2018. Accessed August 10, 2025. https://press.un.org/en/2018/hr5387.doc.htm
62. Rogers R. *Destiny's Landfall: A History of Guam*. University of Hawaiʻi Press; 1995.
63. Soucy D, Janes M, Hall A. State of homelessness: 2024 edition. National Alliance to End Homelessness. August 5, 2024. Accessed April 14, 2025. https://endhomelessness.org/homelessness-in-america/homelessness-statistics/state-of-homelessness
64. Tyndall J, Bond-Smith D, Inafuku R. *The Hawaiʻi Housing Factbook: 2023*. University of Hawaii Economic Research Organization; 2023. Accessed September 28, 2023. https://uhero.hawaii.edu/wp-content/uploads/2023/06/TheHawaiiHousingFactbook.pdf
65. Soaring homeless on CNMI's Saipan. *Radio New Zealand*. July 16, 2019. Accessed September 28, 2023. https://www.rnz.co.nz/international/pacific-news/394489/soaring-homeless-on-cnmi-s-saipan
66. O'Connor J. Volunteers conduct PIT count. *The Guam Daily Post*. January 28, 2023. Accessed September 28, 2023. https://www.postguam.com/news/local/volunteers-conduct-pit-count/article_45e443fa-9e14-11ed-b5bb-0361d9fb3d12.html
67. Petersen G. Indigenous island empires: Yap and Tonga considered. *J Pac Hist*. 2000;35(1):5–27. doi:10.1080/00223340050052275

68. US Census Bureau. 2020 Island Areas Censuses press kit. February 15, 2024. Accessed April 14, 2025. https://www.census.gov/newsroom/press-kits/2021/2020-island-area-census-press-kit.html
69. Ruane MC. Economic development prospects for a small island economy: The case of Guam. *J Econ Econ Educ Res.* 2012;13:15.
70. Ames T. Socio-economic development in Micronesia: A case study of hope and heartbreak in Chuuk, FSM. *Pac Asia Inquiry.* 2011;2(1):195–203. Accessed April 14, 2025. https://www.uog.edu/_resources/files/schools-and-colleges/college-of-liberal-arts-and-social-sciences/pai/pai_195-203.pdf
71. US Bureau of Labor Statistics. US labor force characteristics of Asians, Native Hawaiians, and other Pacific Islanders. May 30, 2024. Accessed August 9, 2025. https://www.bls.gov/blog/2024/u-s-labor-force-characteristics-of-asians-native-hawaiians-and-other-pacific-islanders.htm
72. Office of Minority Health. Native Hawaiian and Pacific Islander health. US Dept of Health and Human Services. Updated June 30, 2025. Accessed August 9, 2025. https://minorityhealth.hhs.gov/native-hawaiian-and-pacific-islander-health
73. Lizama TA. Yo'amte: A deeper type of healing exploring the state of Indigenous Chamorro healing practices. *Pac Asia Inquiry.* 2014;5(1):97–106. Accessed April 14, 2025. https://www.uog.edu/_resources/files/schools-and-colleges/college-of-liberal-arts-and-social-sciences/pai/pai5-lizama-yo-amte.pdf
74. Oneha MF, Spencer M, Bright L, Elkin L, Wong D, Sakurai M. *Ho'oilina Pono A'e*: Integrating Native Hawaiian healing to create a just legacy for the next generation. *Hawaii J Health Soc Welf.* 2023;82(3):72–77. Accessed April 14, 2025. https://hawaiijournalhealth.org/past_issues/hjhsw8203_0072.pdf
75. Ghebreyesus TA. Health is a fundamental human right. World Health Organization. December 10, 2017. Accessed July 6, 2023. https://www.who.int/news-room/commentaries/detail/health-is-a-fundamental-human-right
76. Association of Asian Pacific Community Health Organizations. *The Health of Asian Americans, Native Hawaiians, and Pacific Islanders Served at Health Centers: An Analysis of the 2021 Uniform Data System.* December 2023. Accessed April 14, 2025. https://aapcho.org/wp-content/uploads/2023/12/The-Health-of-Asian-Americans-Native-Hawaiians-and-Pacific-Islanders-Served-at-Health-Centers-An-Analysis-of-the-2021-Uniform-Data-System.pdf
77. Pacific Community. Population. Accessed April 14, 2025. https://sdd.spc.int/topic/population
78. American Hospital Directory. Accessed August 9, 2025. https://www.ahd.com
79. Association of State & Territorial Dental Directors. Territorial & freely associated oral health programs. Accessed August 9, 2025. https://www.astdd.org/territorial-and-jurisdiction-oral-health-programs-federated-states-of-micronesia
80. Pacific Data Hub. SDG 3-Good health and well-being. Pacific Community. Accessed August 9, 2025. https://pacificdata.org/dashboard/sdg-3-good-health-and-well-being
81. Centers for Medicare and Medicaid Services. Re: Medicaid eligibility for COFA migrants. US Dept of Health and Human Services. October 18, 2021. Accessed August 11, 2025. https://www.medicaid.gov/federal-policy-guidance/downloads/sho21005.pdf

82. US Dept of Health and Human Services. Health coverage options for COFA migrants. August 2023. Accessed April 14, 2025. https://www.cms.gov/marketplace/technical-assistance-resources/health-coverage-options-cofa-migrants.pdf
83. Sproat DK. Wai through Kānāwai: Water for Hawaiʻi's streams and justice for Hawaiian communities. *Marquette Law Rev.* 2011;95(1):127–211 Accessed April 14, 2025. https://scholarship.law.marquette.edu/mulr/vol95/iss1/5
84. Parsons C. The Pacific Islands: The front line in the battle against climate change. *Science Matters.* National Science Foundation. May 23, 2022. Accessed April 14, 2025. https://www.nsf.gov/science-matters/pacific-islands-front-line-battle-against-climate
85. McElrath K, Martin M. Bachelor's degree attainment in the United States: 2005 to 2019. US Census Bureau. February 9, 2021. Accessed April 14, 2025. https://www.census.gov/library/publications/2021/acs/acsbr-009.html
86. Teranishi A, Le A, Gutierrez RAE, et al. Native Hawaiians and Pacific Islanders in higher education. APIA Scholars. 2019. Accessed April 14, 2025. https://apiascholars.org/wp-content/uploads/2019/12/NHPI_Report.pdf
87. Singh M, Dunn HH, Burke AM. Revealing the variation in performance of Hawaiʻi's Asian Pacific Islander subgroups on the English Language Arts Smarter Balanced Assessment: Implications for policy and practice. *Int J Educ Res.* 2020;103:101614. doi:10.1016/j.ijer.2020.101614
88. Chatterji R, Yin J. Education policies need to address unique needs of Asian American and Pacific Islander communities. Center for American Progress. January 26, 2022. Accessed April 14, 2025. https://www.americanprogress.org/article/education-policies-need-to-address-the-unique-needs-of-asian-american-and-pacific-islander-communities
89. Ke Kula ʻo Samuel M. Kamakau Laboratory Public Charter School. School profile. Accessed April 14, 2025. https://1.cdn.edl.io/aZU9hWm4oBA58Zbj3DfUGIahU67GXzL30jjtdcLGadFvYTHo.pdf
90. Haw Dept of Nat Res §13-60.9-2. Accessed August 10, 2025. https://dlnr.hawaii.gov/dar/files/2018/04/HAR-13-60.9dr2.pdf
91. Nandwani D, Calvo JA, Tenorio J, Calvo F, Manglona L. Medicinal plants and traditional knowledge in the Northern Mariana Islands. *J Appl Biosci.* 2008;8(2):325–330. Accessed August 10, 2025. https://m.elewa.org/JABS/2008/8(2)/3.pdf
92. First traditional healing course aims to revive cultural wisdom. *Pacific Daily News.* September 25, 2023. Accessed April 14, 2025. https://www.guampdn.com/first-traditional-healing-course-aims-to-revive-cultural-wisdom/article_53d22ce2-5ab2-11ee-ad2e-b3aaa533f15e.html
93. Chief Huråo Academy. Accessed April 14, 2025. https://www.huraoacademy.com
94. Lujan T. Chief Huråo Academy launches preschool. *Guam Daily Post.* August 19, 2018. Accessed April 14, 2025. https://www.postguam.com/entertainment/lifestyle/chief-hur-o-academy-launches-preschool/article_3d507028-a1ee-11e8-8cd1-3b3f907ba6d8.html
95. Cruz-Langas D. A new era of empowerment for Guam's Indigenous youth. *KUAM News.* June 14, 2024. Accessed April 14, 2025. https://www.kuam.com/story/50904505/a-new-era-of-empowerment-for-guams-Indigenous-youth

96. Beans EJ, Fournogerakis D, Gauntlet C, et al. Highly potent, synthetically accessible prostratin analogs induce latent HIV expression in vitro and ex vivo. *Proc Natl Acad Sci USA*. 2013;110(29):11698–11703. doi:10.1073/pnas.1302634110
97. Walker IH. *Waves of Resistance: Surfing and History in Twentieth-Century Hawai'i*. University of Hawai'i Press; 2011.
98. Uperesa L. *Gridiron Capital: How American Football Became a Samoan Game*. Duke University Press; 2022.
99. Voytko L. The highest-paid entertainers 2022. *Forbes*. February 9, 2022. Updated February 9, 2023. Accessed April 14, 2025. https://www.forbes.com/sites/lisettevoytko/2022/02/09/the-highest-paid-entertainers-2022

7

Health Inequities in White European Americans: Key Systems, Root Causes, and the Legacies of Whiteness

Erika Blacksher, PhD, Matt Wray, PhD, MA, and Steven H. Woolf, MD, MPH

INTRODUCTION

In the United States, white people generally have better health and longer lives than people of color. That generalization is attributable to contemporary and historical systems of racial inequity that truncate the life and health prospects of people of color. For more than 400 years, legal, illegal, and extralegal barriers have blocked their social mobility, limited access to health-protective resources, and increased exposure to health hazards and risks.[1-3] This history began with the genocide and displacement of Indigenous people and the enslavement of African Americans during colonization and the establishment of Jim Crow restrictions after Reconstruction, and it continues today with systems and structures that continue to marginalize people of color and compromise their health. These same systems of racial inequity benefit people who are interpreted and classified as "White" (see Box 7-1).[4-10] Since its founding, the United States has placed white European Americans at the pinnacle of a racial hierarchy that confers social, material, and symbolic privileges that generally protect their health and longevity. This racialized social system is described here as *whiteness*, defined as observable and measurable advantages and privileges embedded in interlocking social systems that help sustain the social power and cultural dominance of white European Americans as a social group.[11] Other conceptions of whiteness are discussed in the literature.[12-16] Whiteness is sustained in part by the ideology of *white supremacy*, a system of beliefs that posit the natural superiority of light-skinned ethnoracial groups and that has been perpetuated in the United States through a set of social mechanisms that enabled whites to racially dominate people of color for centuries.

It is important to distinguish between whiteness and white people.[17-20] *White people* are a highly heterogenous population with varying levels of advantage and disadvantage depending on their social location in intersecting power structures (e.g., class, gender,

> **Box 7-1. Who Are *Whites*?**
>
> OMB has long defined *whites* as people "having origins in any of the original peoples of Europe, the Middle East, or North Africa." This category included those who self-identified as white or reported ethnoracial heritages deemed white by the US federal government.[4] On March 28, 2024, the Census Bureau announced a new standalone category for people who identify as MENA, enabling people to report their identities with more accuracy. The previous definition did not correspond perfectly with everyday conceptions of who is white or with conceptions of whiteness discussed in the literature. Many Americans may not view MENA populations as white, and MENA people may neither experience the world as white nor benefit from social and material advantages of those readily identified as white.[5-7] Health inequities within the MENA population therefore are addressed in a separate chapter in this book (see Chapter 5). Health statistics are almost always collected and reported for the OMB category of "White," or "non-Hispanic White," which makes it difficult to distinguish between the health of Americans of European or MENA descent. Studies that do so indicate unique patterns in health for MENA Americans,[8-10] which are not fully generalizable to Americans of European descent, who hereafter we refer to as *white European Americans* or *white(s)*, depending on context.

Note: MENA = Middle Eastern or North African; OMB = US Office of Management and Budget

sexuality). Fine-grained analyses reveal that subgroups of whites have radically different life chances, depending on when, where, and to whom they are born.

Building on new work of scholars from many disciplines, this chapter describes the construction of whiteness from the colonial period to the present, a process that relied on five mechanisms of racial domination and marginalization; significant variation in white European Americans and three root causes—labor and wages, social safety net, and health care—as well as the potential contribution of whiteness; and considerations for action and research that may improve the health of white European Americans and that of all Americans.

PROCESSES OF RACIAL DOMINATION AND MARGINALIZATION AND THE CONSTRUCTION OF *WHITE* AND *WHITENESS*

Whiteness is not only a set of false beliefs about white superiority. It is also a set of processes enacted through social systems and institutions that have enabled white Americans to dominate and marginalize people of color throughout most of this nation's history. Most of these processes work by effectively closing off opportunities for advancement and advantage among people of color while hoarding and reserving resources for whites. These processes may be observed in other nations that are structured by ethnoracial inequality. Some of these processes were first articulated by the political scientist Raul Hilberg in his analysis of anti-Semitism in Europe.[21] Sociologist Loïc Wacquant was the first to combine them into a single analytical framework, calling them "the elementary forms of racial domination."[22(p1)] We refer to them here as categorization, discrimination, segregation, seclusion, and terrorization. The value in identifying and specifying these processes lies in being able to sharpen our analytical focus on a limited set of observable social forces.

Categorization

Categorization refers to the scientific, legal, and cultural process of producing systems of racial and ethnic classification, which sorted and ranked Americans by ancestry, skin color, hair type, and other phenotypical markers of perceived difference. Such differences were presumed to be both biological and immutable, as well as hierarchical. As such, the racial taxonomies developed in the United States were not a product of rigorous scientific observation but rather reflected existing prejudices and ethnocentric biases of the white scientists who produced them. While the science of racial classification was never really settled, the US court system and the US Census imposed binding definitions of who was white and who was not (e.g., the "one drop" rule of hypodescent) and laws were passed based on these nonscientific, commonsense definitions.*[23] These systems of hierarchical classification greatly influenced how white Americans thought and felt about people of color, allowing white supremacist ideology to become much more than a particular set of ethnocentric beliefs and attitudes that symbolically demeaned and dehumanized racial others. The social categorization that followed the cultural logic of white supremacist ideology provided the intellectual, legal, and moral justification for discrimination.

Discrimination

Discrimination refers to the differential treatment of individuals and groups based on group membership. The establishment and legal codification of white as a racial category gave legal cover and rights to whites who sought to treat people of color as less worthy, less deserving, and less capable than themselves, a situation known as de jure or formal discrimination.[25] For example, prior to its amendment after the Civil War, the US Constitution permitted all manner of discrimination against people of color.[26] The 1868 ratification of the Equal Protection Clause of the 14th Amendment made such discrimination unlawful, yet it continued. The lasting power of legal racial discrimination is such that even after the passage of constitutional amendments in the 19th and 20th centuries and federal legislation outlawed specific forms of racial discrimination, many forms of de facto or informal discrimination have endured.[25,27] Over generations, people of color

---

*To take another, more confusing example: the Naturalization Act of 1790 offered citizenship to any "free, white person" without offering a definition for white, and by the late 19th century, immigrants—some of whom documented their Caucasian ancestry—began suing the government to be counted as white. In the vast majority of these "racial prerequisite cases," the plaintiffs—despite their Caucasian genealogy—were denied whiteness and thus denied citizenship.[24]

have been systematically denied access to education, income and wealth accumulation, good jobs, health care, affordable housing, and more—affecting economic and social mobility but also health outcomes.[28] A primary form of discrimination is segregation.

Segregation

Segregation refers to the physical and material separation, voluntary or involuntary, of ethnoracial groups in social spaces. Sometimes the barriers enforcing physical separation were walls, railroad tracks, highways, or other elements of the built environment. Sometimes the barriers were enforced by social customs and habits. For example, following the end of Reconstruction in 1877, Jim Crow laws in the American South relegated Blacks to separate and unequal facilities in nearly all spheres of social life, from housing, to education, to public transportation, to houses of worship, to theaters, and to other public spaces.[29] In all cases, segregation worked effectively to surveil, control, and police the everyday movement of non-white people and to limit the social and physical contact between whites and non-whites. The history of racial segregation in the United States has led to the relative racial isolation of whites in all-white suburbs and rural places and the hyper-concentration of communities of color into poorer and more socially disadvantaged spaces.[30,31] From this legacy of residential racial segregation has followed segregated schools, workplaces, and public spaces of all kinds. Today, highly integrated neighborhoods and communities remain rare in the United States. Segregation has taken many different forms: one of the most of consequential of these is seclusion.

Seclusion

Seclusion refers to a range of practices that result in confining and concentrating specific populations into enclosed or semi-enclosed communities. Among the dominant, they exist as gated communities and wealthy neighborhoods and enclaves. Among the dominated, they take the form of ghettos, reservations, plantations, and camps. Minority populations subject to seclusion are targeted by stigma and held captive in order to allow the majority to better exploit their labor and skills, or to better neutralize any threat they are perceived to pose.*[22] In the United States, the Black urban ghetto and the Native American reservation system are the primary and most enduring examples of seclusive processes at work, while Japanese incarceration camps of World War II serve as a stark reminder that seclusion need not be permanent to have lasting effects. Outside all these spaces of

---

*An often-neglected feature of such places and spaces is that they do not only function as gatekeeping forms of social exclusion and control. In the case of ghettos, they can also serve their residents by becoming sites of protection wherein community-based institutions and social organizations arise that can shield them from the worst abuses of the dominant society.[32]

seclusion, the dominant stand ready to enforce boundaries, order, and subordination through the constant threat of racialized violence, a process we call terrorization.

Terrorization

Terrorization refers to racialized violence—both threats and acts—carried out by majorities against minorities. The various types range from interpersonal intimidation, to lynching and riots, to police brutality and mass incarceration, to ethnic cleansing and genocide. Terrorization has served as the ultimate enforcement of racial domination by whites in the United States. The most disturbing and shameful acts of racial terrorization in US history involve the ethnic cleansing and genocidal conquest of Indigenous Americans, along with centuries of enslavement and murder of Blacks.[33] Yet contemporary forms of racial terrorization (e.g., hate crimes) continue to shape racial interactions throughout the United States today, and are directed not just at Indigenous Americans and Blacks, but Latino, Asian, and Muslim populations as well.[34]

When other processes described here failed to control, contain, and subjugate people of color—or even in cases where some whites merely perceived a threat to white supremacy—racial terror and violence served as a brutal and often lethal reminder that white supremacy was not something that could be contested (even peacefully) by subordinates. When it was, racial terror was directed by whites at individuals, families, and entire communities and offers a compelling explanation for why subject populations complied—at least outwardly—with the dehumanizing categorizations and the daily injustices and insults to their freedom and dignity imposed by discrimination, segregation, and seclusion. To do otherwise was to court imprisonment, violence, torture, or death.

In sum, the five elementary processes proposed by Wacquant allow us to understand the underlying social machinery for producing racial domination and the ongoing marginalization of non-whites. These five different processes of racial domination and marginalization operate in different combinations in different times and places. However, they always involve vast assemblages of people, groups, and organizations all operating under a shared cultural logic—the same basic assumptions about racial and ethnic supremacy—such that decisions and actions need not be dictated by a centralized, top-down bureaucracy, but instead could be carried out from the ground up, as illustrated in the next section.

The Construction of *White* and *Whiteness*

Official racial and ethnic categories like the US Office of Management and Budget definitions have complicated histories in the United States.[35-37] An array of social forces drove their construction and development: capitalist and economic imperatives; ethnic, religious, and cultural nationalisms; white supremacy and (now) discredited racist science;

arcane and illogical legal rulings; popular prejudices; and, not least, social movements and political struggles over social, material, political, and symbolic resources and meanings.[24,38,39] The category of white and the construction of whiteness turned not only on skin color, but also on intersecting notions of class, status, ancestry, property, and freedom.[19,26,40,41]

This identity, formed in Europe over a millennium or more, was one of the major cultural exports of European colonialism.[26,42-44] Northern Europeans, particularly the English, associated lighter, whiter skin with purity, godliness, and Christian piety, valorizing whiteness over blackness.[45] These cultural meanings may have prejudiced Europeans' encounter with colonial Others from the start. For European colonizers in the 16th and 17th centuries, the color-coded symbolism of "whiteness as superior" helped justify the enslavement of darker peoples on plantations and their confinement on reservations (see the Seclusion section earlier), along with the invasion and dispossession of their land and its natural resources and the militarized imposition of colonial rule and genocide (see the Terrorization section earlier).[44,46]

In the American colonies and early republic, white became not just a potent symbol of civilizational superiority, but a highly codified legal and political identity that granted privileges, freedoms, and forms of legal immunity to white male landowners. Whatever the intent of this development of white identity, the practical outcome was a social system that ranked and classified (see the Categorization section earlier) white men in sharp contradistinction to Blacks, Indigenous people, and women of all races—who were viewed as inferior in all respects. This racialized social system protected white property, taken from Indigenous peoples and built on the labor of enslaved Africans, and the economic interests of the white elite.[47,48]

The progression from *white* as a symbol of civilizational superiority to *whiteness* as a legal and political materialization of near absolute power over other racial groups reached its high point in the antebellum American South. The Civil War marked the first historical turning point against whiteness, particularly the power to enslave, when the Emancipation Proclamation (1863) and Constitutional Amendments of the Reconstruction Era (1865-1877) began to formally recognize the full humanity of non-whites in both policy and law.

White backlash against the political and social advancement of non-whites was swift and violent (more terrorization).[49-51] Some whites sought new legal and extralegal ways to maintain white racial domination. Jim Crow laws—which restricted the rights of Blacks to vote, work, and get an education—enabled whites, particularly in the South, to maintain a superior social, economic, and political status.[16,29] In the words of W. E. B. Du Bois, these laws effectively paid even the poorest whites a "psychological wage" that gave them a sense of moral superiority over non-whites, thereby dissuading poor whites from making common cause or seeking solidarity with their economic peers because they were persons of color (see the Discrimination section earlier).[29,52,53]

Massive immigration in the 19th and early 20th centuries, primarily from Europe, but also from Asia, posed cultural and legal confusion about who counted as white. With few exceptions, only those deemed white by law could be eligible for US citizenship through naturalization, making questions over who would be classified as white of acute national importance and the subject of intensive study by racial scientists of the day, nearly all of whom were avid advocates of the new science of eugenics.[54,55] Their answers formed the evidentiary base for multiple legal rulings that strengthened the boundaries of the white category, restricting it to those already deemed by law and popular opinion to belong. Eugenics provided the rationale for the exclusionary immigration laws of 1924 and justified the involuntary sterilization of disabled or poor whites deemed biologically inferior and socially unfit for procreation.[11,56–58] Within a decade, many of these same laws were adopted in Germany, forming the legal foundation of Nazi racial hygiene and segregationist policies that led directly to the Holocaust.[59,60] In subsequent years, compulsory sterilization and medical experimentation in the United States also targeted Black and Latina women.[61–64]

Despite its power to subjugate and subordinate, whiteness in America is not a story of unwavering racial domination of whites over people of color. White supremacy, as both a political ideology and as a set of interlinked mechanisms embedded in America's key social institutions, began to lose its footing in the mid-20th century.[65] The end of World War II in 1945 unleashed two forces that challenged the meaning of whiteness and brought greater opportunities and social mobility to non-whites. The first was the discrediting of eugenics and scientific racism in the wake of the Holocaust. The horrors of racial extermination camps and scientific justification of genocide were deemed crimes against humanity and immoral. White Americans began to join non-white Americans in denouncing and resisting white supremacy.[65,66] For example, prosecutors and judges at the Nuremberg Trials denounced not just the terrors of Nazi murder but also racial hygiene and marriage laws, the segregation and ghettoization of ethnic minorities, and the racial logic of Aryan supremacy.[67]

The second major force challenging postwar whiteness was the ascendant Civil Rights and Black Freedom movements. Led by Black Americans, this massive social movement unsettled the racialized social order, and not just in the South. Progressive whites in the North and Midwest joined the movement as allies. Moreover, tangible economic and political gains were ushered in by Supreme Court rulings like *Brown v Board of Education* (1954) and the passage of the federal Civil Rights Acts of 1957, 1960, and 1964, the last of which prohibited discrimination on the basis of race, color, religion, sex, and national origin. Together, these acts targeted racial inequality in voting, labor markets, schools, and public accommodations and transportation. These federal policy changes both incited violent white backlash to racial desegregation in the South and inspired progressive white Americans to join movements for racial equality. Commenting on this period, philosopher Charles Mills noted that while formal, juridical white supremacy had come to an end, it was immediately replaced by a regime of de facto discrimination sustained in part by ongoing white racial resentment.[25]

A political commitment to racial equity was codified by a 1961 Presidential Executive Order that directed the federal government to take "affirmative action" to ameliorate racial discrimination. By the 1970s, state and federal policies supporting quotas and affirmative action became commonplace.[68] Indeed, these postwar decades coincided with a rising tide of intergenerational economic security and social mobility for many Americans of all colors. The G. I. Bill paved the way for hundreds of thousands of veterans' college degrees, professional careers, and homeownership. Steady jobs that offered good wages that could support a family could be had even by those without a college degree, benefits that accrued disproportionately to white men and their families.[69] Yet, union practices hostile to non-whites and women, along with discriminatory practices in the housing market that persisted even after redlining was outlawed in 1968, continued to limit the social mobility of people of color.[70,71]

Just as the newfound commitment to racial equality and broad acceptance of multiculturalism were taking hold in the 1980s, a rival political movement, which some scholars call neoliberalism,[72,73] began to make serious gains in both the United States and abroad. Framed in economic and political terms (e.g., free markets, austerity, small government, deregulation, individual rights), by the 1990s neoliberal rhetoric mobilized white resentment against racial minorities, whom they perceived as the primary beneficiaries of government programs.[74-77] The eventual result was a neoliberal political order whose imperatives were to globalize markets and labor, dissolve unions, and eliminate social safety nets in the name of economic restructuring and austerity.[78] Social scientists studying the long-term effects of neoliberalism often argue that among its chief consequences have been unchecked economic inequality and a concomitant limiting of life chances for all but the most privileged class.[79]

Around this same time, a "colorblind" racial ideology—the idea that race should not determine a society's treatment of people—became normative, tapping into American ideals of equal opportunity and hewing to neoliberalism's spirit of individualism. The refrain, "I don't see color," seeped into the white public's consciousness, forging a more covert form of racism that obscured centuries of white privilege and ignored entrenched racial inequities.[69,80] By the 1990s, the national conversation about racial equity shifted to the value of "multiculturalism" in workplaces, schools, and communities,[81] which by the 2000s was replaced with rhetoric and practices of "diversity, equity, and inclusion (DEI)."

A logic of cultural difference guided these movements. The central demand was equal recognition for people of color, women, lesbian, gay, bisexual, transgender, queer, and questioning (LGBTQ+) individuals and other marginalized identities, not economic equality,[82] making them compatible with capitalism and neoliberalism.[78] The upshot was a lexicon of social justice that sidelined class as a category of social analysis and class politics as a platform for economic justice for all and amplified identity-based difference and politics.[20,83,84] How, if at all, white identities fit within this logic of cultural and racial difference remains unclear.[83,85] But it may be implicated in the resurrection of a virulent form of white identity. In recent years, some white insurrectionist leaders and elected politicians have openly embraced old ideologies of white supremacy, stoked fears of "replacement theory," and boldly advocated a return to whites-only public spaces and to closing US borders to non-white immigrants,[86] often doing so by mobilizing white class resentment against multicultural elites.

Postwar America opened up a conscious renegotiation of white American identity and whiteness. A resurgent white supremacist ideology and identity began to appear in the mid-1990s, as the advent of the internet offered new avenues for dissemination and circulation of old ideas as well as provided powerful means for recruitment and social networking for racist elements of the Far Right.[87,88] Racial resentment and race hatred, having been confined to the margins after Civil Rights, was now reentering mainstream politics and discourse, most prominently in the form of the Tea Party, which flourished in the wake of the 2008 presidential election.[89] One result is that the racial status of white Americans is a topic now hotly contested by whites themselves, with a resulting political polarization among whites that may drive election cycles for a generation or more to come.[16,90,91]

HEALTH DISPARITIES IN WHITE EUROPEAN AMERICANS: EPIDEMIOLOGY AND ROOT CAUSES

Systemic racism has compromised the health status of communities of color for generations and maintained deep, persistent disparities with the generally superior health status of white European Americans. However, white European Americans are a large and highly heterogenous population, and their health varies dramatically between rich and poor, educated and uneducated, and other subgroups differentially situated at the crossroads of advantage and disadvantage. For all the social, material, and psychological advantages that accompany whiteness, it should not be conceptualized as a monolith of privilege.[92,93]

As is the case for everyone, disparities in the health of white European Americans are attributable to root causes that shape opportunities for health and health risks. Extensive research demonstrates that social and material resources embedded in social, economic, and environmental conditions—such as education, income, occupation, health care, housing, transportation, and safety—shape health outcomes.[94,95] Macro-social structures, such as public policies and spending, the law, and economic and labor market trends in turn influence the availability of and access to these conditions. This multilevel ecosystem of structures, conditions, and resources drives the production and distribution of health at the population level (Figure 7-1).[96]

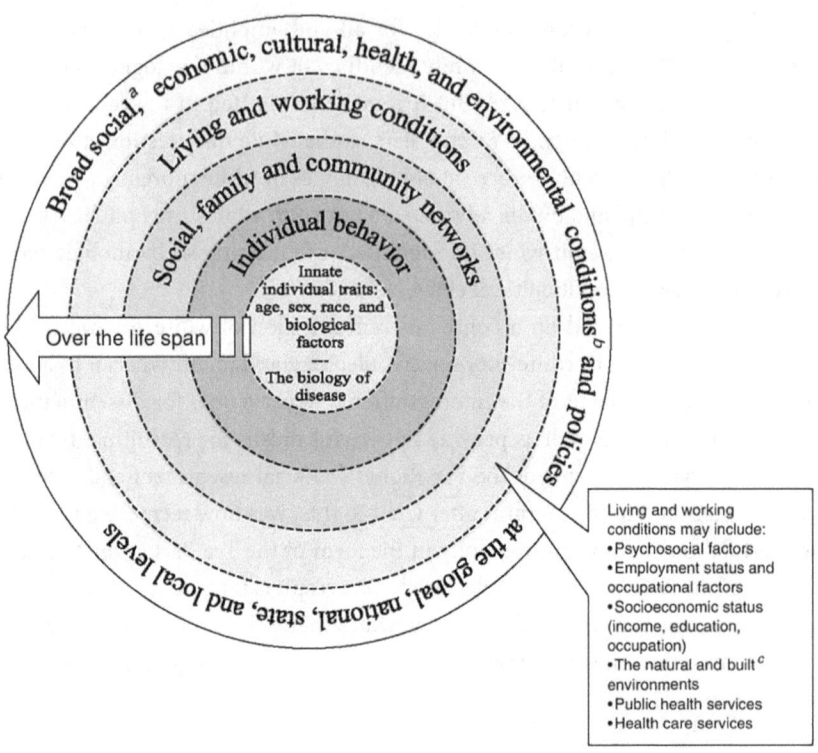

Source: Institute of Medicine.[96] Reprinted with permission of National Academies Press.
[a]Social conditions include, but are not limited to, economic inequality, urbanization, mobility, cultural values, attitudes, and policies related to discrimination, and intolerance on the basis of race, gender, and other differences.
[b]Other conditions at the national level might include major sociopolitical shifts, such as recession, war, and governmental collapse.
[c]The built environment includes transportation, water and sanitation, housing, and other dimensions of urban planning.

Figure 7-1. Socioecological Model

Absent from this ecosocial model of health are the power relations that determine the range of possible social conditions and distribute populations into those conditions.[97–99] They determine not only the range of opportunities and socioeconomic resources available to different populations but also the social relations to which people are exposed. Interlocking systems of power at the macro level (e.g., structural racism, colonialism, capitalism, patriarchy, heterosexism) oppress some to the benefit of others.

These systems of power may not be easily seen but they are powerfully felt. They differentially expose people at the micro level to various forms of harm from disrespect and discrimination to exclusion and extermination,[100] all of which have health implications. With the notable exception of skin color, other sources of social differentiation and domination that shape the life chances of all Americans also shape the health prospects of white European Americans. Their health chances turn not only on advantages they hold in a socially constructed racial hierarchy but also on their location in social systems that sort and stratify human value on the basis of class origin, education, income, wealth, sexual orientation, gender, geography, and more.[101-105] Being white does not protect the mind and body from adverse childhood experiences, intergenerational poverty, chronic socioeconomic stress, poor quality schools, domestic and community violence, unsafe housing, environmental toxins, structural sexism, or ableism. These social conditions and relations get under the skin,[99,106,107] even if that skin is white.[108]

The pathways from social conditions to poor health can take a variety of routes. Some are more direct than others, as when people lack the health care they need to survive. Others are more indirect, as when the brain responds to chronic stress by activating the adrenal gland, triggering the release of cortisol and other stress hormones that, over time, can harm the body. The potential health consequences of chronic stress include immune disorders and inflammation, atherosclerosis, coronary heart disease, preterm birth, cognitive impairment, premature mortality, and more.[109-113]

Examples of White Health Disparities

Health disparities exist within the white population and, for some subgroups of whites, a "white health advantage" compared with Blacks and American Indians/Alaska Natives is much smaller than many might presume or nonexistent. Health disparities within the white population are nontrivial and highly variable across the United States. In 2023, the death rate among non-Hispanic white people in West Virginia was 77% higher than among white people in Hawai'i.[114] During 2019-2023, in Marlboro County, South Carolina, the risk that white adults aged 40 to 64 years might die from heart disease was more than 16 times higher than in Marin County, California.[115]

As is the case for other racial groups, health outcomes are highly dependent on social class. For example, a recent study found that the probability of white adults aged 25 to 64 years dying in the next 34 years was 24% lower among incorporated white business owners than among white workers. Those not in the labor force (e.g., due to disability, retirement, or domestic responsibilities) were 148% more likely to die.[105]

White European Americans with less education, low-wage and precarious employment, and limited or no wealth experience more adverse health outcomes than those higher on the socioeconomic ladder. For example, white adults living in poverty are more than five times as likely to report poor health status than those with the most income.[116] A study based on national data collected from death certificates found that life expectancy among white women with 0 to 11 years of education was about 10 years shorter than white women with 16 or more years of education.[101]

The health of white European Americans is particularly poor in geographic areas with longstanding intergenerational poverty. White European Americans living in six states—Alabama, Georgia, Kentucky, Mississippi, Tennessee, and West Virginia—generally

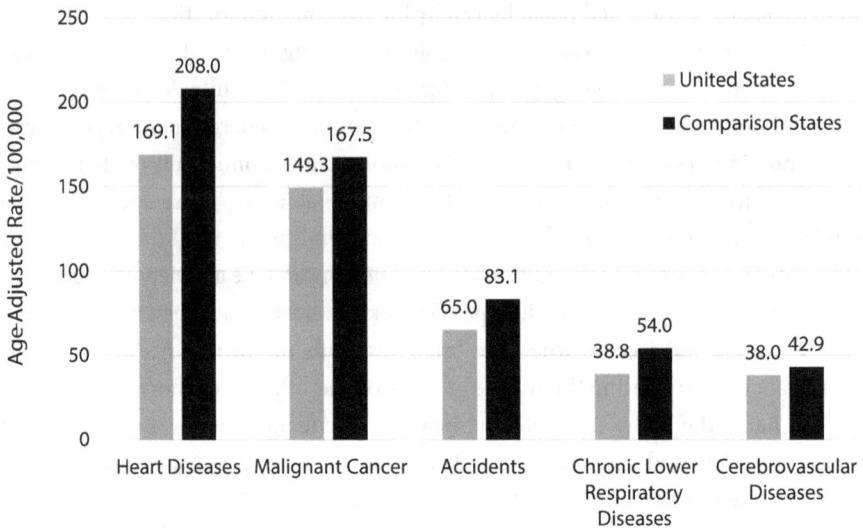

Source: Based on data from Centers for Disease Control and Prevention.[114]
Note: Comparison states include Alabama, Georgia, Kentucky, Mississippi, Tennessee, and West Virginia.

Figure 7-2. Mortality Rates for the 5 Leading Causes of Death Among Non-Hispanic White Populations: Comparison States Vs. United States, 2023

experience the shortest life expectancy and higher rates of disease, injury, and mortality than those elsewhere (Figure 7-2).[114] In 2023, four out of 10 (41.2%) white adults in West Virginia were obese and in 2022, one out of five (21.9%) white adults in Kentucky described their health as fair or poor.[117]

Living in rural America also contributes to poor health. Compared with white European Americans in urban counties, those in rural counties generally experience worse health outcomes—greater disease, injury, and disability—than white European Americans living in suburban or urban settings. This "rural health penalty" has increased over time.[118] In 2020, the all-cause mortality rate among whites in rural counties was 21% higher than in large metropolitan counties, up from 7% in 1999.[119] This rural health penalty is notable among white European American youth: rural counties experience the highest infant mortality rates, the highest suicide rate at ages 10 to 24 years, the highest homicide rate among infants and children below age 15, and the highest death rate from motor vehicle accidents at ages 10 to 24 years.[120] Rural areas also experience higher rates of chronic disease from the leading causes of death among middle-aged and older adults (e.g., malignant cancer, circulatory disease, chronic lower respiratory disease, chronic liver disease, suicide).

When health data are compared by racial group in aggregate, the superior health of higher income and higher educated whites obscures very poor health for low-income whites who lack college and high school degrees. For the most socially disadvantaged, little to no "white health advantage" may exist. For example, in 2019 to 2023 in Alabama, the

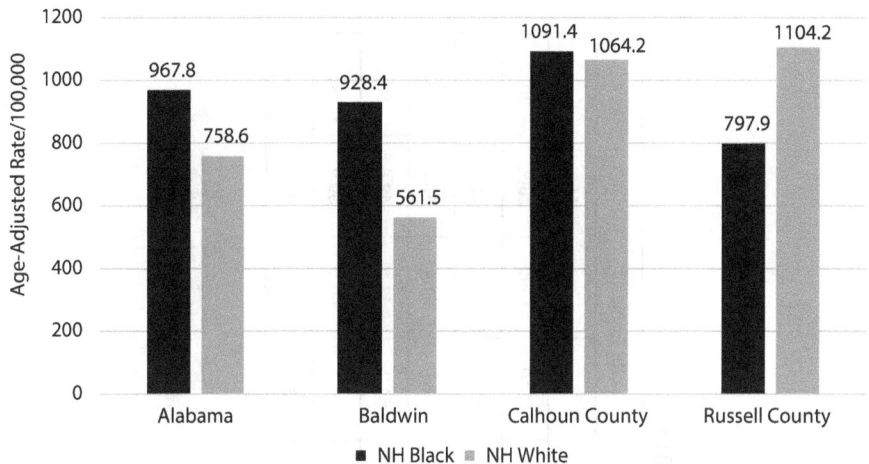

Source: Based on data from National Institute on Minority Health and Health Disparities.[115]
Note: NH = non-Hispanic.

Figure 7-3. Age-Adjusted Mortality by Race, Ages 40–64 Years: Alabama and Selected Counties, 2019–2023

probability of Black adults aged 40 and older dying prematurely (<65 years) was 967.8 per 100,000, 28% higher than among white adults of the same age statewide (758.6/100,000). However, the disparity between Black and white mortality rate differed considerably at the county level. While the Black mortality rate was 65% higher than in the white population in Baldwin County, Alabama, adjacent to Mobile, it was only 3% higher in Calhoun County, home to Anniston (Figure 7-3).[115] In Russell County, Alabama, which borders Georgia, the mortality rate in white adults aged 40 to 64 years was 28% higher than in the Black population.

There are other examples. A study based on national data collected from death certificates found that life expectancy among 25-year-old Black women with 0 to 11 years of education was higher than among white women with the same age and level of education, the latter of whom experienced a 3-year decline in life expectancy, as seen in Table 7-1.[101]

The white population has generally poorer health than Hispanic/Latino and Asian Americans who, for example, experience longer life expectancy (Figure 7-4)[121] as well as lower prevalence rates for many forms of disease and injury.[122]

Root Causes of White Health Disparities

Socioeconomic status and resources are root causes of health disparities in all populations, including white European Americans. Population health theory and voluminous evidence demonstrate that socioeconomic resources are causally implicated in the

Table 7-1. Life Expectancy (Y) at Age 25 by Race, Gender, and Educational Attainment: United States, 1990–2010

| Education (y) | NH White | | | | | | | NH Black | | | | | |
| | Women | | | Men | | | Women | | | Men | | |
	1990	2000	2010	1990	2000	2010	1990	2000	2010	1990	2000	2010
0–11	54.0	51.5	50.9	46.0	45.2	45.4	49.9	49.5	51.8	39.6	42.2	45.5
12	55.1	55.6	55.9	48.7	50.0	50.5	49.2	50.4	52.7	41.4	43.9	46.5
13–15	55.2	56.0	56.7	49.7	52.3	52.8	49.6	51.6	54.2	43.1	48.6	50.9
≥16	56.5	58.7	60.2	52.1	54.9	57.3	51.8	54.5	56.5	46.5	50.4	54.1
Total	55.4	55.8	56.9	49.3	51.1	52.5	50.8	51.6	54.0	42.2	45.3	48.5

Source: Sasson.[101] Reprinted under the terms of the CC BY license (https://creativecommons.org/licenses/by/4.0).

Note: NH = non-Hispanic.

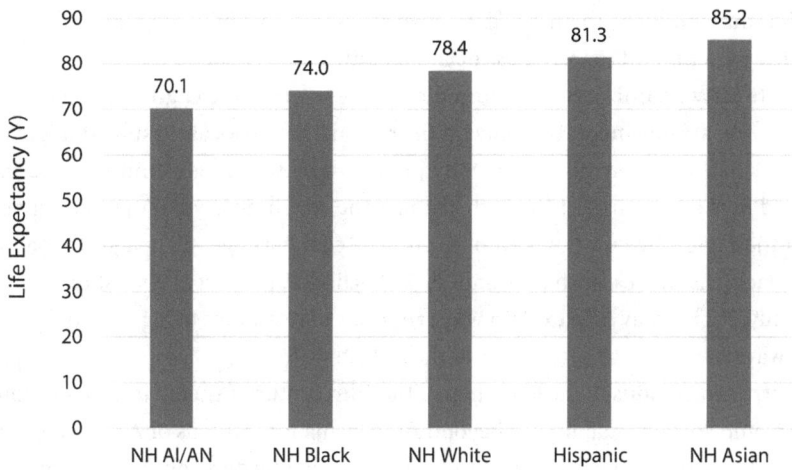

Source: Based on data from Arias et al.[121]
Note: AI/AN = American Indian or Alaska Native; NH = non-Hispanic.

Figure 7-4. Life Expectancy by Race/Ethnicity: United States, 2023

production and distribution of health, functioning as "fundamental causes" of health inequalities.[123,124] The importance of education and income to health, including the health of white European Americans, has grown over time in the United States.[125,126] Three areas of US policy drive white health disparities: labor and wages, the social safety net, and health care.

Labor and Wages

Since its founding, the United States has favored the interests of capital over labor. There have been periods of progressive government action to protect people's health and well-being, such as New Deal policies, the War on Poverty, the Great Society, and Civil Rights legislation.[78] But the pendulum tends always to swing back to the interests of those with capital and power.

This history is reflected in the health outcomes of white European Americans, past and present. Take, for example, the longstanding poor health documented in white Appalachians. The original settlers took control of most of the Appalachian Mountain range from central Pennsylvania southwest to Georgia after the Trail of Tears and other federal acts of Indian Removal. Their dominance gave way to transnational coal producers who acquired tens of thousands of acres of land and the rights to all natural resources. The region became a "sacrifice zone" where the Northeast and Midwest extracted resources and maximized profits for investors, who did not reinvest in the land

and labor that produced them, an "extractive economy" that blights a region's human and ecological systems and exacerbates social inequities.[127]

Despite early unionization and periodic displays of union strength, exploitative working and living arrangements prevailed in the region, leaving locals to subsist in poverty.[128] As unions declined, sometimes violently put down by the US government, and mining dwindled in the latter half of the 20th century, the coal industry built public support for coal in the region by curating and marketing a "coal heritage" campaign that appealed to Appalachians' values, such as economic self-reliance, property ownership, male labor, and family.[128] This may help explain why eruptions of resistance to big coal in Appalachia have always given way to acceptance of the industry.[129]

Government actions in the latter half of the 20th century ushered in greater economic precarity and social instability far beyond Appalachia for millions of Americans, including white European Americans. A web of US governmental decisions (e.g., union busting, tax cuts for the wealthy), policies (e.g., trade agreements such as the 1992 North American Free Trade Agreement, welfare reforms such as the 1996 Personal Responsibility and Work Opportunity Act), and labor trends (e.g., the gig economy) reflected the rise of neoliberalism (see The Construction of White and Whiteness section earlier) that globalized markets and labor, privatized the economy, and redistributed income and wealth upward to the economic elite.[76–78,130–132]

Deindustrialization, the dissolution of unions, and the transition from an industrial economy to a knowledge economy transformed the US labor market. Workers were moved from factories to offices and laboratories and made a four-year college degree a prerequisite for many jobs and a marker of social status.[133] While some Americans made this transition by getting a college degree or more advanced training and entered the middle class, others could not. People of all races were left behind, particularly people of color, but also working-class white European Americans. Many had grown accustomed to stable manufacturing jobs with good benefits and the possibility of career advancement. They now had had to fall back on less desirable jobs, often in the service industry, that paid less and offered fewer, if any, benefits.

Wages for available jobs often failed to keep pace with inflation and the rising cost of living. Minimum wage laws, where they existed, were set too low to keep families out of poverty. Expenses for basic needs such as nutritious food, housing, transportation, and childcare became increasingly unaffordable, especially for low-income households. Escalating health care costs dramatically outpaced inflation, compelling people to defer care or take on medical debt (see the Health Care System section later). The costs of living were acute for families of limited means, forcing many to work multiple jobs, including women who often shouldered the dual responsibilities of caregiving and outside work. Social mobility became exceedingly difficult for those with limited education. When adjusted for inflation, workers with a high school diploma made 2.7% less in 2017 than they would have in 1979; workers with no high school diploma made almost 10% less.[134]

The 21st century brought another major change to labor: a shift from standard employment arrangements involving a contract, rights, and benefits to precarious employment as an independent contractor.[135] Big companies transitioned from employing a stable, full-time workforce, in which labor shared in gains, to outsourcing operations to cut labor costs.[136] While this "gig" work may be advantageous for the highly skilled and well compensated, workers without a college degree now deliver people's food or walk dogs to make ends meet.[137] Millions of good jobs with living wages, benefits, regular hours, security, and social connections have been replaced by precarious jobs unprotected by minimum wage regulations, overtime rules, unemployment insurance, and workers' compensation.[135] Compared with other high-income countries, the United States stands out for the high percentage of its workforce (~25%) doing low-wage work.[135] Most low-wage workers lack access to benefits that typically accompany higher wage work done by those with a college education, such as health insurance, sick pay, paid vacation, and retirement accounts.

These flexible employment arrangements increase the rate of unemployment and underemployment and shift risk and expenses (e.g., for health insurance and copayments, car expenses, and retirement savings) from employers and companies to individuals and their families.[134,138] These ostensibly flexible job arrangements are often not that flexible, and ultimately offer only part-time work.[135] The United States ranks at the bottom among Organisation for Economic Co-operation and Development countries on numerous indicators of worker protections for temporary work arrangements.[139]

This transformation in work arrangements and wages affected all racial groups, including white European Americans, particularly those lacking a college or high school degree. However, whites who had been middle or working class, or who were from families that once enjoyed working-class or middle-class stability and respectability, may have been experiencing such hardships for the first time (see the Whiteness section later).

Social Safety Net

The United States tolerates among the highest levels of adult and childhood poverty in countries with developed economies.[140] Studies show that millions of Americans live in "deep poverty," defined as less than $2 a day, a standard long thought relevant only to low-income countries.[141,142] Despite the myth that "poverty happens to other people," the majority of Americans experience poverty in their lifetimes, including whites.[143] Although people of color are disproportionately represented among the poor, whites still account for more than 40% of the total number of poor people in the United States.[144]

The nation lacks a comprehensive, federally guaranteed safety net and millions of Americans do not apply or receive benefits for which they are eligible.[145] The system is fragmented, application procedures are complicated, and the stigma associated with welfare programs is potent.[134,143] Although welfare spending has increased considerably over the past several decades, much of it never reaches those who need it.[134] In 1996, when the Aid to Families with Dependent Children program was replaced by Temporary Assistance for Needy Families (TANF), states were given block grants and broad flexibility in how to use the money. Many states use the dollars for purposes other than direct income support for poor families.[146] In 2020, only 22 cents of every dollar budgeted for TANF went directly to poor families.[134] States spent the money on a wide range of other programs, such as job training, financial literacy programs, juvenile justice administration, marriage support and counseling initiatives, abstinence-only sex education, and anti-abortion crisis pregnancy centers.[134] States are allowed to roll TANF dollars over from year to year rather than keeping children and adults out of poverty, and dollars that do reach the people in need go disproportionately to health care (e.g., Medicaid), rather than keeping them out of poverty and free of disease.[134]

Much of the assistance offered to low-income Americans goes untapped by those who need it. Only 25% of families who qualify for TANF apply for it; 20% of parents eligible for Medicaid and the Children's Health Insurance program do not enroll; and during the Great Recession (2007–2009) only 10% of Americans drew unemployment.[134e] Each year, billions of dollars go unclaimed: by one estimate, $17.3 billion in Earned Income Tax Credit dollars; $13.4 billion in food stamp benefits; $62.2 billion in government health insurance; $9.9 in unemployment insurance; and $38.9 billion in Supplemental Security Income go unclaimed.[134]

The United States also stands out among high-income countries for lacking programs that help keep workers in the labor force, such as guaranteed paid leave.[147] Employers might grant such leave voluntarily, but it varies in duration and generosity. Part-time and low-wage workers are far less likely to receive any such benefits. Income assistance exists, but people have to be poor enough to qualify for some mix of cash and in-kind assistance.

Health Care System

The health care system contributes to health inequities through multiple pathways, among them barriers to access (e.g., costs) and delays and discrimination in delivering timely and effective care. Although health is shaped by the social determinants of health and health care accounts for only 10% to 20% of health outcomes,[148] health care services or the lack thereof play a central role in almost every disease and affect all ethnoracial groups, including white European Americans. Primary and specialty care, hospitals and emergency departments, emergency medical services and trauma centers, and mental health and substance abuse services determine morbidity and mortality rates from acute emergencies, chronic diseases, mental illness, addiction disorders, and survival from attempted suicide or homicide.

The lack of universal access to health care in the United States and the over-reliance on employer-based health insurance adversely affect health outcomes,[149] as do exorbitant out-of-pocket costs for copayments, prescription medications, and medical supplies. Health inequities experienced by the white population and other ethnoracial groups have much to do with its cost. In Nebraska in 2023, for example, more than one out of five (21%) respondents reported medical cost burden (costs accounting for >10% of annual income).[150] Out-of-pocket costs pose an economic burden even for those who are insured under employer-based commercial plans or public programs such as Medicare and Medicaid. A 2017 survey found that 17% of white people were in debt for medical bills, owing an average of $12,310,[151] and a more recent 2022 study reported that 37% of white adults carry medical debt.[152]

Economic downturns also reduce access to care. A previous generation of white workers enjoyed reliable health insurance among the benefits of union jobs. Workers who lost jobs when the manufacturing sector collapsed in the 1970s and 1980s and who experienced stagnant or decreasing incomes and rising poverty rates faced mounting cost burdens for health care, housing, childcare, and more. Costly health care is untenable for uninsured or underinsured people, who are more likely to forgo care due to costs. Medical costs pose an even greater barrier in areas with high poverty rates, such as Appalachia. In 2023, approximately 12% of white adults in Alabama, Mississippi, and Georgia said they could not get needed medical care because of costs.[150]

Although low-income individuals are eligible for Medicaid, the threshold for eligibility varies by state. Eligibility was expanded under the Affordable Care Act, but a number of states opposed Medicaid expansion, removing health care options for many low-income families in those states, white families included (Figure 7-5).[153]

Cost is not the only barrier to health care. Shortages in medical, dental, and behavioral health providers and in hospitals, laboratories, and other facilities can limit access to care, as can lack of resources and transportation to travel to other areas. People who do not own automobiles, who cannot afford or access public transportation, or who have little time because of (often multiple) jobs and family duties are often unable to seek medical care and face even greater challenges in obtaining regular follow-up for chronic diseases. Distance is a particular challenge for people in rural areas, where hospitals are often scarce and poorly funded, and specialists are located in faraway cities and suburbs. For example, in the extremely rural state of Wyoming in 2023, 21% of white respondents reported not having a regular doctor.[150] Between 2010 and 2021, financial pressures caused the closure of 136 rural hospitals[154] and today hundreds more are at risk of closing.[155]

Finally, victims of trauma (e.g., drug overdoses, attempted suicide, firearm injuries, motorists involved in traffic accidents), especially in rural areas, often do not survive because of delays in receiving emergency care or in getting transported to trauma centers.[156] One study reported that 29% of rural patients were initially transported to major trauma centers compared with 89% of urban patients.[157]

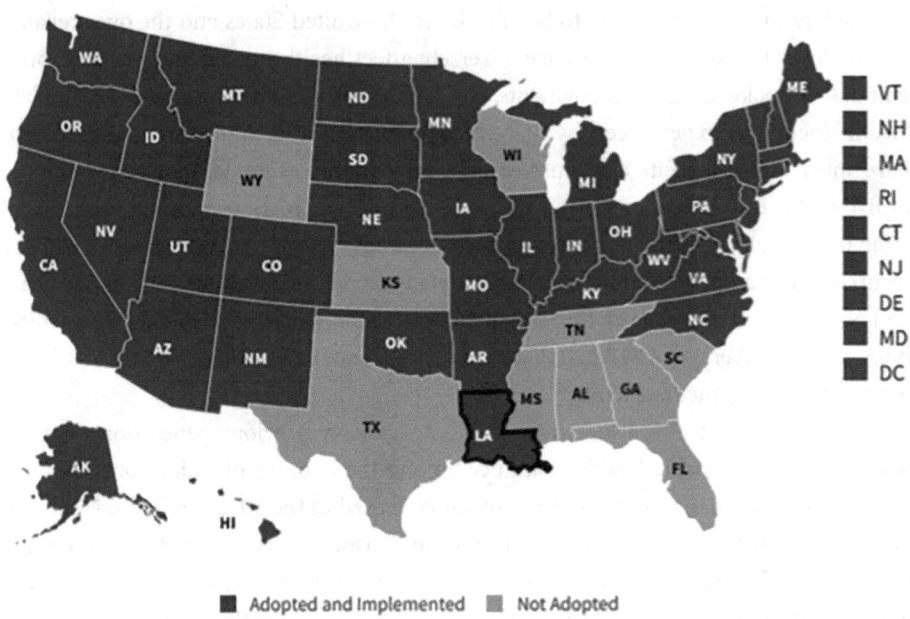

Source: Reprinted from Kaiser Family Foundation.[155]

Figure 7-5. States That Have Adopted Medicaid Expansion: United States, 2025

The impact of prolonged economic precarity and chronic socioeconomic deprivation compromises people's minds and bodies, no matter their race. However, one promising area of new research has begun to investigate the health of whites through a prism of whiteness, investigating how whiteness influences whites' policy preferences, which help shape US economic conditions, as well as how they register socioeconomic hardship.

Whiteness

In addition to the social determinants of health just described, whiteness has been proposed as a potential contributor to health disparities in the white population, but the supporting evidence is nascent. Whiteness studies in population health to date are relatively few and preliminary in nature.[158-165] However, this chapter discusses this important emerging area of study for two reasons. First, the racial category "white" has been inadequately investigated as a racial category in population health research. The meanings, realities, and potential health implications of being white have yet to be fully conceptualized and studied. Instead, the racial category white has functioned primarily as a referent or norm against which to compare the health of other ethnoracial groups. Used in this way, the category may help to maintain false and racist ideas about white superiority.

Second, research on the potential harmful effects of whiteness may enable more complete explanations of health disparities among white European Americans. An intersectional turn in population health posits that health disparities cannot be adequately explained or remedied by examining health outcomes one analytic category at a time—such as race *or* class *or* gender *or* sexuality.[166] Studies must instead examine how these structures operate together (e.g., race *and* class *and* gender) because they act jointly in the world, shaping lived realities and the meaning people make of it.[167,168] For example, explaining the absolute decline in life expectancy of low-education white women noted above will require elucidating the meaning and consequences of living as a white woman without a high school diploma in the late 20th century. An explanation will need to attend to the likely interplay not only of class (poor, low education) and gender (female) but also race (whiteness). Similarly, the longstanding poor health among white people in Appalachia reflects not only the effects on the mind and body of grinding poverty but also the ways whiteness shapes the experience and meaning of impoverishment and the persistence of a "white trash" stigma associated with being white, rural, and poor.[11]

Malat and colleagues have advanced the first comprehensive framework of whiteness in population health, central to which is the idea of racial capitalism.[161] *Racial capitalism* holds that capitalism relies on the differentiation of human value and exploitation of land and labor to extract profit and accumulate wealth, and that these are inseparable from racialization and racism.[169,170] Because US capitalism evolved in concert with racialized systems (e.g., slavery, settler colonialism, Jim Crow), Malat et al. argue that recognizing the linkages between whiteness and capitalism will help elucidate "the paradox of whites' poor health on selected indicators, despite their many advantages in the racialized social system."[161(p148)] They posit that whiteness shapes US economic conditions in ways that limit the health potential of all Americans, including white European Americans.

Malat et al. identify several pathways through which whiteness may impact the health of whites: societal conditions, individual social characteristics and experiences, and psychosocial responses.[162] The history and ideology of whiteness—which turn on the creation of racial categories and supporting white supremacist narratives—contribute to inequitable social conditions, which in turn affect individual social characteristics and experiences that mediate psychosocial responses.

One primary way whiteness may contribute to inequitable social conditions is opposition to social policies. Public support for social policies can turn on attitudes and prejudices about the groups perceived to benefit.[171,172] Experimental studies have shown that explicit specification of African American as a racial category or racial cues (e.g., images) can activate attributions of individual responsibility (e.g., for crime, poverty, and poor health) and weaken support for social responsibility and programs.[173-175] Studies have also shown that opposition among whites to the Affordable Care Act and past health care legislation was based on overt or covert racial prejudice.[162,176,177] Politicians who opposed Medicaid expansion were motivated in part by racist concerns that benefits would accrue to people of color.[176, 178-180] One can infer, given the extensive evidence of the health benefits of Medicaid expansion,[181] that racially motivated opposition compromised health outcomes and may have caused excess deaths, including in the white population.

Drawing on critical race theory, some whiteness studies also posit that opposition to social programs based on economic or moral grounds (e.g., austerity, free markets, individualism, liberty) is implicitly racist, because such opposition upholds structural racism and perpetuates racial inequity.[80] For example, in focus groups, Metzl found that concerns expressed by whites on a range of issues—Medicaid expansion, the repeal of the Affordable Care Act, taxes, and gun policy—often lacked any explicit mention of race or racial animus.[162] Instead those concerns were couched in economic or moral terms (e.g., austerity, free markets, personal responsibility). Yet, Metzl finds whiteness at work in these justifications, because they are often tinged with racial subtext about deservingness and perpetuate racial inequity.

Psychosocial responses to economic and social hardship are another potential pathway under investigation. As white expectations for success have been dashed by decades of declining social and economic mobility among working-class and middle-income whites, they may register these conditions not only as a threat to their well-being and that of their families, but also to their social or racial status, leading them to long for a "better past."[161] Survey data document the prevalence of this narrative, with more than half of white Americans reporting that discrimination against whites is a serious problem.[182,183] The psychosocial upshot, studies hypothesize, is a racial or social threat response that can lead to poor health via biological and behavioral mechanisms, such as depression, anger, and prolonged stress that leads to chronic disease, suicide, and substance misuse.[163] A recent scoping review found 12 studies suggesting that actual or perceived threats to social position can adversely impact the health of some whites, just as they do in other racial and ethnic groups.[165] Languishing associated with economic deprivation and status loss predicts mortality, and some research suggests the effect may be stronger in whites than in Blacks.[184]

Other psychosocial responses may also be at work. For example, research has found that socially advantaged groups have less capacity to adapt to adversity.[185] Whereas Blacks, who have long faced great socioeconomic hardship, may be more likely to attribute adversity to structural explanations and find positive meaning in adversity (e.g., redemption), whites may be more likely to blame Black and brown people or to blame themselves.[161] Both attributions of blame reflect ideologies of individualism and meritocracy, which can harm the health of people no matter their race.[186]

Whiteness studies in population health parallel scholarship in a wide array of other disciplines that, while not focused on health, provide additional conceptual footing for this work. For example, Desmond describes American capitalism as an unregulated, extractive, and exploitative market economy that originated on slave labor plantations and today produces extreme inequality, poverty, and widespread misery.[187] Hohle argues that neoliberal imperatives (e.g., privatization, deregulation, dissolution of unions, tax cuts for the wealthy) pivot on a "white-private/black-public binary."[188(p4)] McGhee traces the paucity of US public goods—from universal health care to quality public schools and infrastructure—to a racist "zero-sum" mindset.[69]

Whether and to what degree whiteness may be implicated in white health disparities remains to be demonstrated. Any answer to the question will depend on how whiteness is conceptualized and operationalized. There is no consensus on the question of what whiteness is, and conceptual models will need to address intersectional heterogeneity within the white population. Another nontrivial challenge to the field is developing measures that can accurately plumb what whites believe and why. Critical race theories and whiteness frameworks putatively resolve some of the key issues by interpreting the ideologies of capitalism, meritocracy, and individualism themselves as racist. But in empirical studies, theory needs to be supported by measures sensitive enough to distinguish between beliefs grounded in racial prejudice and beliefs grounded in economic or moral principles that on their face are race-free (e.g., austerity, small government, personal responsibility, liberty).[189] Ideas, emotions, and attitudes are notoriously difficult to observe and measure; how and to what extent they might motivate or dictate actions, behaviors, and policy preferences—much less their effect on health outcomes—are even harder to discern.

The five structural processes of racial domination and marginalization (categorization, discrimination, segregation, seclusion, and terrorization) delineated earlier, however, are more amenable to measurement. If operationalized for the context of population health, these processes could provide alternative or additional evidence about the role of whiteness in shaping white health disparities. Keeping the focus on structures, rather than individuals, might also help support a sense of shared responsibility for positive social action in the here and now.[190]

CONSIDERATIONS FOR ACTION AND FURTHER RESEARCH

Many population health investments that would prevent disease and support health in white European Americans would also support the health of all Americans. Among the most important steps toward health equity is to address the legacy of systemic racism, which continues to perpetuate inequities in health and other dimensions of well-being. Antiracism efforts are working to reduce segregation, dismantle policies and structures that have operated for generations to limit opportunities based on race, and apply an equity lens to promote more inclusive policies.

A commitment to racial equity should include an intentional approach to population health investments that protects against inadvertently exacerbating racial inequities in health. *Proportionate universalism*, for example, recommends making universal investments at the structural level to promote overall health and targeted investments in subpopulations that are proportionate to the level of disadvantage.[191] This approach could help ensure that population health policy can meet the health needs of all vulnerable communities no matter their color, while reducing the chances that such investments exacerbate inequities rooted in race, class, gender, and other systems of marginalization. Moving the needle on health equity for all ethnoracial groups will require population health investments in all three policy arenas discussed in this chapter.

Labor and Wages

Equipping workers with competitive skills for 21st century jobs should be a priority. Investing in education from pre-K and secondary education through college and vocational schools is critical. The revitalization of unions and a labor movement that protects workers of all races and genders would help secure livable wages, paid leave, affordable health insurance coverage, secure retirements, and social mobility for workers' children.[192]

Strategies to promote economic development and job creation are also vital, especially in communities that have suffered from chronic disinvestment. Priorities include community infrastructure such as ensuring food security, providing affordable housing and public transportation, creating built environments that encourage physical activity and ease stress, addressing the root causes of crime and violence, and reducing vulnerability to severe weather and climate change. Rural communities need investments in infrastructure (e.g., broadband), to attract economic opportunity.

Social Safety Net

Strengthening the social safety net would protect the health and well-being of those set back by serious illness, economic downturns, and catastrophic events such as the COVID-19 pandemic and increasingly common extreme weather events. A first priority should be to help millions of families enroll in programs for which they are eligible but do not apply for. A second should be making permanent the Earned Income Tax Credit (EITC) and expanding its eligibility criteria, as occurred during the COVID-19 pandemic. While some states have made the tax credit permanent, most states have let it sunset. The EITC lifts millions of families out of poverty, improves health outcomes, and supports child development.[193,194] Affordable housing solutions and support for poor and low-income families should also be prioritized. Unlike spending growth in other social programs, housing aid has plummeted to its lowest level in a quarter century.[195]

None of these priorities can occur in the absence of political will, which requires broad public support. Building public support for anti-poverty programs in a nation that valorizes self-reliance, individualizes responsibility, and stigmatizes poverty is a complex challenge. Solutions will need to take many forms, from communication campaigns that destigmatize poverty by showing that it can and does afflict millions of Americans of all ethnoracial groups for reasons beyond individual control to intersectionally diverse anti-poverty social movements such as the Poor People's Campaign.[196]

Health Care

States that have resisted the opportunity under the Affordable Care Act should expand Medicaid. Medicaid expansion increases health care coverage, access, and utilization among low-income adults.[197] Controlling health care and prescription drug costs, reducing provider shortages, and bringing resources and services (e.g., federally qualified health centers) to underserved areas should also be prioritized. This includes medical, dental, and other health services, notably behavioral and public health services that have been chronically underfunded.

Policies and programs should address addiction disorders, misuse of drugs and alcohol, depression, and suicidality, which have contributed to rising midlife mortality among all ethnoracial groups.[198] Priorities include a comprehensive approach to combating the opioid epidemic, supporting naloxone distribution and medication-assisted treatment initiatives for opioid addiction, strengthening mental health and substance abuse services (especially in low-income and rural communities), and sensible firearm policies.

Making these policies priorities at the federal, state, and local levels will not be easy. Americans are divided, and trust of institutions, experts, and one another is at a historic low.[199] Many communities are working to reweave their social fabric and strengthen civic connection in partnership with faith-based and other community organizations to advance opportunity and well-being of all.[200] But much more research and social experimentation are needed to understand how to build shared purpose on population health challenges across race, place, culture, and political ideology. The pandemic amplified a long and contentious debate in America about who is responsible for health and what, if any, health protections we owe one another.[201] Solid facts and tested policy solutions alone cannot improve the nation's health. Americans need also to trust those facts and solutions, and for that they need to trust one another.

REFERENCES

1. Braveman PA, Arkin E, Proctor D, Kauh T, Holm N. Systemic and structural racism: Definitions, examples, health damages, and approaches to dismantling. *Health Aff.* 2022;41(2):171–178. doi:10.1377/hlthaff.2021.01394
2. Jones CP. Levels of racism: A theoretic framework and a gardener's tale. *Am J Public Health.* 2000;90(8):1212–1215. doi:10.2105/ajph.90.8.1212
3. Bailey ZD, Krieger N, Agénor M, Graves J, Linos N, Bassett MT. Structural racism and health inequities in the USA: Evidence and interventions. *Lancet.* 2017;389(10077):1453–1463. doi:10.1016/S0140-6736(17)30569-X
4. US Office of Management and Budget. 1997 standards for maintaining, collecting, and presenting federal data on race and ethnicity. 1997. Accessed April 15, 2025. https://spd15revision.gov/content/spd15revision/en/history/1997-standards.html

5. Chaney KE, Sanchez DT, Saud L. White categorical ambiguity: Exclusion of Middle Eastern Americans from the white racial category. *Soc Psychol Pers Sci*. 2021;12(5):593–602. doi:10.1177/1948550620930546
6. Maghbouleh N. From white to what? MENA and Iranian American non-white reflected race. *Ethn Racial Stud*. 2020;43(4):613–631. doi:10.1080/01419870.2019.1599130
7. Maghbouleh N, Schachter A, Flores RD. Middle Eastern and North African Americans may not be perceived, nor perceive themselves, to be white. *Proc Natl Acad Sci USA*. 2022;119(7):e2117940119. doi:10.1073/pnas.2117940119
8. Dallo FJ, Kindratt TB. Disparities in chronic disease prevalence among Non-Hispanic whites: Heterogeneity among foreign-born Arab and European Americans. *J Racial Ethn Health Disparities*. 2016;3(4):590–598. doi:10.1007/s40615-015-0178-8
9. Kindratt TB, Dallo FJ, Zahodne LB, Ajrouch KJ. Cognitive limitations among Middle Eastern and North African immigrants. *J Aging Health*. 2022;34(9–10):1244–1253. doi:10.1177/08982643221103712
10. Read JG, West JS, Kamis C. Immigration and health among non-Hispanic whites: The impact of arrival cohort and region of birth. *Soc Sci Med*. 2020;246:112754. doi:10.1016/j.socscimed.2019.112754
11. Wray M. *Not Quite White: White Trash and the Boundaries of Whiteness*. Duke University Press; 2006.
12. Hartigan J Jr. Establishing the fact of whiteness. *Am Anthropol*. 1997;99(3):495–505. doi:10.1525/aa.1997.99.3.495
13. Hartigan J Jr. *Race in the 21st Century: Ethnographic Approaches*. Oxford University Press; 2010.
14. Katznelson I. *When Affirmative Action Was White: An Untold History of Racial Inequality in Twentieth-Century America*. W. W. Norton & Company; 2005.
15. Daniels J, Schulz AJ. Constructing whiteness in health disparities research. In: Schulz AJ, Mullings L, eds. *Gender, Race, Class, & Health: Intersectional Approaches*. Jossey-Bass; 2006:89–127.
16. Eyerman R. *The Making of White American Identity*. Oxford University Press; 2022.
17. Hartigan, J Jr. *Odd Tribes: Toward a Cultural Analysis of White People*. Duke University Press; 2005.
18. Hartigan J Jr. *Racial Situations: Class Predicaments of Whiteness in Detroit*. Princeton University Press; 1999.
19. Brander Rasmussen B, Klinenberg E, Nexica IJ, Wray M, eds. *The Making and Unmaking of Whiteness*. Duke University Press; 2001.
20. Wray M, Newitz A, eds. *White Trash: Race and Class in America*. Routledge; 1997.
21. Hilberg R. *The Destruction of the European Jews*. Rev ed. Holmes & Meier; 1985:142–147.
22. Wacquant L. *Racial Domination*. John Wiley & Sons; 2024.
23. Hollinger DA. The one drop rule & the one hate rule. *Daedalus*. 2005;134(1):18–28. doi:10.1162/0011526053124424
24. Haney Lopez I. *White by Law: The Legal Construction of Race*. 10th Anniv ed. New York University Press; 2006.
25. Mills CW. *The Racial Contract*. Cornell University Press; 1997.
26. Painter NI. *The History of White People*. W. W. Norton & Company; 2010.

27. Richard R. What have we—De facto racial isolation or de jure segregation?. *Hum Rights*. 2014;40(3):8–10. Accessed April 15, 2025. https://www.jstor.org/stable/26408465
28. Williams DR, Lawrence JA, Davis BA. Racism and health: Evidence and needed research. *Annu Rev Public Health*. 2019;40:105–125. doi:10.1146/annurev-publhealth-040218-043750
29. Du Bois WEB. *Black Reconstruction in America*. Harcourt, Brace and Co.; 1935.
30. Massey DS, Denton NA. Trends in the residential segregation of Blacks, Hispanics, and Asians: 1970-1980. *Am Sociol Rev*. 1987;52(6):802–825. doi:10.2307/2095836
31. Massey DS, Tannen J. A research note on trends in Black hypersegregation. *Demography* 2015;52(3):1025–1034. doi:10.1007/s13524-015-0381-6
32. Suttles GD. *The Social Order of the Slum: Ethnicity and Territory in the Inner City*. University of Chicago Press; 1968.
33. Tolnay SE, Beck EM. *A Festival of Violence: An Analysis of Southern Lynchings, 1882–1930*. University of Illinois Press; 1995.
34. Cunningham D, Lee H, Ward G. Legacies of racial violence: Clarifying and addressing the presence of the past. *Ann Am Acad Pol Soc Sci*. 2021;694(1):8–20. doi:10.1177/00027162211022712
35. Harawa NT, Ford CL. The foundation of modern racial categories and implications for research on Black/white disparities in health. *Ethn Dis*. 2009;19:209–217. Accessed April 15, 2025. https://ethndis.org/archive/files/ethn-19-02-209.pdf
36. Humes K, Hogan H. Measurement of race and ethnicity in a changing, multicultural America. *Race Soc Prob*. 2009;1:111–131. doi:10.1007/s12552-009-9011-5
37. Zuberi T. *Thicker than Blood: How Racial Statistics Lie*. New ed. University of Minnesota Press; 2001.
38. Omi M, Winant H, *Racial Formation in the United States: From the 1960s to the 1990s*. Routledge; 1994.
39. Smedley A. *Race in North America: Origin and Evolution of a Worldview*. 2nd ed. Westview Press; 1999.
40. Harris CI. Whiteness as property. *Harvard Law Rev*. 1993;106;8:1707–1791. Accessed April 15, 2025. https://harvardlawreview.org/print/no-volume/whiteness-as-property
41. Isenberg N. *White Trash: The 400-Year Untold History of Class in America*. Viking Press; 2016.
42. Horsman R. *Race and Manifest Destiny: The Origins of American Racial Anglo-Saxonism*. Harvard University Press; 1981.
43. Takaki R. The Tempest in the wilderness: The racialization of savagery. *J Am Hist*. 1992;79(3):892–912. doi:10.2307/2080792
44. Fredrickson GM. *Racism: A Short History*. Rev ed. Princeton University Press; 2002.
45. Jordan WD. *White Over Black: American Attitudes Toward the Negro 1550–1812*. University of North Carolina Press; 1968.
46. Morgan ES. *American Slavery, American Freedom*. W. W. Norton & Company; 1975.
47. Allen TW. *The Invention of the White Race. Vol 2*. Verso; 1994.
48. Marx A. *Making Race and Nation: A Comparative Analysis of the United States, South Africa and Brazil*. Cambridge University Press; 1998.
49. Foner E. Reconstruction revisited. *Rev Am Hist*. 1982;10(4):82–100. doi:10.2307/2701820
50. Gates HL Jr. *Stony the Road: Reconstruction, White Supremacy, and the Rise Of Jim Crow*. Penguin Publishing; 2020.

51. Equal Justice Initiative. *Reconstruction in America: Racial Violence after the Civil War, 1865-1876*. 2020. Accessed April 15, 2025. https://eji.org/report/reconstruction-in-america
52. Roediger D. *The Wages of Whiteness: Race and the Making of the American Working Class*. Verso; 1991.
53. Feagin JR. *Racist America: Roots, Current Realities, and Future Reparations*. Routledge; 2000.
54. Haller MH. *Eugenics: Hereditarian Attitudes in American Thought*. Rutgers University Press; 1963.
55. Turda M. Race, science, and eugenics in the twentieth century. In: Bashford A, Levine P, eds. *The Oxford Handbook of The History of Eugenics*. Oxford University Press; 2010:62-79.
56. Rafter NH, ed. *White Trash: The Eugenic Family Studies, 1877-1919*. Northeastern University Press; 1988.
57. Cohen A. *Imbeciles: The Supreme Court, American Eugenics, and the Sterilization of Carrie Buck*. Penguin; 2017.
58. Lombardo PA. *Three Generations, No Imbeciles: Eugenics, the Supreme Court, and Buck v Bell*. Johns Hopkins University Press; 2022.
59. Kevles DJ. *In the Name of Eugenics: Genetics and the Uses of Human Heredity*. Alfred A. Knopf; 1985.
60. Ordover N. *American Eugenics: Race, Queer Anatomy, and the Science of Nationalism*. University of Minnesota Press; 2003.
61. Axelsen DE. Women as victims of medical experimentation: J. Marion Sims' surgery on slave women, 1845-1850. *Sage*. 1985;2(2):10-13.
62. Roberts D. *Killing the Black Body: Race, Reproduction, and the Meaning of Liberty*. Vintage Books; 2014.
63. Gutiérrez ER, Fuentes L. Population control by sterilization: The cases of Puerto Rican and Mexican-origin women in the United States. *Latino(a) Res Rev*. 2009;7(3):85-100.
64. Skloot R. *The Immortal Life of Henrietta Lacks*. Broadway Paperbacks; 2017.
65. Winant, H. *The World is a Ghetto: Race and Democracy since World War II*. Basic Books; 2001.
66. Morris AD. *The Origins of The Civil Rights Movement*. Simon and Schuster; 1984.
67. Proctor R. *Racial Hygiene: Medicine Under the Nazis*. Harvard University Press; 1988.
68. Anderson TH. *The Pursuit of Fairness: A History of Affirmative Action*. Oxford University Press; 2004.
69. McGhee H. *The Sum of Us: What Racism Costs Everyone and How We Can Prosper Together*. One World; 2021.
70. Roediger D. What if labor were not white and male? Recentering working-class history and reconstructing debate on the unions and race. *Int Labor Work Class Hist*. 1997;51:72-95. doi:10.1017/S014754790000199X
71. Rothstein R. *The Color of Law: A Forgotten History of How Our Government Segregated America*. Liveright; 2017.
72. Harvey D. *A Brief History of Neoliberalism*. Oxford University Press; 2007.
73. Navarro V. Neoliberalism as a class ideology; or, the political causes of the growth of inequalities. *Int J Health Serv*. 2007;37(1):47-62. doi:10.2190/AP65-X154-4513-R520
74. Feagin, J. *White Party, White Government: Race, Class, and US Politics*. Routledge: 2012.

75. McGirr L. *Suburban Warriors: The Origins of the New American Right.* Rev ed. Princeton University Press; 2015.
76. MacLean N. *Democracy in Chains: The Deep History of the Radical Right's Stealth Plan for America.* Penguin Books; 2017.
77. Appelbaum B. *The Economists' Hour: False Prophets, Free Markets, and the Fracture of Society.* Bay Back Books; 2019.
78. Gerstle G. *The Rise and Fall of the Neoliberal Order: America and the World in the Free Market Era.* Oxford University Press; 2022.
79. Ganti T. Neoliberalism. *Annu Rev Anthropol.* 2014;43:89–104. doi:10.1146/annurev-anthro-092412-155528
80. Bonilla-Silva E. *Racism Without Racists: Color-Blind Racism and the Persistence of Racial Inequality in America.* Rowman & Littlefield; 2003.
81. Kymlicka W. The rise and fall of multiculturalism? New debates on inclusion and accommodation in diverse societies. *Int Soc Sci J.* 2010;61(199):97–112. doi:10.1111/j.1468-2451.2010.01750.x
82. Fraser N, Honneth A, eds. Golb J, Ingram J, Wilke C, trans. *Redistribution or Recognition? A Political Philosophical Exchange.* Verso; 2003.
83. Coole D. Is class a difference that makes a difference? *Radical Philosophy.* 1996;77:17-25.
84. Sayer A. *The Moral Significance of Class.* Cambridge University Press; 2005.
85. Blacksher E. Shrinking poor White life spans: Class, race, and health justice. *Am J Bioeth.* 2018;18(10):3–14. doi:10.1080/15265161.2018.1513585
86. Bonilla-Silva E. *White Supremacy and Racism in the Post-Civil Rights Era.* Lynne Rienner Publishers; 2001.
87. Simi P, Futrell R. Cyberculture and the endurance of White power activism. *J Polit Milit Sociol.* 2006;34(1):115–142. Accessed April 15, 2025. https://www.jstor.org/stable/45294188
88. Blee KM, Futrell R, Simi P. *Out of Hiding: Extremist White Supremacy and How It Can Be Stopped.* Routledge; 2023.
89. Willer R, Feinberg M, Wetts R. Threats to racial status promote Tea Party support among white Americans. Available at SSRN 2770186. Published 2016.
90. Gest J. *The New Minority: White Working Class Politics in an Age of Immigration and Inequality.* Oxford University Press, 2016.
91. Jardina A. *White Identity Politics.* Cambridge University Press; 2019.
92. Levine-Rasky C. Intersectionality theory applied to whiteness and middle-classness. *Soc Identities.* 2011;17(2):239–253. doi:10.1080/13504630.2011.558377
93. Wray, M. A typology of white people in America. In: Kindinger, E. Schmidtt, M. eds. *The Intersections of Whiteness.* Routledge; 2019:38-52.
94. World Health Organization. Closing the gap in a generation: Health equity through action on the social determinants of health—Final Report of the Commission on Social Determinants of Health. 2008. Accessed April 15, 2025. https://www.who.int/publications/i/item/WHO-IER-CSDH-08.1
95. Woolf SH, Braveman P. Where health disparities begin: The role of social and economic determinants—and why current policies may make matters worse. *Health Aff (Millwood).* 2011;30(10):1852–1859. doi:10.1377/hlthaff.2011.0685

96. Institute of Medicine (US) Committee on Assuring the Health of the Public in the 21st Century. Understanding population health and its determinants. In: Institute of Medicine (US) Committee on Assuring the Health of the Public in the 21st Century. *The Future of the Public's Health in the 21st Century*. National Academies Press; 2002;46–95.
97. Jones CP, Jones CY, Perry GS, et al. Addressing the social determinants of children's health: A cliff analogy. *J Health Care Poor Underserved*. 2009;20(suppl 4):1–12. doi:10.1353/hpu.0.0228. PMID: 20168027
98. Beckfield J. *Political Sociology and the People's Health*. Oxford University Press; 2018.
99. Krieger N. Measures of racism, sexism, heterosexism, and gender binarism for health equity research: From structural injustice to embodied harm—An ecosocial analysis. *Annu Rev Public Health*. 2020;41:37–62. doi:10.1146/annurev-publhealth-040119-094017
100. Fraser N. Social justice in the age of identity politics: Redistribution, recognition, and participation. In: Fraser N, Honneth A, eds. Golb J, Ingram J, Wilke C, trans. *Redistribution or Recognition? A Political Philosophical Exchange*. Verso; 2003:7–109.
101. Sasson I. Trends in life expectancy and lifespan variation by educational attainment: United States, 1990–2010. *Demography*. 2016;53(2):269–293. doi:10.1007/s13524-015-0453-7
102. Banks J, Marmot M, Oldfield Z, Smith JP. Disease and disadvantage in the United States and in England. *JAMA*. 2006;295(17):2037–2045. doi:10.1001/jama.295.17.2037
103. Braveman PA, Kumanyika S, Fielding J, et al. Health disparities and health equity: The issue is justice. *Am J Public Health*. 2011;101(suppl 1):S149–S155. doi:10.2105/AJPH.2010.300062
104. Institute of Medicine Committee on Understanding and Eliminating Racial and Ethnic Disparities in Health Care; Smedley BD, Stith AY, Nelson AR, eds. *Unequal Treatment: Confronting Racial and Ethnic Disparities in Health Care*. National Academies Press; 2003.
105. Eisenberg-Guyot J, Finsaas MC, Prins SJ. Dead labor: Mortality inequities by class, gender, and race/ethnicity in the United States, 1986–2019. *Am J Public Health*. 2023;113(6):637–646. doi:10.2105/AJPH.2023.307227
106. Geronimus AT, Bound J, Waidmann TA, et al. Weathering, drugs, and whack-a-mole: Fundamental and proximate causes of widening education inequity in US life expectancy by sex and race, 1990–2015. *J Health Soc Behav*. 2019;60(2):222–239. doi:10.1177/0022146519849932
107. Villarosa L. *Under the Skin: The Hidden Toll of Racism on American Lives and on the Health of Our Nation*. Doubleday; 2022.
108. Geronimus AT, Pearson JA, Linnenbringer E, et al. Race/ethnicity, poverty, urban stressors and telomere length in a Detroit community-based sample. *J Health Soc Behav*. 2015;56(2):199–224. doi:10.1177/0022146515582100
109. McEwen BS, Gianaros PJ. Central role of the brain in stress and adaptation: Links to socioeconomic status, health, and disease. *Ann NY Acad Sci*. 2010;1186:190–222. doi:10.1111/j.1749-6632.2009.05331.x
110. Gu HF, Tang CK, Yang YZ. Psychological stress, immune response, and atherosclerosis. *Atherosclerosis*. 2012;223(1):69–77. doi:10.1016/j.atherosclerosis.2012.01.021
111. Redmond N, Richman J, Gamboa CM, et al. Perceived stress is associated with incident coronary heart disease and all-cause mortality in low- but not high-income participants in the Reasons for Geographic and Racial Differences in Stroke study. *J Am Heart Assoc*. 2013;2(6):e000447. doi:10.1161/JAHA.113.000447

112. Steptoe A, Kivimäki M. Stress and cardiovascular disease: An update on current knowledge. *Annu Rev Public Health.* 2013;34:337-354. doi:10.1146/annurev-publhealth-031912-114452
113. Sabbath EL, Mejía-Guevara I, Noelke C, Berkman LF. The long-term mortality impact of combined job strain and family circumstances: A life course analysis of working American mothers. *Soc Sci Med.* 2015;146:111-119. doi:10.1016/j.socscimed.2015.10.024
114. National Center for Health Statistics. CDC WONDER multiple cause of death files, 2018-2023. Centers for Disease Control and Prevention. Accessed August 10, 2025. http://wonder.cdc.gov/ucd-icd10-expanded.html
115. National Institute on Minority Health and Health Disparities. HDPulse: An ecosystem of minority health and health disparities resources. US Dept of Health and Human Services. Accessed August 10, 2025. https://hdpulse.nimhd.nih.gov
116. National Center for Health Statistics. *Health, United States, 2019.* Centers for Disease Control and Prevention; 2021. Accessed April 15, 2025. https://www.ncbi.nlm.nih.gov/books/NBK569306
117. Centers for Disease Control and Prevention. BRFSS prevalence & trends data. Updated July 19, 2023. Accessed August 8, 2025. https://www.cdc.gov/brfss/brfssprevalence
118. National Academies of Sciences, Engineering, and Medicine; Health and Medicine Division; Board on Population Health and Public Health Practice; Roundtable on Population Health Improvement; Nicholson A, ed. *Population Health in Rural America in 2020: Proceedings of a Workshop.* National Academies Press; 2021.
119. Curtin SA, Spencer MR. Trends in death rates in urban and rural areas: United States, 1999-2019. *NCHS Data Brief.* 2021;(417):1-8. Accessed April 15, 2025. https://www.cdc.gov/nchs/data/databriefs/db417.pdf
120. National Center for Health Statistics. CDC WONDER underlying cause of death files, 1999-2020. Centers for Disease Control and Prevention. Accessed June 10, 2024. http://wonder.cdc.gov/ucd-icd10.html
121. Arias E, Xu JQ, Kochanek K. United States life tables, 2023. *Natl Vital Stat Rep.* 2025;74(6):1-63. doi:10.15620/cdc/174591
122. National Center for Health Statistics. *Health, United States, 2020-2021: Annual Perspective.* Centers for Disease Control and Prevention; 2023. doi:10.15620/cdc:122044
123. Link BG, Phelan J. Social conditions as fundamental causes of disease. *J Health Soc Behav.* 1995;Spec No:80-94. Accessed April 15, 2025. https://core.ac.uk/reader/77145022
124. Adler NE, Rehkopf DH. US disparities in health: Descriptions, causes, and mechanisms. *Annu Rev Public Health.* 2008;29:235-252. doi:10.1146/annurev.publhealth.29.020907.090852
125. Cutler DM, Lleras-Muney A. Understanding differences in health behaviors by education. *J Health Econ.* 2010;29(1):1-28. doi:10.1016/j.jhealeco.2009.10.003
126. Chetty R, Stepner M, Abraham S, et al. The association between income and life expectancy in the United States, 2001-2014. *JAMA.* 2016;315(16):1750-1766. doi:10.1001/jama.2016.4226
127. Grassroots Global Justice Alliance. Extractive economy. June 8, 2020. Accessed August 8, 2025. https://ggjalliance.org/program-activities/extractive-economy
128. Lewin PG. "Coal is not just a job, it's a way of life": The cultural politics of coal production in Central Appalachia. *Soc Prob.* 2019;66(1):51-68. doi:10.1093/socpro/spx030

129. Gaventa J. *Power and Powerlessness: Quiescence and Rebellion in an Appalachian Valley*. University of Illinois Press; 1980.
130. Stiglitz J. The price of inequality. *New Perspect Q*. 2013;30(1):52–53. doi:10.1111/npqu.11358
131. Mayer J. *Dark Money: The Hidden History of the Billionaires Behind the Rise of the Radical Right*. Knopf Doubleday Publishing; 2016.
132. Wu T *The Curse of Bigness: Antitrust in the New Gilded Age*. Columbia Global Reports; 2018.
133. Reich RB. *The Work of Nations: Preparing Ourselves for 21st Century Capitalism*. Knopf Doubleday Publishing; 2010.
134. Desmond M. *Poverty, by America*. Crown Publishing; 2023.
135. Thelen K. The American precariat: US capitalism in comparative perspective. *Perspect Polit*. 2019;17(1):5–27. doi:10.1017/S1537592718003419
136. Weil D. *The Fissured Workplace: Why Work Became So Bad for So Many and What Can Be Done to Improve It*. Harvard University Press; 2014.
137. Smith A. Gig work, online selling and home sharing. Pew Research Center. November 17, 2016. Accessed April 15, 2025. https://www.pewresearch.org/internet/2016/11/17/gig-work-online-selling-and-home-sharing
138. Hacker JS. *The Great Risk Shift*. Oxford University Press; 2006.
139. Organisation for Economic Co-operation and Development. The New OECD Employment Protection Legislation Indicators for Temporary Contracts. November 2021. Accessed August 8, 2025. https://www.oecd.org/content/dam/oecd/en/data/datasets/indicators-of-employment-protection/OECD-EPLIndicators-TemporaryContracts.pdf
140. Denk O, Hagemann RP, Lenain P, Somma V. *Inequality and Poverty in the United States: Public Policies for Inclusive Growth*. Organisation for Economic Co-operation and Development; 2022. doi:10.1787/5k46957cwv8q-en
141. Smith C, Chandy L. How poor are America's poorest? US $2 a day poverty in a global context. Brookings Institution. August 26, 2014. Accessed April 15, 2025. https://www.brookings.edu/articles/how-poor-are-americas-poorest-u-s-2-a-day-poverty-in-a-global-context
142. Shaefer HL, Edin K. Rising extreme poverty in the United States and the response of federal means-tested transfer programs. *Soc Serv Rev*. 2013;87(2):250–268. doi:10.1086/671012
143. Rank MR. *Confronting Poverty: Economic Hardship in the United States*. Sage Publications; 2021.
144. Shrider EA, Creamer J. Poverty in the United States, 2022. US Census Bureau. September 12, 2023. Accessed April 15, 2025. https://www.census.gov/library/publications/2023/demo/p60-280.html
145. Giannarelli L, Minton S, Wheaton L, Knowles S. A safety net with 100 percent participation: How much would benefits increase and poverty decline? Urban Institute. August 2023. Accessed April 15, 2025. https://www.urban.org/research/publication/safety-net-100-percent-participation
146. Azevedo D, Safawi A. To promote equity, states should invest more TANF dollars in basic assistance. Center on Budget and Policy Priorities. January 12, 2022. Accessed April 15, 2025. https://www.cbpp.org/research/income-security/to-promote-equity-states-should-invest-more-tanf-dollars-in-basic
147. Kaiser Family Foundation. Paid leave in the US. December 17, 2021. Accessed April 15, 2025. https://www.kff.org/womens-health-policy/fact-sheet/paid-leave-in-u-s

148. Hood CM, Gennuso KP, Swain GR, Catlin BB. County health rankings: Relationships between determinant factors and health outcomes. *Am J Prev Med*. 2016;50(2):129–135. doi:10.1016/j.amepre.2015.08.024
149. Wilper AP, Woolhandler S, Lasser KE, McCormick D, Bor DH, Himmelstein DU. Health insurance and mortality in US adults. *Am J Public Health*. 2009;99(12):2289–2295. doi:10.2105/AJPH.2008.157685
150. State Health Access Data Assistance Center. Percent of adults with no personal doctor. 2023. Accessed April 15, 2025. https://statehealthcompare.shadac.org/map/120/percent-of-adults-with-no-personal-doctor-by-race-ethnicity-2011-to-2020#40/32/157
151. Bennett N, Eggleston J, Mykyta L, Sullivan B. 19% of US households could not afford to pay for medical care right away. US Census Bureau. April 7, 2021. Accessed April 15, 2025. https://www.census.gov/library/stories/2021/04/who-had-medical-debt-in-united-states.html
152. Lopes L, Kearney A, Montero A, Hamel L, Brodie M. Health care debt in the US: The broad consequences of medical and dental bills. Kaiser Family Foundation. Jun 16, 2022. Accessed April 15, 2025. https://www.kff.org/report-section/kff-health-care-debt-survey-main-findings
153. Kaiser Family Foundation. Status of state Medicaid expansion decisions. April 9, 2025. Accessed April 15, 2025. https://www.kff.org/status-of-state-medicaid-expansion-decisions
154. American Hospital Association. Rural hospital closures threaten access: Solutions to preserve care in local communities. September 2022. Accessed April 15, 2025. https://www.aha.org/system/files/media/file/2022/09/rural-hospital-closures-threaten-access-report.pdf
155. Center for Healthcare Quality & Payment Reform. Rural hospitals at risk of closing. March 2025. Accessed April 15, 2025. https://ruralhospitals.chqpr.org/downloads/Rural_Hospitals_at_Risk_of_Closing.pdf
156. Jarman MP, Castillo RC, Carlini AR, Kodadek LM, Haider AH. Rural risk: Geographic disparities in trauma mortality. *Surgery*. 2016;160(6):1551–1559. doi:10.1016/j.surg.2016.06.020
157. Newgard CD, Fu R, Bulger E, et al. Evaluation of rural vs urban trauma patients served by 9-1-1 emergency medical services. *JAMA Surg*. 2017;152(1):11–18. doi:10.1001/jamasurg.2016.3329
158. Fujishiro K. Is perceived racial privilege associated with health? Findings from the Behavioral Risk Factor Surveillance System. *Soc Sci Med*. 2009;68(5):840–844. doi:10.1016/j.socscimed.2008.12.007
159. Kwate NO, Goodman MS. An empirical analysis of white privilege, social position and health. *Soc Sci Med*. 2014;116:150–160. doi:10.1016/j.socscimed.2014.05.041
160. Lee Y, Muennig P, Kawachi I, Hatzenbuehler ML. Effects of racial prejudice on the health of communities: A multilevel survival analysis. *Am J Public Health*. 2015;105(11):2349–2355. doi:10.2105/AJPH.2015.302776
161. Malat J, Mayorga-Gallo S, Williams DR. The effects of whiteness on the health of whites in the USA. *Soc Sci Med*. 2018;199:148–156. doi:10.1016/j.socscimed.2017.06.034
162. Metzl JM. *Dying of Whiteness: How the Politics of Racial Resentment Is Killing America's Heartland*. Basic Books; 2019.
163. Siddiqi A, Sod-Erdene O, Hamilton D, Cottom TM, Darity W Jr. Growing sense of social status threat and concomitant deaths of despair among whites. *SSM Popul Health*. 2019;9:100449. doi:10.1016/j.ssmph.2019.100449

164. Rambotti S. Examining the association between racialized economic threat and white suicide in the United States, 2000–2016. *J Health Soc Behav*. 2022;63(3):375–391. doi:10.1177/00221465211069873
165. Efird CR, Bennett F, Metzl JM, Siddiqi A. Perceived status threat and health among white Americans: A scoping review. *SSM Popul Health*. 2022;21:101326. doi:10.1016/j.ssmph.2022.101326
166. Schulz A, Mullings L, eds. *Gender, Race, Class, & Health: Intersectional Approaches*. Jossey-Bass; 2006.
167. Bowleg L. The problem with the phrase women and minorities: Intersectionality—An important theoretical framework for public health. *Am J Public Health*. 2012;102(7):1267–1273. doi:10.2105/AJPH.2012.300750
168. Bauer GR. Incorporating intersectionality theory into population health research methodology: Challenges and the potential to advance health equity. *Soc Sci Med*. 2014;110:10–17. doi:10.1016/j.socscimed.2014.03.022
169. Melamed J. Racial capitalism. *Crit Ethn Stud*. 2015;1(1):76–85. doi:10.5749/jcritethnstud.1.1.0076
170. Robinson C. *Black Marxism: The Making of the Black Radical Tradition*. University of North Carolina Press; 1983.
171. Morone JA. Enemies of the people: The moral dimension to public health. *J Health Polit Policy Law*. 1997;22(4):993–1020. doi:10.1215/03616878-22-4-993
172. Nelson TE, Kinder DR. Issue frames and group-centrism in American public opinion. *J Polit*. 1996;58(4):1055–1078. doi:10.2307/2960149
173. Iyengar S. Framing responsibility for political issues: The case of poverty. *Polit Behav*. 1990;12(1):19–40. doi:10.1007/BF00992330
174. Iyengar S. Framing responsibility for political issues. *Ann Am Acad Pol Soc Sci*. 1996;546(1):59–70. doi:10.1177/0002716296546001006
175. Gollust SE, Lynch J. Who deserves health care? The effects of causal attributions and group cues on public attitudes about responsibility for health care costs. *J Health Polit Policy Law*. 2011;36(6):1061–1095. doi:10.1215/03616878-1460578
176. Tesler M. The spillover of racialization into health care: How President Obama polarized public opinion by racial attitudes and race. *Am J Polit Sci*. 2012;56(3):690–704. doi:10.1111/j.1540-5907.2011.00577.x
177. Quadagno J. Why the United States has no national health insurance: Stakeholder mobilization against the welfare state, 1945–1996. *J Health Soc Behav*. 2004;45(suppl):25–44. Accessed April 15, 2025. https://www.jstor.org/stable/3653822
178. Henderson M, Hillygus DS. The dynamics of health care opinion, 2008–2010: Partisanship, self-interest, and racial resentment. *J Health Polit Policy Law*. 2011;36(6):945–960. doi:10.1215/03616878-1460533
179. Grogan CM, Park SE. The racial divide in state Medicaid expansions. *J Health Polit Policy Law*. 2017;42(3):539–572. doi:10.1215/03616878-3802977
180. Fording R, Patton D. Medicaid expansion and the political fate of the governors who support it. *Policy Stud J*. 2019;47(2):274–299. doi:10.1111/psj.12311

181. Mazurenko O, Balio CP, Agarwal R, Carroll AE, Menachemi N. The effects of Medicaid expansion under the ACA: A systematic review. *Health Aff (Millwood)*. 2018;37(6):944–950. doi:10.1377/hlthaff.2017.1491

182. Jones RP, Cox D, Cooper B, Lienesch R. *Anxiety, Nostalgia, and Mistrust: Findings from the 2015 American Values Survey*. Public Religion Research Institute; 2015. Accessed April 15, 2025. https://www.prri.org/research/survey-anxiety-nostalgia-and-mistrust-findings-from-the-2015-american-values-survey

183. Robert Wood Johnson Foundation. Discrimination in America: Experiences and views. October 24, 2017. Accessed April 15, 2025. https://www.rwjf.org/en/insights/our-research/2017/10/discrimination-in-america--experiences-and-views.html

184. Assari S, Burgard S, Zivin K. Long-term reciprocal associations between depressive symptoms and number of chronic medical conditions: Longitudinal support for Black–white health paradox. *J Racial Ethn Health Disparities*. 2015;2(4):589–597. doi:10.1007/s40615-015-0116-9

185. Keyes CL. The Black–white paradox in health: Flourishing in the face of social inequality and discrimination. *J Pers*. 2009;77(6):1677–1706. doi:10.1111/j.1467-6494.2009.00597.x

186. Kwate NO, Meyer IH. The myth of meritocracy and African American health. *Am J Public Health*. 2010;100(10):1831–1834. doi:10.2105/AJPH.2009.186445

187. Desmond, M. In order to understand the brutality of American capitalism, you have to start on the plantation. *New York Times*. August 14, 2019. Accessed April 15, 2025. https://www.nytimes.com/interactive/2019/08/14/magazine/slavery-capitalism.html

188. Hohle R. *Race and the Origins of American Neoliberalism*. Routledge; 2015.

189. Feldman S, Huddy L. Racial resentment and white opposition to race-conscious programs: Principles or prejudice? *Am J Pol Sci*. 2005;49(1):168–183. doi:10.2307/3647720

190. Young IM. *Responsibility for Justice*. Oxford University Press; 2011.

191. Benach J, Malmusi D, Yasuo Y, Martinez JM. A new typology of policies to tackle health inequalities and scenarios of impact based on Rose's population approach. *J Epidemiol Community Health*. 2013;67(3):286–291. doi:10.1136/jech-2011-200363

192. Freeman R, Han E, Madland D, Duke B. Bargaining for the American dream: What unions do for mobility. Center for American Progress. September 9, 2015. Accessed April 15, 2025. https://www.americanprogress.org/article/bargaining-for-the-american-dream

193. Troller-Renfree SV, Costanzo MA, Duncan GJ, et al. The impact of a poverty reduction intervention on infant brain activity. *Proc Natl Acad Sci USA*. 2022;119(5):e2115649119. doi:10.1073/pnas.2115649119

194. Centers for Disease Control and Prevention. Earned income tax credits: Interventions addressing the social determinants of health. 2021. Accessed February 10, 2024. https://archive.cdc.gov/#/details?url=https://www.cdc.gov/policy/hi5/taxcredits/index.html

195. DeParle J. As need rises, housing aid hits lowest level in nearly 25 years. *New York Times*. December 19, 2023. Accessed August 10, 2025. https://www.nytimes.com/2023/12/19/us/politics/housing-aid-rent-costs.html

196. Poor People's Campaign: A National Call for Moral Revival. Homepage. Accessed August 8, 2025. https://www.poorpeoplescampaign.org

197. Glied SA, Weiss MA. Impact of the Medicaid coverage gap: Comparing states that have and have not expanded eligibility. Commonwealth Fund. September 11, 2023. Accessed August 10, 2025. https://www.commonwealthfund.org/publications/issue-briefs/2023/sep/impact-medicaid-coverage-gap-comparing-states-have-and-have-not
198. National Academies of Sciences, Engineering, and Medicine; Mullan Harris K, Majmundar MK, Becker T, eds. *High and Rising Mortality Rates Among Working-Age Adults*. National Academies Press; 2021.
199. Pew Research Center. Public trust in government: 1958–2023. June 24, 2024. Accessed April 15, 2025. https://www.pewresearch.org/politics/2023/09/19/public-trust-in-government-1958-2023
200. Fallows JM, Fallows D. *Our Towns: A 100,000-Mile Journey Into the Heart of America*. Pantheon Books; 2018.
201. Reiser SJ. Responsibility for personal health: A historical perspective. *J Med Philos*. 1985;10(1): 7–17. doi:10.1093/jmp/10.1.7

8

Cross-Cutting Solutions to Address Structural Racism to Advance Health Equity

Marshall H. Chin, MD, MPH, Tyson H. Brown, PhD, and Anna Ricklin, MHS

INTRODUCTION

This book underscores actionable solutions that would open the doors to opportunity for health for all in the United States. In many previous studies, the National Academies have shown ways that structural racism, discrimination, systemic segregation, poverty, and cumulative disadvantage are causal drivers of poor health and health inequities in the United States.[1-3] Some policies have caused intergenerational harm to *communities*, defined as populations and places having common cultural or ethnic ties, racialized experiences, or geographic boundaries. These harms continue to impede optimal health today. Besides the toll on people's lives, racial and ethnic health inequities cause great economic costs. Combining excess medical care expenditures, lost labor market productivity, and the value of excess premature death, economic costs to the United States were estimated to be $421 to $451 billion in 2018.[4] Reversing these negative impacts and achieving a healthy United States for all will require bold, decisive, and intentional action involving multiple sectors, systems, and branches of government.[5,6]

Evidence suggests that we can begin dismantling barriers to a healthy life by increasing socioeconomic opportunity, investing in community infrastructure, and providing equitable access to high-quality health care and education. The systematic, structural, and cultural barriers to long, healthy lives outlined in this book are interdependent and lead to cascading impacts on health across populations, and "efforts to remedy structural oppression and its deleterious effects should account for its multilevel, multifaceted, interconnected, systemic, and intersectional nature."[6(p36)] Thus, an array of bold policy bundles—not just a single fix—are necessary to lead to constructive changes. Moreover, we can foster a sense of shared responsibility and collaboration by intentionally designing and implementing key actions in genuine partnership with impacted communities. A collaborative approach improves the health of all populations by ensuring that policy solutions resonate with community values and express respect for members of the communities.[2]

This chapter summarizes key actionable solutions by identifying common themes across the preceding chapters. Some solutions could be enacted now, and some are more aspirational. We abstracted excerpts of relevant information with select citations. We encourage readers to visit the previous chapters for the full context and justification for the recommended actionable solutions. We also acknowledge that providing detailed recommendations for every sector goes beyond the scope of this project. We provide key general recommendations for actionable solutions, examples, and references for further details and exploration.

A CONCEPTUAL MODEL TO GUIDE STRUCTURAL AND SYSTEMIC SOLUTIONS THAT ADDRESS UNDERLYING CAUSES OF POOR HEALTH

The only way to address racism's many tentacles and the systematic nature of racial oppression is to move upstream from individual health behaviors and examine how systems differentially enable and constrain the health of whole communities that are often segregated by both race and income.

–Keels et al., Chapter 3

Structural and systemic problems require structural and systemic solutions. We need targeted and cross-cutting actions that remove barriers to access US opportunity structures, which include systems, resources, and connections that enable people to reach their full potential. Solutions should dismantle the obstacles that have been built and perpetuated through policies to create unequal access to opportunities. These solutions can guide us into a future where everyone has access to a healthy life and the conditions that protect and support health. A conceptual model serves as a guide to the summary of actionable solutions in this chapter (Figure 8-1) and is explained in the next two sections.

Root Causes of Poor Health and Health Inequities

Underlying causes of poor health are often shared across multiple communities and populations and go beyond access to high-quality health care.[7] Grounded in power and hierarchy, the root causes of poor health for many communities are structural and systemic racism, imperialism, and unfettered capitalism.[8-11] These systems of oppression influence our daily interactions and health-related actions, and they are shaped by and shape cultural norms, beliefs, and values. These systems must be considered from intersectional and transnational perspectives and throughout the life course.[12]

A plethora of research provides evidence that stressors rooted in chronic disadvantage across identities and their cumulative effects have a direct impact on health.

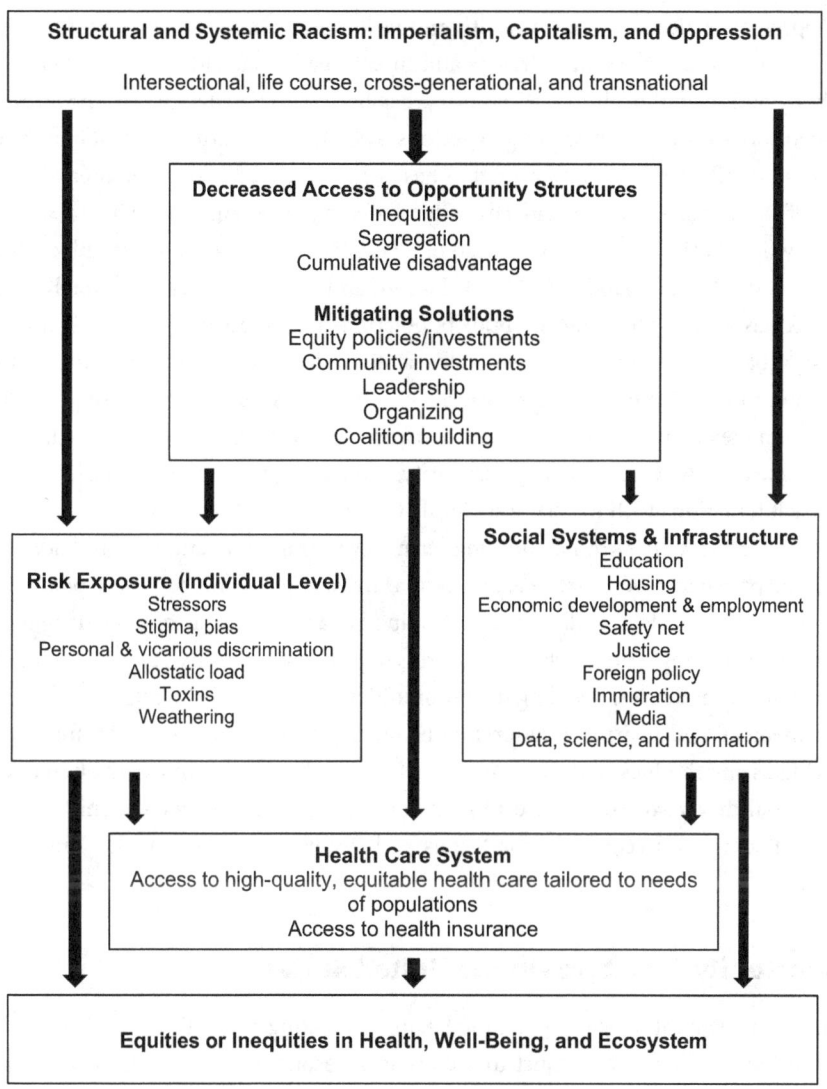

Figure 8-1. Conceptual Model: Structural and Systemic Racism's Impact on Health Equity/Inequity

These stressors include decreased or lack of access to opportunity structures such as quality health care, housing, education, and economic vitality. Stressors also include individual-level risk exposures, such as experiences with bias, discrimination, marginalization, and oppression based on race, ethnicity, immigration, socioeconomic status, gender, and sexual orientation.[13-15] In other words, social and environmental factors rooted in structural racism, hierarchies of human value, and power play a significant role in one's wellness over the lifespan and across generations.

Oppressive experiences harm health and well-being. One example is weathering, in which repeated racism-related stresses and threats lead to cascading harmful effects on the body and overall health.[7,16] Weathering has been associated with chronic stress and elevated cortisol levels over prolonged periods, known as allostatic load, that in turn leads to systemic inflammation. Inflammation has been associated with a heightened risk for onset of chronic diseases that unnecessarily burden many people in the United States.[17-21] People who identify as American Indian or Alaska Native (AI/AN), Asian, Black, Native Hawaiian or Pacific Islander (NH/PI), Latino, and Middle Eastern or North African (MENA), as well as economically poor populations regardless of their racial, ethnic, or ancestral background in the United States, statistically experience more chronic stress. Common to the disproportionate patterns of chronic disease among these populations are systemic exposure to discrimination, marginalization, low educational attainment, job insecurity, low wages, housing insecurity, food insecurity, and more-frequent-than-average interactions with the criminal legal system, among other stressors.

These stressors are chronic and long term—even transgenerational—and add to the increased prevalence of obesity, cardiovascular disease, and cancer in these populations. Chronic stress can also cause unhealthy coping behaviors (e.g., alcohol or drug misuse, smoking, overeating) and psychological stress (e.g., depression, anxiety) and their potentially fatal consequences. Residing in communities plagued by disinvestments that create food, medical, and pharmacy deserts, poor quality housing, and high unemployment, individuals and families struggle to meet basic needs. These situations are often referred to as social drivers or social determinants of health, as they create chronically disadvantaged social and economic conditions and significant barriers to US opportunity structures.

Opportunity Structures in the United States

Structural racism influences population health by creating and maintaining a racial hierarchy of human value and unjust distribution of resources, characterized by inequitable access to US opportunity structures.[22] The mechanisms of structural racism include, among other things, discriminatory policies and practices and cultural biases. Structural racism determines who has access to beneficial resources. It also operates across social systems and institutions that impact health, including education, employment, economic development, housing, community infrastructure, justice, immigration, and the media. Consequently, the unequal distribution of resources creates inequities in social systems that directly impact health. For example, minoritized racial and ethnic populations are more likely to live in housing near waste dumping sites, environmental toxins, and pollution, which can increase the risk of cancer and asthma. Inequities in social systems can also indirectly impact health through inadequate access to the health care system. A key example is that low-paying jobs are more likely to offer no health insurance benefits or poor-quality health insurance. Underinsurance creates barriers to accessing high-quality health care tailored to meet the medical and social needs of racially minoritized populations, ultimately leading to health inequities.

Dismantling barriers at the root of US opportunity structures will require an all-hands-on-deck approach to correct the inequitable distribution of access to resources in society. Federal, state, and local levels of government and civil society need to understand and eliminate the threads of segregation, poverty, and discrimination across systems and sectors evident in policies, practices, and culture today to create a new American health compact with all people living in the United States.[23] Leadership, organizing, and coalition building can mitigate the effects of structural racism and proactively improve opportunities for good health and healthy ecosystems. Below are highlighted cross-cutting solutions that address the root causes of poor health, with specific examples selected from the different chapters.

ACTIONABLE SOLUTIONS

The impact of colonization on AI/AN populations is profound. For over 500 years, Euro-American culture has been imposed on AI/AN populations . . . the intersection of structural barriers, cultural misalignment of services and programs, and social determinants of health have resulted in some of the worst health disparities in the nation. Structural barriers include racism, marginalization, poverty, unemployment, and unequal access to health care, healthy and traditional foods, and adequate housing.

–Warne et al., Chapter 1

Residential segregation enables the spatial allocation of resources . . . systems of residential segregation buttress systems of economic oppression.

–Keels et al., Chapter 3

This section highlights some solutions that, if implemented, could have cascading impacts across systems and populations. The systems covered are data, science, and information; health care; economic infrastructure, safety net, labor and employment; education; justice and civil rights law; media; immigration and foreign policy; and Indigenous sovereignty. Please refer to the population chapters in this book for a full description of actionable solutions by population.

Data, Science, and Information

While disaggregation of the NH/PI and Asian categories is helpful, the definition created by the OMB directive does little to acknowledge the heterogeneity of the vastly diverse peoples, languages, cultures, worldviews, and demographics that are combined into the NH/PI category. It is therefore imperative that disaggregation of Oceanic cultural identities within the federal NH/PI designation be promoted along with disaggregation from the Asian category. Data gaps will continue to persist as long as OMB and Census categorizations fail to acknowledge the granular realities that are rendered statistically invisible when combined into a seemingly homogenous grouping.

– Fitisemanu, Jr. et al., Chapter 6

Population health research often omits key systems and contextual intersections of history, race and ethnicity, and institutional power, reducing the importance of social and political determinants and the accumulation of disadvantages over the life course.

–Zambrana et al., Chapter 4

Data, science, and information are imperative to understand how and why some populations are experiencing optimal health and others are not. One challenge with the study of health equity lies in our reliance on race and ethnicity as identifiers, which grossly aggregate large and different subpopulations while masking data and outcomes. For example, the terms "Hispanic" and "Asian" cover large, heterogenous populations with origins across the globe and different levels of health risks. Moreover, when a small racial group (NH/PI) is combined with a larger racial group (Asian) to create a category called Asian American and Pacific Islander, the status of the large group skews the data and masks the status of the smaller group.[24] In collecting census information, the US Office of Management and Budget (OMB) has forced data into six (seven as of 2024) racial/ethnic categories—American Indian or Alaska Native, Asian, Black or African American, Middle Eastern or North African, Native Hawaiian or Pacific Islander, Latino, and White. OMB sets the standards that federal agencies like the US Census Bureau should adopt, and many nonfederal agencies have also adopted the classification. However, historically, the basis for categorization schemes for race and ethnicity has not been universally accepted by institutions nor understood by the lay public and has been weaponized to discriminate against and dehumanize groups (e.g., who was designated as Black during Reconstruction and Jim Crow; Chinese Exclusion Act of 1882).

In addition, broad categories do not account for within-group variability, such as variation across ethnicity or intersectional social and environmental differences, all of which contribute to one's identity, life experiences, and health. For example, MENA people have until recently been categorized as white by OMB, but experience a higher prevalence of diabetes, cardiovascular disease, and cancer than their white counterparts, a disparity that is hidden by their integration into the white racial group. Responding to advocacy from MENA communities, OMB announced a new MENA category that will allow for the disaggregation of people who identify as MENA from people who identify as white.

Actionable solutions should include making the scientific data collection process more equitable, particularly in including meaningful categories for marginalized populations.

Scientists should work to make the invisible visible; that is, no population should be considered too small to matter when categorizing data. This should also include the disaggregation of scientific data into more granular racial and ethnic categories and across more intersectional factors that can impact equity, such as gender and class. When partnering with communities, scientists and researchers should redistribute and/or share power in research question development, methods, data collection, and dissemination of research findings. A summary of actionable solutions for data, science, and information follow:

- Data categorization
  - Disaggregate race/ethnicity data into more granular categories (e.g., specific Asian and Latino ethnicities).[25-30]
  - Create meaningful categories that accurately capture heterogenous lived experiences (e.g., separate Asians and NH/PIs and collect ethnicity data for them).[31]
- Scientist–community partnerships
  - Facilitate coalition building and organizing by partnering with communities.[2]
  - Embrace the diversity of experiences and potential solutions specific to each community's opportunities and constraints, using new and innovative research methods and building on participatory action research.[27,32]

Health Care

The health care sector—including primary and specialty care as well as behavioral, dental, and population health services—could have more direct and positive effects on health if access and quality were equitably distributed across places and populations in the United States. These efforts should be prioritized using the principles of *proportionate universalism*, with greater investments made in populations and communities with greater needs.

The root causes of limited access to health care, a key driver of health inequities, lie not only in the health care sector (e.g., physician shortages, unaffordable health insurance) but also in other sectors. For example, low educational attainment generally leads to low wages and employment in jobs that do not offer health insurance or time off work to seek care. Other examples include housing insecurity and poor public transportation, which geographically limits those seeking care from hospitals or clinics.

Variable quality of care is another cause of inequities in health outcomes. Health care quality can be improved for all by tailoring it to the needs of diverse US populations. Health inequities can be identified by improving the collection of race/ethnicity and other social identity data and stratifying clinical performance metrics by these social factors. Root cause analysis can identify the etiology of these inequities, and interventions should address those causes. For example, high blood pressure might be difficult to control because of the unaffordability of medications, poor communication and mistrust, culturally blind dietary recommendations, food deserts, inadequate infrastructure for caring for patients with limited English proficiency, or insufficient monitoring and follow-up of patients. In addition, the media shapes our perceptions of people from different backgrounds, influencing how health care providers interact with patients (see later). The United States needs to change the financing of health care to expand access to care and reform payment policies to support and incentivize equitable, high-quality care and equitable outcomes.[33]

Explicit efforts generally are not made to identify and root out structures, policies, and regulations in the health care system, including in financing and payment, that have been shaped by racism and other intersectional systems of oppression (e.g. sexism, homophobia, classism, ableism).[1,34-36] For example, the fundamental design, underfinancing, and state variation in resourcing of the Medicaid program are rooted in the racial politics of the 1960s, with lasting effects to the present day.[37,38] Today's multi-tiered financing and payment systems create perverse incentives for health care delivery organizations to limit care for underresourced, marginalized, and minoritized racial/ethnic populations, such as patients with Medicaid insurance.[39,40] Payment disparities also create financial barriers to locating facilities in geographic areas populated with high percentages of patients with Medicaid insurance, including predominantly poor neighborhoods with minoritized racial/ethnic populations.[40]

Actionable solutions should include ensuring access to health care and implementing policies that support and incentivize equitable health care that is tailored to meet the needs of all populations.[33,41] See Table 8-1 for a more expansive list of potential solutions.[1,2,35,42-76]

Economic Infrastructure, Safety Net, Labor/Employment

Inadequately resourced school systems coupled with unfair employment practices and lack of health care access stifle access to an opportunity structure of stable employment, family economic stability, and intergenerational mobility.

–Zambrana et al., Chapter 4

Socioeconomic status and resources are root causes of health disparities in all populations, including white European Americans. Population health theory and voluminous evidence demonstrate that socioeconomic resources are causally implicated in the production and distribution of health, functioning as "fundamental causes" of health inequalities.

–Blacksher et al., Chapter 7

Strengthening the United States' economic infrastructure for people disadvantaged by imposed restrictions on access to resources should be a key policy focus, as resource scarcity has cascading effects on health. Marginalized communities suffer from a lack of good schools, jobs that pay livable wages, and capital investments in community

Table 8-1. Health Care: Actionable Solutions

Health Care Action	Actionable Solution
Ensure access to health care	Redesign health care financing to expand access to care for marginalized populations.[1,35,42-45]
	Expand Medicaid and individual non-group market health insurance.[46]
	Expand support for health insurance navigators and assisters.[47,48]
	Increase requirements for employers to offer health insurance, including increasing the enrollment of small businesses in public insurance options.[49,50]
	Eliminate barriers to insurance based on immigration status.[51,52]
	Repeal any public charge laws that consider a noncitizen's probability of depending on the government for subsistence when determining whether to grant a green card or visa.[53]
	Increase Medicaid reimbursement rates so that health care delivery organizations have support and incentives to care for Medicaid beneficiaries rather than limit their care.[46]
Implement policies supporting and incentivizing equitable health care tailored to meet the needs of all populations	Support health care services that are patient-, family-, and community-centered, including proactive engagement of patients, families, and caregivers during care.[1,54-56]
	Clarify requirements and increase enforcement of language access in all health care programs and services, including ensuring access to qualified health care interpreters and translations of written materials.[54,57,58]
	Expand the role of community health workers and patient advisors to mitigate access, cultural, and structural barriers to health care systems.[59]
	Increase health workforce diversity and ensure federally funded training and diversity programs create sustainable employment opportunities for underrepresented groups.[60-64]
	Increase cultural humility and health equity training for health care professionals and staff.[65]
	Strengthen mental health and substance use disorder services to meet patients where they are.[66-68]
	Address health-related social needs such as food insecurity, housing insecurity, and transportation, and structural, social drivers of health.[55,68]
	Reform payment systems to support and incentivize overall wellness, disease prevention, and care specifically tailored to meet the medical and social needs of all populations.[69,70]
	Provide more funding and support to underresourced health care delivery organizations that frequently provide uncompensated or undercompensated care serving marginalized racial/ethnic communities.[2]
	Increase racial/ethnic diversity in the health care workforce, as well as patient-provider racial/ethnic concordance, colocated community health care services/whole-person care, team-based care, and care delivery in the language of preference.[69]
	Improve representation in clinical trials and research.[71]
	Develop sustainable models for value-based payment and alternative payment models that reward high-quality, equitable care and outcomes and social return on investment.[72-74]
	Encourage public and private payers, accreditation organizations, and monitoring agencies to include and prioritize health equity metrics.[72-74]
	Focus on structural changes to systems rather than perceived deficits of individuals (e.g. increase after-hours appointment availability for "nonadherent" patients who miss appointments because they cannot get time off from work).[1,75]
	Prevent and mitigate racial and ethnic bias in health care algorithms.[76]

infrastructure. A US economic infrastructure that provides opportunity to all, as well as labor and safety net investments, would provide access to the necessary resources to live a healthy life, build savings for the long term, and accumulate generational health and wealth. Put simply, economic development and investments are public health interventions.[77] Strengthening sustainable economic development, particularly in communities that need it most, will lead to a healthier America.

Actionable solutions should include measures of investments into economic infrastructure, safety nets for marginalized communities, and labor/employment. These solutions should also include investments in youth and families to prevent incarceration, create job opportunities, and improve reentry programs for formerly incarcerated individuals to transition successfully to the community.

- Economic infrastructure investments
    - Invest in economic development, food security, affordable housing, public transportation, and rural broadband.[2,78]
    - Create built environments that promote physical activity, ease stress, enhance green space, and reduce vulnerability to severe weather and climate change.[2,79]
    - Invest in renewable energy infrastructure, particularly in the Oceanian territories and Freely Associated States, to benefit all generations.[80,81]
    - Rebalance public investments from incarceration and detention to strengthening communities and families.[67,82]
    - Address economic harms of the past by providing economic and land reparations.[83–85]
    - Rectify the racial wage gap and wealth divide.[86,87]
    - Increase access to home ownership.[88,89]
    - Increase access to banks and lending institutions in marginalized communities.[90,91]
    - Increase representation of people from a diverse range of races and ethnicities in leadership across sectors, including government, academia, and health care.[63,64]
- Safety net investments for marginalized communities
    - Increase enrollment of those eligible for assistance programs and expand access to overlooked marginalized groups.[92]
    - Design assistance programs to encourage financial security, savings, and economic advancement.[92–94]
    - Support subsidies for childcare and reduce student loan debt (see Education section for more).[95]
- Labor/employment investments
    - Develop and enforce fair working conditions for low-wage workers.[96–98]

- Expand paid family leave.[99,100]
- Increase the federal minimum wage, with built-in cost of living increases.[101]
- Make the Earned Income Tax Credit permanent and expand eligibility.[94,102]
- Protect the right to unionize.[103]
- Increase training for 21st-century jobs.[86]
- Expand educational opportunities for trade jobs.[86]
- Improve access to job benefits like health insurance in the gig economy.[1,92,104]

Education

Educational equity for low-income Latinos is a life course investment that begins with access to high-quality early childhood education: a K–12 experience that prepares students for college careers, postsecondary education, and access to lifelong learning opportunities. The lack of access, outreach, and high rates of disenrollment and dropouts of Mexican and Puerto Rican youth in federal and state education programs calls for increased accountability of funding priorities to ensure equitable access to monetary, recreational, and academic skill-building programs.

–Zambrana et al., Chapter 4

High-quality education is a driving factor in socioeconomic status and is not equally distributed across all populations and communities in the United States. Socioeconomic status, in turn, predicts health outcomes. Education opens the door to life opportunities, predicting employment and home ownership, whereas inadequate education predicts adverse outcomes such as early pregnancy, delinquency, and crime. Investing in quality education leads to increased wealth accumulation, social mobility, access to health insurance, and improved health. Additionally, the United States can and should do more to help underrepresented populations pursue careers in health science, health care, and public health careers to improve workforce diversity.

Actionable solutions should focus on reforming the educational system to make it more accessible to underrepresented populations, eliminating barriers to high-quality education, and investing in educational pipelines to professional career opportunities.

- Education
    - Restructure how education is financed to eliminate inequities.[105]
    - Improve the quality of schooling from early childhood through postsecondary education for all.[106]
    - Reduce student loan debt.[107]
    - Increase investments in education scholarships for students across underrepresented populations.[108]
    - Incorporate accurate histories of minoritized racial/ethnic populations into general educational curricula.[109,110]

- Pipelines into professional careers
    - Invest in community colleges and vocational schools as pathways to good-paying employment, including the trades.[86]
    - Invest in educational pipelines into the health and science, technology, engineering, and mathematics professions for students from underrepresented populations.[61,106]

Justice and Civil Rights Law

Incarceration is much more than an individual experience; its costs are borne collectively. This means examining how mass incarceration and mass police surveillance go far beyond directly affecting the health of individuals with [criminal legal system] contact to having spillover effects that harm the health of romantic partners and their infants and older children.

–Keels et al., Chapter 3

The legal system is rooted in structural racism. For example, Black people experience disproportionately higher rates of police stops, arrests, and convictions and are at a higher risk of experiencing police brutality. The resulting trauma extends beyond the individual. Incarceration removes a parent from a child's life and increases the financial and caregiving burden to the rest of the family. Incarceration also removes human capital and social and economic resources from the neighborhood, further exacerbating systemic inequities. Dismantling systemic racism in the criminal legal system would improve equity in social systems and health.

Additionally, civil rights are under attack and must be bolstered. To create actionable solutions, reforms are needed in the criminal legal system, including requiring mandatory collection and reporting of racial and ethnic data for all stops and searches of motorists and pedestrians, creating an independent committee to review and respond to racial profiling complaints, and allowing those who have been targets of profiling to get legal relief. Public reporting processes to look for, mitigate, and eliminate implicit and structural biases in criminal prosecutions, convictions, and sentencing would play a key role in accountability in transforming biased systems.[111]

Actionable solutions should also focus on civil rights laws, including stopping the erosion of civil rights funding and restoring disparate impact and discriminatory effects discrimination claims. Barriers to voting, such as additional documentation requirements for voter registration and voting, limits on mail-in ballots, and limits on times and places for early and same-day voting, should be removed. A summary of key actionable solutions follows:

- Criminal legal system
    - Ban racial profiling and prevent over-policing.[82,111]
    - Develop routine public reporting databases.[82,112]
    - Fund preschool programs and public schools.[113]
    - Implement sensible firearm policy.[114-116]
- Civil rights laws
    - Increase civil rights funding.[117]
    - Create systems and databases to monitor violations of civil rights.[118]
    - Restore disparate impact and discriminatory effects discrimination claims.[118,119]
    - Remove barriers to voting.[10,120]

Media

Despite the religious, racial, cultural, and ethnic diversity of the region, US media has created a homogenizing Arab or MENA look, and those who fit that profile are potential targets of Islamophobic acts, whether they are from the MENA population or not. . . . Arabs and those from the MENA region are uniformly portrayed as Muslim, and Islam is portrayed as an uncivilized and violent religion, used to racialize anyone perceived as Muslim as inferior to white Americans.

–Ajrouch et al., Chapter 5

Asian Americans were (and still are) impacted by anti-Asian rhetoric and misinformation related to the [COVID-19] pandemic in the media, particularly about the origins of the virus. . . . Such media stories awakened long-standing associations of Asian bodies with invasive illness and disease. . . . Also, following 9/11, South Asians were targeted in incidents of street violence as well as federal policy and media reports. . . . Asian Americans faced racist rhetoric, scapegoating, and a surge of targeted attacks and violence related to the COVID-19 pandemic.

–Sharif et al., Chapter 2

The media has an important role in informing the public about the populations in this book, impacting different groups' access to the opportunity structures in the United States and even exposing them to overt threats to their health and safety. Specifically, media can perpetuate harmful stereotypes or provide accurate and nuanced depictions of what it means to be part of a particular community in the United States. Public perceptions are shaped by what is seen and heard through various media platforms and associated networks. Negative perceptions about a particular group of people can be perpetuated, but fortunately, so can positive perceptions, thus providing an opportunity to change the culture.

Actionable solutions include working with news, media, and the entertainment industry to implement media and communications plans that combat the stereotyping of minoritized groups, destigmatize poverty, and promote the accurate narrative that health equity benefits all rather than being a zero-sum game. Key recommendations include the following:

- Promote accurate representative narratives of heterogeneous communities rather than narratives that use harmful stereotypes.[109,110,121,122]
- Increase representation in the media/entertainment workforce, including content creators.[121,122]
- Counter the representations that members of particular populations are harmful and problematic.[30,110,123,124]
- Counter the myth that whites are superior to others.[125]
- Highlight that poor and disadvantaged whites benefit from equitable social and health care policies.[126]

Immigration and Foreign Policy

[A]ttention to US foreign policy illustrates how the Arab/MENA case is uniquely tied to global political developments that can alter the profile and selectivity of MENA immigrants in different eras.

–Ajrouch et al., Chapter 5

Following the US loss in the Vietnam War in 1975, hundreds of thousands of Southeast Asian refugees . . . resettled in the United States and elsewhere from Vietnam, Laos, and Cambodia. A disproportionate number of these political refugees had limited education and fewer marketable skills, which marginalized them to the bottom segments of the labor market.

–Sharif et al., Chapter 2

Depending on their place of origin/residence, NH/PIs can fall under various immigration statuses. . . . The decades-long struggle to reinstate Medicaid eligibility for Micronesians from [Compact of Free Association] signatory nations is just one example of how the immigration system privileges certain legal statuses over others, and how these distinctions directly contribute to inequitable access to health services.

– Fitisemanu Jr., et al., Chapter 6

The US immigration and foreign policy systems have an unequal effect on the treatment and health of people from certain populations and countries. In particular, biases in these policies directed at immigrants adversely affect access to the opportunity structures in the United States through mechanisms such as pathways to citizenship and perceived security risks. These effects are further compounded by racism, as illustrated throughout history among each of the populations.

Actionable solutions should focus on reforming the immigration system and protecting immigrant communities from adverse foreign policies, such as providing pathways to citizenship for immigrants (including Deferred Action for Childhood Arrivals [DACA] youth), preserving family reunification, and expanding employment-based opportunities for immigrants.

- Immigration
    - Provide pathways to citizenship and remove barriers to citizenship.[127,128]
    - Relieve immigrant visa backlogs.[127]
    - Eliminate English-only laws and promote language access in voting and all public services.[129]
- Foreign Policy
    - Address policies such as the USA PATRIOT Act that create unfair "national security risk" biases against populations such as MENA and Chinese Americans.[130,131]

Indigenous Sovereignty

In addition to health, education, and economic systems, cross-cutting and foundational issues include protecting and valuing intact ecosystems and preserving traditional knowledges by fostering intergenerational relationships with elders and knowledge bearers. The aim should be to include AI/AN peoples in all levels of health systems, including systems that protect and value intact ecosystems, intergenerational relationships, and include fully funding health systems, in addition to improving economic opportunities to include education and training.

–Warne et al., Chapter 1

The overemphasis on health disparities and inequities is demoralizing and fails to uplift the incredible assets of Oceania peoples who continue to persist, innovate, and advance despite statistical invisibility, dismal health indicators, and disproportionate burden of disease. The same legacy of resilient perseverance, Indigenous ingenuity, and oneness of people/land that sustained NH/PI societies through military occupation, cultural genocide, and colonial imperialism are unique, untapped strengths that can bolster efforts to improve, change, and/or replace systemic structures that prevent NH/PIs from achieving optimal health.

– Fitisemanu Jr., et al., Chapter 6

Colonization, genocide, and forced assimilation have caused great harm to Indigenous peoples in the territory currently known as the United States. Yet great assets, strengths, and expertise are present in AI/AN and NH/PI peoples. The principle of *sovereignty*—the authority of Indigenous peoples to govern themselves—is a key component of solutions to improve health equity and the health of land and water ecosystems.

Actionable solutions related to Indigenous sovereignty should include reforms across land and ecosystems, health care, economic investments, education, and data. Solutions should include the full funding of the Indian Health Service (IHS), which, according to the IHS Budget Formulation Committee and the National Indian Health Board, would (in 2023) require $49.8 billion, a 10-fold increase in funding.[132] See Table 8-2 for a more expansive list of actionable solutions regarding Indigenous sovereignty.[45,80,81,91,109,133–147]

Table 8-2. Indigenous Sovereignty: Actionable Solutions

System	Actionable Solution
Land and ecosystem	Remove/revise policies that prohibit customary usage and access to ancestral lands and waters by lineal descendants of traditional custodians and residents.[133,134]
	Include Indigenous peoples in all levels of systems that protect and value intact ecosystems and intergenerational relationships and that address climate change.[135-137]
	Increase funding opportunities for sustainable economic development and renewable energy infrastructure in all Oceania territories and FAS.[80,81]
Health care	Fully fund IHS.[45]
	Provide culturally safe and respectful care that understands the historical perspectives, childhood and intergenerational trauma, and circumstances unique to Indigenous peoples.[134]
	Support traditional healing practices.[133]
	Improve coordination across IHS/Tribal/urban Indian health programs and public/private sector health systems.[45]
	Develop an available, accessible, affordable, and competent workforce that integrates community voices and AI/AN traditions into culturally sensitive care.[138]
	Incorporate midwives, social workers, mental health counselors, doulas, AI/AN traditional healers, knowledge bearers, birth workers and peers, community health workers, and physician extenders into the care of Indigenous people.[139]
	Expand digital access and telehealth in resource-limited areas to supplement existing care resources (but not act as a substitute for care) and to provide sufficient resources to these areas.[139]
Economics	Invest in economic infrastructure in AI/AN and NH/PI communities. Promoting banking, business development, wireless internet, and economic sovereignty on reservations, Hawai'i, and US Pacific Island territories is necessary to promote wellness in Indigenous communities.[91,140]
	Implement culturally rooted and sustainable community-based management systems.[141]
	Approach economic development as a public health intervention.[140]
	Develop a system to protect and value intact ecosystems.[133,134]

(Continued)

Table 8-2. (Continued)

System	Actionable Solution
Education	Incorporate accurate AI/AN and NH/PI history and cultural values into general educational curricula; culturally competent education should be reflected in both curricula and personnel.[109,142]
	Provide funding and resources to facilitate the universal teaching of Indigenous languages and decolonized history in public schools in the state of Hawai'i, the US territories of Guam and American Samoa, CNMI, and the signatory nations of COFA.[143]
	Invest in AI/AN and NH/PI schools and Tribal colleges.[144]
	Foster intergenerational relationships with elders and knowledge-bearers.[136,137]
Data	Ensure Tribal data sovereignty and ownership and control of data.[145]
	Disaggregate the NH/PI category from the broader Asian category; disaggregate Tribal data.[146,147]

Note: AI/AN = American Indian or Alaska Native; COFA = Compact of Free Association; CNMI = Commonwealth of the Northern Marianas Islands; FAS = Freely Associated States; IHS = Indian Health Service; NH/PI = Native Hawaiian or Pacific Islander.

CONCLUSION

Americans widely support giving everyone a fair and just opportunity for health—part of the classic American dream.[148] Yet, structural racism prevents many minoritized racial and ethnic groups from accessing opportunity structures in fields such as education, employment, economic development, and health care that give people a fair chance for health and well-being. Health inequities exact a heavy toll on the lives and daily experiences of marginalized people, at a staggering economic cost to the country. However, health inequities resulting from structural racism are not inevitable. A series of conscious policy decisions have embedded racism in opportunity structures, so we can enact policies that intentionally root out racist structures, rules, regulations, and procedures that unfairly prevent everyone from having a chance for health and well-being. Far from being a zero-sum game, health equity for minoritized racial and ethnic groups and other marginalized populations benefits everyone. All racial and ethnic groups, including poor and disadvantaged whites, benefit from equitable social and health care policies, and the United States benefits economically when we do not waste the contributions and productivity of every American. We all hope our children and the next generation will live in a world where they can reach their full potential. We can shatter the constraints of structural racism and together create a future where everyone has a fair opportunity for productive, healthy lives.

REFERENCES

1. National Academies of Sciences, Engineering, and Medicine; Nass SJ, Amankwah FK, DeVoe JE, Benjamin GC, eds. 2024. *Ending Unequal Treatment: Strategies to Achieve Equitable Health Care and Optimal Health for All*. National Academies Press; 2024.
2. National Academies of Sciences, Engineering, and Medicine; Baciu A, Negussie Y, Geller A, et al., eds. *Communities in Action: Pathways to Health Equity*. National Academies Press; 2017.
3. National Academies of Sciences, Engineering, and Medicine; Geller AB, Polsky DE, Burke SP, eds. *Federal Policy to Advance Racial, Ethnic, and Tribal Health Equity*. National Academies Press; 2023.
4. LaVeist TA, Pérez-Stable EJ, Richard P, et al. The economic burden of racial, ethnic, and educational health inequities in the US. *JAMA*. 2023;329(19):1682–1692. doi:10.1001/jama.2023.5965
5. Michener J. Racism, power, and health equity: The case of tenant organizing. *Health Aff (Millwood)*. 2023;42(10):1318–1324. doi:10.1377/hlthaff.2023.00509
6. Brown TH, Homan P. The future of social determinants of health: Looking upstream to structural drivers. *Milbank Q*. 2023;101(suppl 1):36–60. doi:10.1111/1468-0009.12641
7. Simons RL, Lei MK, Klopack E, Beach SRH, Gibbons FX, Philibert RA. The effects of social adversity, discrimination, and health risk behaviors on the accelerated aging of African Americans: Further support for the weathering hypothesis. *Soc Sci Med*. 2021;282:113169. doi:10.1016/j.socscimed.2020.113169
8. Michener J, Ford TN. Racism and health: Three core principles. *Milbank Q*. 2023;101(S1):333–355. doi:10.1111/1468-0009.12633
9. Jahn JL, Zubizarreta D, Chen JT, et al. Legislating inequity: Structural racism in groups of state laws and associations with premature mortality rates. *Health Aff (Millwood)*. 2023;42(10):1325–1333. doi:10.1377/hlthaff.2023.00471
10. Brown TH, Homan P. Structural racism and health stratification: Connecting theory to measurement. *J Health Soc Behav*. 2024;65(1):141–160. doi:10.1177/00221465231222924
11. Lantz PM, House JS, Lepkowski JM, Williams DR, Mero RP, Chen J. Socioeconomic factors, health behaviors, and mortality: Results from a nationally representative prospective study of US adults. *JAMA*. 1998;279(21):1703–1708. doi:10.1001/jama.279.21.1703
12. Homan P, Brown TH, King B. Structural intersectionality as a new direction for health disparities research. *J Health Soc Behav*. 2021;62(3):350–370. doi:10.1177/00221465211032947
13. Adler NE, Newman K. Socioeconomic disparities in health: Pathways and policies. *Health Aff (Millwood)*. 2002;21(2):60–76. doi:10.1377/hlthaff.21.2.60
14. Solar O, Irwin A. *A Conceptual Framework for Action on the Social Determinants of Health*. World Health Organization; 2010. Accessed August 5, 2025. https://www.who.int/publications/i/item/9789241500852
15. Brown TH, Hargrove TW, Homan P, Adkins DE. Racialized health inequities: Quantifying socioeconomic and stress pathways using moderated mediation. *Demography*. 2023;60(3):675–705. doi:10.1215/00703370-10740718
16. Geronimus AT, Hicken M, Keene D, Bound J. 'Weathering' and age patterns of allostatic load scores among Blacks and whites in the United States. *Am J Public Health*. 2006;96(5):826–833. doi:10.2105/AJPH.2004.060749

17. Miller HN, LaFave S, Marineau L, Stephens J, Thorpe RJ Jr. The impact of discrimination on allostatic load in adults: An integrative review of literature. *J Psychosom Res.* 2021;146:110434. doi:10.1016/j.jpsychores.2021.110434
18. Duru OK, Harawa NT, Kermah D, Norris KC. Allostatic load burden and racial disparities in mortality. *J Natl Med Assoc.* 2012;104(1–2):89–95. doi:10.1016/s0027-9684(15)30120-6
19. Forde AT, Crookes DM, Suglia SF, Demmer RT. The weathering hypothesis as an explanation for racial disparities in health: A systematic review. *Ann Epidemiol.* 2019;33:1–18.e3. doi:10.1016/j.annepidem.2019.02.011
20. Joseph JJ, Golden SH. Type 2 diabetes and cardiovascular disease: What next?. *Curr Opin Endocrinol Diabetes Obes.* 2014;21(2):109–120. doi:10.1097/MED.0000000000000044
21. Braveman P, Gottlieb L. The social determinants of health: It's time to consider the causes of the causes. *Public Health Rep.* 2014;129(suppl 2):19–31. doi:10.1177/00333549141291S206
22. Christopher GC. Truth, racial healing, and transformation: Creating public sentiment. *Health Equity.* 2021;5(1):668–674. doi:10.1089/heq.2021.29008.ncl
23. Indian Health Service. IHS and Alaska Tribal Health Compact successfully complete fiscal year 2024 negotiations. Press release. June 8, 2023. Accessed August 5, 2025. https://www.ihs.gov/newsroom/pressreleases/2023-press-releases/ihs-and-alaska-tribal-health-compact-successfully-complete-fiscal-year-2024-negotiations
24. Muramatsu N, Chin MH. Asian, Native Hawaiian, and Pacific Islander populations in the US—Moving from invisibility to health equity. *JAMA Netw Open.* 2024;7(5):e2411617. doi:10.1001/jamanetworkopen.2024.11617
25. US Dept of Health and Human Services. *Data Disaggregation Resource Guide: Advancing Equity for Asian American, Native Hawaiian, and Pacific Islander Communities in COVID-19 Response Efforts.* US Dept of Health and Human Services; 2023. Accessed August 10, 2025. https://vaccineresourcehub.org/download-files/3219
26. Yi SS, Kwon SC, Suss R, et al. The mutually reinforcing cycle of poor data quality and racialized stereotypes that shapes Asian American health. *Health Aff (Millwood).* 2022;41(2):296–303. doi:10.1377/hlthaff.2021.01417
27. Islam NS, Khan S, Kwon S, Jang D, Ro M, Trinh-Shevrin C. Methodological issues in the collection, analysis, and reporting of granular data in Asian American populations: Historical challenges and potential solutions. *J Health Care Poor Underserved.* 2010;21(4):1354–1381. doi:10.1353/hpu.2010.0939
28. Errisuriz VL, Zambrana RE, Parra-Medina D. Critical analyses of Latina mortality: Disentangling the heterogeneity of ethnic origin, place, nativity, race, and socioeconomic status. *BMC Public Health.* 2024;24(1):190. doi:10.1186/s12889-024-17721-9
29. Nicole W. Paradox lost? The waning health advantage among the US Hispanic population. *Environ Health Perspect.* 2023;131(1):12001. doi:10.1289/EHP11618
30. Naber N. Ambiguous insiders: An investigation of Arab American invisibility. *Ethn Rac Stud.* 2000;23(1):37–61. doi:10.1080/014198700329123
31. Shimkhada R, Scheitler AJ, Ponce NA. Capturing racial/ethnic diversity in population-based surveys: Data disaggregation of health data for Asian American, Native Hawaiian, and Pacific Islanders (AANHPIs). *Popul Res Policy Rev.* 2021;40(1):81–102. doi:10.1007/s11113-020-09634-3

32. Pulido L. A critical review of the methodology of environmental racism research. *Antipode.* 2006;28:142–59. doi:10.1111/j.1467-8330.1996.tb00519.x
33. Chin MH, Dale K, Hernández-Cancio S. Reforms to support the health care industry to address adverse health-related social factors. *JAMA Netw Open.* 2024;7(10):e2440439. doi:10.1001/jamanetworkopen.2024.40439
34. Bailey ZD, Krieger N, Agénor M, Graves J, Linos N, Bassett MT. Structural racism and health inequities in the USA: Evidence and interventions. *Lancet.* 2017;389(10077):1453–1463. doi:10.1016/S0140-6736(17)30569-X
35. Cook SC, Todić J, Spitzer S, et al. Opportunities for psychologists to advance health equity: Using liberation psychology to identify key lessons from 17 years of praxis. *Am Psychol.* 2023;78(2):211–226. doi:10.1037/amp0001126
36. Singletary KA, Chin MH. What should anti-racist payment reform look like? *AMA J Ethics* 2023;25(1):55–66. doi:10.1001/amajethics.2023.55
37. Illicit history-2-Medicaid vs states' rights ft. Jamila Michener. The Michael Brooks Show. June 26, 2019. Accessed August 6, 2025. https://www.youtube.com/watch?v=ZRtakJsEc74
38. Nolen LT, Beckman AL, Sandoe E. How foundational moments in Medicaid's history reinforced rather than eliminated racial health disparities. *Health Affairs Forefront.* September 1, 2020. doi:10.1377/forefront.20200828.661111
39. Eschliman BH, Pham HH, Navathe AS, Dale KM, Harris J. The role of payment and financing in achieving health equity. *Health Serv Res.* 2023;58(suppl 3):311–317. doi:10.1111/1475-6773.14219
40. Chisolm DJ, Dugan JA, Figueroa JF, et al. Improving health equity through health care systems research. *Health Serv Res.* 2023;58(suppl 3):289–299. doi:10.1111/1475-6773.14192
41. Fernandez A, Chin MH. Keep your eyes on the prize: Focusing on health care equity. *N Engl J Med.* 2024;390(19):1733–1736. doi:10.1056/NEJMp2400424
42. Berwick DM. Salve lucrum: The existential threat of greed in US health care. *JAMA.* 2023;329(8):629–630. doi:10.1001/jama.2023.0846.
43. Chin MH. Uncomfortable truths—What COVID-19 has revealed about chronic-disease care in America. *N Engl J Med.* 2021;385(18):1633–1636. doi:10.1056/NEJMp2112063
44. Health Care Payment Learning and Action Network Health Equity Advisory Team. *Advancing Health Equity Through APMs: Guidance on Social Risk Adjustment.* 2022. Accessed August 6, 2025. https://web.archive.org/web/20250623113904/http://hcp-lan.org/workproducts/APM-Guidance/Advancing-Health-Equity-Through-APMs-Social-Risk-Adjustment.pdf
45. Warne D, Frizzell LB. American Indian health policy: Historical trends and contemporary issues. *Am J Public Health.* 2014;104(suppl 3):S263–S267. doi:10.2105/AJPH.2013.301682.
46. Jaffe S. NYC guarantees health care to all. *The Lancet.* 2019;393(10169):e3–e4. doi:10.1016/S0140-6736(19)30157-6
47. Pear R. Trump officials slash grants that help consumers get Obamacare. *New York Times.* July 10, 2018. Accessed August 5, 2025. https://www.nytimes.com/2018/07/10/us/politics/trump-affordable-care-act.html
48. Myerson R, Li H. 2022. Information gaps and health insurance enrollment: Evidence from the Affordable Care Act Navigator Programs. *Am J Health Econ.* 2022;8(4):477–505. doi:10.1086/721569

49. Branch B, Conway D. Health insurance coverage by race and Hispanic origin: 2021. US Dept of Commerce, US Census Bureau. November 2022. Accessed August 5, 2025. https://www.census.gov/content/dam/Census/library/publications/2022/acs/acsbr-012.pdf
50. Wilper AP, Woolhandler S, Lasser KE, McCormick D, Bor DH, Himmelstein DU. Health insurance and mortality in US adults. *Am J Public Health* 2009;99(12):2289–2295. doi:10.2105/AJPH.2008.157685
51. Ommerborn MJ, Ranker LR, Touw S, Himmelstein DU, Himmelstein J, Woolhandler S. Assessment of immigrants' premium and tax payments for health care and the costs of their care. *JAMA Netw Open.* 2022;5(11):e2241166. doi:10.1001/jamanetworkopen.2022.41166
52. Ku L. Who pays for immigrants' health care in the US? *JAMA Netw Open.* 2022;5(11):e2241171. doi:10.1001/jamanetworkopen.2022.41171
53. Huynh N. Public charge: An injustice and its chilling effects on AAPI and low-income communities. *Asian American Policy Review* (blog). October 5, 2020. Accessed August 5, 2025. https://studentreview.hks.harvard.edu/public-charge-an-injustice-and-its-chilling-effects-on-aapi-and-low-income-communities
54. Zambrana RE, Torres-Burgos D, Carvajal DN. Expert perspectives on effective community-based pediatric healthcare for low-income Latino families: Persistent issues over time. *J Racial Ethn Health Disparities.* 2022;9(3):1051–1061. doi:10.1007/s40615-021-01044-1
55. National Academies of Sciences, Engineering, and Medicine. *Integrating Social Care into the Delivery of Health Care: Moving Upstream to Improve the Nation's Health.* National Academies Press; 2019.
56. O'Kane M, Agrawal S, Binder L, et al. An equity agenda for the field of health care quality improvement. *NAM Perspect.* 2021:10.31478/202109b. doi:10.31478/202109b
57. Jang Y, Kim MT. Limited English proficiency and health service use in Asian Americans. *J Immigr Minor Health.* 2019;21(2):264–270. doi:10.1007/s10903-018-0763-0
58. Muramatsu N, Chin MH. Battling structural racism against Asians in the United States: Call for public health to make the "invisible" visible. *J Public Health Manag Pract.* 2022;28(suppl 1):S3–S8. doi:10.1097/PHH.0000000000001411
59. Shiro AG, Reeves RV. Latinos often lack access to healthcare and have poor health outcomes. here's how we can change that. Brookings Institution. September 25, 2020. https://www.brookings.edu/articles/latinos-often-lack-access-to-healthcare-and-have-poor-health-outcomes-heres-how-we-can-change-that
60. Islas IG, Brantley E, Portela Martinez M, Salsberg E, Dobkin F, Frogner BK. Documenting Latino representation in the US health workforce. *Health Aff (Millwood).* 2023;42(7):997–1001. doi:10.1377/hlthaff.2022.01348
61. Cooper LA, Hill MN, Powe NR. Designing and evaluating interventions to eliminate racial and ethnic disparities in health care. *J Gen Intern Med.* 2002;17(6):477–486. doi:10.1046/j.1525-1497.2002.10633.x
62. Saha S, Komaromy M, Koepsell TD, Bindman AB. Patient-physician racial concordance and the perceived quality and use of health care. *Arch Intern Med.* 1999;159(9):997–1004. doi:10.1001/archinte.159.9.997
63. Lee TH, Volpp KG, Cheung VG, Dzau VJ. 2021. Diversity and inclusiveness in health care leadership: Three key steps. *NEJM Catalyst.* 2021;2(3). doi:10.1056/CAT.21.0166

64. Dzau VJ, Lee TH. Confronting racial disparities in C-suite health care leadership. *NEJM Catalyst.* 2021:2(6). doi:10.1056/CAT.21.0449
65. Guillaume G, Robles J, Rodríguez JE. Racial concordance, rather than cultural competency training, can change outcomes. *Fam Med.* 2022;54(9):745–746. doi:10.22454/FamMed.2022.633693
66. Hodgkinson S, Godoy L, Beers LS, Lewin A. Improving mental health access for low-income children and families in the primary care setting. *Pediatrics.* 2017;139(1):e20151175. doi:10.1542/peds.2015-1175
67. Nowotny KM, Belknap J, Lynch S, DeHart D. Risk profile and treatment needs of women in jail with co-occurring serious mental illness and substance use disorders. *Women Health.* 2014;54(8):781–795. doi:10.1080/03630242.2014.932892
68. Escobar-Galvez I, Yanouri L, Herrera CN, Callahan JL, Ruggero CJ, Cicero D. Intergenerational differences in barriers that impede mental health service use among Latinos. *Pract Innov.* 2023;8(2):116–130. doi:10.1037/pri0000204
69. National Academies of Sciences, Engineering, and Medicine; Robinson SK, Meisnere M, Phillips RL Jr., McCauley L, eds. *Implementing High-Quality Primary Care: Rebuilding the Foundation of Health Care.* National Academies Press; 2021.
70. National Academy of Medicine; Pham H, Chesney M, Chisolm D, et al., eds. 2024. *Valuing America's Health: Aligning to Reward Better Health and Well-Being.* National Academies Press; 2024.
71. National Academies of Sciences, Engineering, and Medicine; Bibbins-Domingo K, Helman A, eds. *Improving Representation in Clinical Trials and Research: Building Research Equity for Women and Underrepresented Groups.* National Academies Press; 2022.
72. Health Care Payment Learning and Action Network Health Equity Advisory Team. 2021. *Advancing Health Equity Through APMs: Guidance for Equity-Centered Design and Implementation.* 2021. Accessed August 5, 2025. https://hcp-lan.org/workproducts/APM-Guidance/Advancing-Health-Equity-Through-APMs.pdf
73. Health Care Payment Learning and Action Network Health Equity Advisory Team. *Guidance for Health Care Entities Partnering with Community-Based Organizations: Addressing Health-Related Social Needs in Alternative Payment Models.* 2023. Accessed August 5, 2025. https://hcplan.org/workproducts/APM-Guidance/HEAT-CBO-Partnership-Guidance.pdf
74. Health Care Payment Learning and Action Network Health Equity Advisory Team. *Value of Health Care Redefined: Social Return on Investment.* 2024. Accessed August 5, 2025. https://hcplan.org/wp-content/uploads/2024/11/HCPLAN-Social-ROI-Publication_vFinal.pdf
75. Bukstein DA, Friedman A, Gonzalez Reyes E, Hart M, Jones BL, Winders T. Impact of social determinants on the burden of asthma and eczema: Results from a US patient survey. *Adv Ther.* 2022;39(3):1341–1358. doi:10.1007/s12325-021-02021-0
76. Chin MH, Afsar-Manesh N, Bierman AS, et al. Guiding principles to address the impact of algorithm bias on racial and ethnic disparities in health and health care. *JAMA Netw Open.* 2023;6(12):e2345050. doi:10.1001/jamanetworkopen.2023.45050
77. Marmot M, Buss P. An economics of health for all. *BMJ.* 2023;381:1178. doi:10.1136/bmj.p1178
78. Post C. *The American Road to Capitalism: Studies in Class-Structure, Economic Development and Political Conflict, 1620–1877.* Brill; 2011.

79. Office of Disease Prevention and Health Promotion. Social determinants of health. Healthy people 2030. US Dept of Health and Human Services. Accessed August 5, 2025. https://health.gov/healthypeople/priority-areas/social-determinants-health
80. Ames T. Socio-economic development in Micronesia: A case study of hope and heartbreak in Chuuk. *Pac Asia Inquiry.* 2011;2(1):195–203. Accessed August 5, 2025. https://www.uog.edu/_resources/files/schools-and-colleges/college-of-liberal-arts-and-social-sciences/pai/pai_195-203.pdf
81. Ruane MCM. Economic development prospects for a small island economy: The case of Guam. *J Econ Econ Educ Res.* 2012;13:15–24. Accessed August 5, 2025. https://www.alliedacademies.org/articles/economic-development-prospects-for-a-small-island-economy-the-case-of-guam.pdf
82. Wildeman C, Wang EA. Mass incarceration, public health, and widening inequality in the USA. *Lancet.* 2017;389(10077):1464–1474. doi:10.1016/S0140-6736(17)30259-3
83. Francis DV, Hamilton D, Mitchell TW, Rosenberg NA, Stucki BW. Black land loss: 1920–1997. *AEA Pap Proc.* 2022;112:38–42. doi:10.1257/pandp.20221015
84. Darity W Jr., Mullen AK, Slaughter M. The cumulative costs of racism and the bill for Black reparations. *J Econ Persp.* 2022;36(2):99–122. doi:10.1257/jep.36.2.99
85. Feagin JR. *Racist America: Roots, Current Realities, and Future Reparations.* Routledge; 2000.
86. Freeman R, Han E, Madland D, Duke B. Bargaining for the American dream: What unions do for mobility. Center for American Progress. September 9, 2015. https://www.americanprogress.org/article/bargaining-for-the-american-dream
87. Eisenberg-Guyot J, Keyes KM, Prins SJ, et al. Wage theft and life expectancy inequities in the United States: A simulation study. *Prev Med.* 2022;159:107068. doi:10.1016/j.ypmed.2022.107068
88. Fowle MZ. Racialized homelessness: A review of historical and contemporary causes of racial disparities in homelessness. *Hous Policy Debate.* 2022;32(6):940–967. doi:10.1080/10511482.2022.2026995
89. Fan Q, Nogueira L, Yabroff KR, Hussaini SMQ, Pollack CE. Housing and cancer care and outcomes: A systematic review. *J Natl Cancer Inst.* 2022;114(12):1601–1618. doi:10.1093/jnci/djac173
90. Fletcher MLM. *American Indian Tribal Law.* Aspen Publishing; 2020.
91. Federal Deposit Insurance Corporation. 2023 FDIC National Survey of Unbanked and Underbanked Households. Updated November 14, 2024. Accessed August 5, 2025. https://www.fdic.gov/household-survey
92. Institute of Medicine (US) Committee on Health Insurance Status and Its Consequences. *America's Uninsured Crisis: Consequences for Health and Health Care.* National Academies Press; 2009.
93. Hacker JS. *The Great Risk Shift: Why American Jobs, Families, Health Care and Retirement Aren't Secure—And How We Can Fight Back.* Oxford University Press; 2006.
94. Desmond M. *Poverty, by America.* Crown Publishing; 2023.
95. Remor I, Raza R. Stabilizing child care supply through a new funding mechanism. The Urban Institute. October 2021. Accessed August 5, 2025. https://researchconnections.org/sites/default/files/132586.pdf
96. Oberg C, Hodges HR, Gander S, Nathawad R, Cutts D. The impact of COVID-19 on children's lives in the United States: Amplified inequities and a just path to recovery. *Curr Probl Pediatr Adolesc Health Care.* 2022;52(7):101181. doi:10.1016/j.cppeds.2022.101181

97. Khattar R, Vela J, Roque L. Latino workers continue to experience a shortage of good jobs. Center for American Progress. 2022. Accessed August 6, 2025. https://www.americanprogress.org/article/latino-workers-continue-to-experience-a-shortage-of-good-jobs/
98. Cherlin AJ. *Labor's Love Lost: The Rise and Fall of the Working-Class Family in America*. Russell Sage Foundation; 2014.
99. Taylor JK. Structural racism and maternal health among Black women. *J Law Med Ethics*. 2020;48(3):506–517. doi:10.1177/1073110520958875
100. Howell EA. Reducing disparities in severe maternal morbidity and mortality. *Clin Obstet Gynecol*. 2018;61(2):387–399. doi:10.1097/GRF.0000000000000349
101. Economic Policy Institute. The impact of raising the minimum wage to $15 by 2025, by congressional district: Mapping the impact of the Raise the Wage Act of 2021 on workers. January 28, 2021. Accessed August 6, 2025. https://www.epi.org/publication/minimum-wage-to-15-by-2025-by-congressional-district
102. Troller-Renfree SV, Costanzo MA, Duncan GJ, et al. The impact of a poverty reduction intervention on infant brain activity. *Proc Natl Acad Sci USA*. 2022;119(5):e2115649119. doi:10.1073/pnas.2115649119
103. González N, Galdámez M. More than solidarity: How labor unions preserved Latino jobs. UCLA Latino Policy & Politics Institute. September 6, 2021. Accessed August 6, 2025. https://latino.ucla.edu/wp-content/uploads/2021/09/More-than-Solidarity-How-Labor-Unions-Preserved-Latino-Jobs-1.pdf
104. Smith A. Gig work, online selling and home sharing. Pew Research Center. November 17, 2016. Accessed August 6, 2025. https://www.pewresearch.org/internet/2016/11/17/gig-work-online-selling-and-home-sharing
105. National Research Council; Ladd HF, Chalk R, Hansen JS, eds. *Equity and Adequacy in Education Finance: Issues and Perspectives*. National Academies Press; 1999.
106. Zambrana RE, Hurtado S. *The Magic Key: The Educational Journey of Mexican Americans from K-12 to College and Beyond*. University of Texas Press; 2015.
107. Scott-Clayton J, Li J. Black-white disparity in student loan debt more than triples after graduation. *Evidence Speaks Rep*. 2016;2(3). Accessed August 6, 2025. https://www.brookings.edu/articles/black-white-disparity-in-student-loan-debt-more-than-triples-after-graduation
108. Stern GM. Tuition-free college in New Mexico. *Hispanic Outlook on Education Magazine*. June 2022. Accessed August 6, 2025. https://www.hispanicoutlook.com/articles/tuition-free-college-new-mexico
109. Haozous EA. Native America 101—Why are health researchers teaching high school history? *Res Nurs Health*. 2023;46(3):279–281. doi:10.1002/nur.22311
110. Contreras F, Rodriguez J. Investing in educational equity for Latinos: How accountability, access, and systemic inequity shape opportunity. In: Murillo EG Jr., Delgado Bernal D, Morales S, et al., eds. *Handbook of Latinos and Education: Theory, Research, and Practice*. Routledge; 2021:103–113.
111. Kasravi N, Meyers CT II, Dockins-Miller I, Oliver E. Born suspect: Stop-and-frisk abuses and the continued fight to end racial profiling in America. National Association for the Advancement of Colored People. September 15, 2014. Accessed August 6, 2025. https://search.issuelab.org/resource/born-suspect-stop-and-frisk-abuses-and-the-continued-fight-to-end-racial-profiling-in-america.html

112. Massoglia M, Pridemore WA. Incarceration and health. *Ann Rev Sociol.* 2015;41:291–310. doi:10.1146/annurev-soc-073014-112326
113. Lee H, Wildeman C. Assessing mass incarceration's effects on families. *Science.* 2021;374:277–281. doi:10.1126/science.abj7777
114. National Academies of Sciences, Engineering, and Medicine; Alper J, French M, Wojtowicz A. *Health Systems Interventions to Prevent Firearm Injuries and Death: Proceedings of a Workshop.* National Academies Press; 2019.
115. National Research Council; Wellford CF, Pepper JV, Petrie CV, eds. *Firearms and Violence: A Critical Review.* National Academies Press; 2005.
116. Institute of Medicine, National Research Council; Leshner AI, Altevogt BM, Lee AF, McCoy MA, Kelley PW, eds. *Priorities for Research to Reduce the Threat of Firearm-related Violence.* National Academies Press; 2013.
117. Kemp B, Grumbach JM, Montez JK. US state policy contexts and physical health among midlife adults. *Socius.* 2022;8. doi:10.1177/23780231221091324
118. Roberts JL, Eichner H. Disability rights in health care dodge a bullet. *JAMA Health Forum.* 2022;3(6):e221353. doi:10.1001/jamahealthforum.2022.1353
119. *Students for Fair Admissions v. President and Fellows of Harvard College*, 600 US __ (2023).
120. Homan PA, Brown TH. Sick and tired of being excluded: Structural racism in disenfranchisement as a threat to population health equity. *Health Aff (Millwood).* 2022;41(2):219–227. doi:10.1377/hlthaff.2021.01414
121. Hicken MT, Miles L, Haile S, Esposito M. Linking history to contemporary state-sanctioned slow violence through cultural and structural racism. *Ann Am Acad Pol Soc Sci.* 2021;694(1):48–58. doi:10.1177/00027162211005690
122. Michaels EK, Lam-Hine T, Nguyen TT, Gee GC, Allen AM. The water surrounding the iceberg: Cultural racism and health inequities. *Milbank Q.* 2023;101(3):768–814. doi:10.1111/1468-0009.12662
123. Petersen W. Success story, Japanese-American style. *New York Times*, January 9, 1996. Accessed August 6, 2025. https://www.nytimes.com/1966/01/09/archives/success-story-japaneseamerican-style-success-story-japaneseamerican.html
124. Alsultany E. *Arabs and Muslims in the Media: Race and Representation after 9/11.* New York University Press; 2012.
125. Naber NS. Imperial whiteness and the diasporas of empire. *Am Q.* 2014;66(4):1107–1115. doi:10.1353/aq.2014.0068
126. Sasson I. Trends in life expectancy and lifespan variation by educational attainment: United States, 1990–2010. *Demography.* 2016;53(2):269–293. doi:10.1007/s13524-015-0453-7
127. National Immigration Forum; Calderin G. 2023. Eliminating the naturalization backlog. National Immigration Forum. May 11, 2023. Accessed August 6, 2025. https://immigrationforum.org/article/eliminating-the-naturalization-backlog
128. Iyer D. *We Too Sing America: South Asian, Arab, Muslim, and Sikh Immigrants Shape Our Multiracial Future.* The New Press; 2017.
129. Yam K. Georgia's Asian American voter rates hit record high. How voting bill threatens progress. *NBC News.* March 31, 2021. Accessed August 6, 2025. https://www.nbcnews.com/news/asian-america/asian-american-voter-rates-georgia-hit-record-high-how-voting-n1262682

130. Yaccino S, Preston J, Santora M. Wisconsin shooter identified as US Army veteran. *New York Times.* August 6, 2012. Accessed August 6, 2025. https://web.archive.org/web/20120806192801/http://www.nytimes.com/2012/08/07/us/army-veteran-identified-as-suspect-in-wisconsin-shooting.html?pagewanted=all
131. American Civil Liberties Union. Surveillance under the USA/PATRIOT Act. October 23, 2001. Accessed August 6, 2025. https://www.aclu.org/documents/surveillance-under-usapatriot-act
132. The National Tribal Budget Formulation Workgroup. *Building Health Equity With Tribal Nations: The National Budget Formulation Workgroup's Recommendations on the Indian Health Service Fiscal Year 2023 Budget.* 2021. Accessed April 2, 2025. https://www.nihb.org/wp-content/uploads/2025/01/FY-2023-Tribal-Budget-Formulation-Workgroup-Recommendations-Vol-1.pdf
133. Ahmed F, Zuk AM, Tsuji LJS. The impact of land-based physical activity interventions on self-reported health and well-being of Indigenous adults: A systematic review. *Int J Environ Res Public Health.* 2021;18(13):7099. doi:10.3390/ijerph18137099
134. Evans-Campbell T. Historical trauma in American Indian/Native Alaska communities: A multilevel framework for exploring impacts on individuals, families, and communities. *J Interpers Violence.* 2008;23(3):316–338. doi:10.1177/0886260507312290
135. Hansen T. Kill the land, kill the people: There are 532 superfund sites in Indian country. *ICT News.* June 17, 2014. Accessed August 6, 2025. https://ictnews.org/archive/kill-the-land-kill-the-people-there-are-532-superfund-sites-in-indian-country
136. Deloria V Jr., Lytle CM. *American Indians, American Justice.* University of Texas Press; 2012.
137. Thornton R. *American Indian Holocaust and Survival: A Population History since 1492.* University of Oklahoma Press; 1997.
138. Association of American Medical Colleges. Diversity in medicine: Facts and figures 2019. 2019. Accessed August 6, 2025. https://www.aamc.org/data-reports/workforce/data/figure-15-percentage-full-time-us-medical-school-faculty-race/ethnicity-2018
139. Sharma G, Kelliher A, Deen J, et al. Status of maternal cardiovascular health in American Indian and Alaska Native individuals: A scientific statement from the American Heart Association. *Circ Cardiovasc Qual Outcomes.* 2023;16(6):e000117. doi:10.1161/HCQ.0000000000000117
140. National Center for American Indian Enterprise Development. Accessed August 6, 2025. https://www.ncaied.org
141. Dick A (Kwaxsistalla Wathl'thla), Sewid-Smith D (Mayanilth), Recalma-Clutesi K (Oqwilowgwa), Deur D (Moxmowisa), Turner NJ (Galitsimġa). 'From the beginning of time': The colonial reconfiguration of native habitats and Indigenous resource practices on the British Columbia coast. *Facets.* 2022;7:543–570. doi:10.1139/facets-2021-0092
142. Journell W. An incomplete history: Representation of American Indians in state social studies standards. *J Am Indian Educ.* 2009;48(2):18–32. Accessed April 2, 2025. https://www.jstor.org/stable/24398743
143. Lutz EL. Saving America's endangered languages. *Cult Surv Q.* 2007;31(2). Accessed April 2, 2025. https://www.culturalsurvival.org/publications/cultural-survival-quarterly/saving-americas-endangered-languages
144. Redvers N, Reid P, Carroll D, et al. Indigenous determinants of health: a unified call for progress. *Lancet.* 2023;402(10395)7–9. doi:10.1016/s0140-6736(23)01183-2

145. LaFrance J, Nichols R. Reframing evaluation: Defining an Indigenous evaluation framework. *Can J Program Eval.* 2008;23(2):13–31. doi:10.3138/cjpe.23.003
146. Haozous EA, Lee J, Soto C. Urban American Indian and Alaska Native data sovereignty: Ethical issues. *Am Indian Alsk Native Ment Health Res.* 2021;28(2):77–97. doi:10.5820/aian.2802.2021.77
147. Rainie SC, Rodriguez-Lonebear D, Martinez A. Policy brief: Indigenous data sovereignty in the United States. Native Nations Institute, University of Arizona. 2017. Accessed April 2, 2025. https://nnigovernance.arizona.edu/policy-brief-indigenous-data-sovereignty-united-states
148. Carman KG, Chandra A, Miller C, et al. *Development of the Robert Wood Johnson Foundation National Survey of Health Attitudes: Description and Top-Line Summary Data.* RAND Corporation; 2016. Accessed August 6, 2025. https://www.rand.org/pubs/research_reports/RR1391.html

Contributors

Nadia N. Abuelezam, ScD is a leading epidemiologist on patient- and community-centered Arab and Middle Eastern and North African (Arab/MENA) American health research. She is the 1855 associate professor of family medicine at Michigan State University College of Human Medicine. Her work aims to use novel data streams and community-driven insights to highlight the health needs of historically excluded patients and Arab/MENA American community members. Dr. Abuelezam holds her doctorate in epidemiology from the Harvard T. H. Chan School of Public Health.

Fuimaono Nia Aitaoto, PhD, MPH, MS is a public health practitioner and community-based research and principal consultant for the Pacific Islander Center of Primary Care Excellence at the Association of Asian Pacific Community Health Organizations. Her research portfolio includes breast and cervical cancer screening, diabetes prevention and management, health policy, social and cultural drivers of health, and traditional medicine. She also provides training, technical assistance, and support to ministries of health, departments of health, community health centers, and nonprofit organizations in Hawai'i, the continental United States, American Sāmoa, the Commonwealth of the Northern Mariana Islands, the Federated States of Micronesia, Guam, the Republic of the Marshall Islands, and the Republic of Palau.

Kristine J. Ajrouch, PhD is a research professor in the Research Center for Group Dynamics at the University of Michigan's Institute for Social Research, where she codirects the Michigan Center for Contextual Factors in Alzheimer's Disease. As a sociologist and gerontologist, she examines health outcomes and disparities over the life course, dedicated to understanding variation within and between groups. She attends to culture as a key context in which to better understand the link between social inequalities and health. For over 25 years, her research has focused on the health of Middle Eastern and Arab American populations. Dr. Ajrouch's current work addresses social aspects of Alzheimer's disease, where she is leading efforts to establish prevalence levels among Middle Eastern and Arab Americans.

Ignatius Bau, JD has served as a consultant on Asian American and Native Hawaiian/Pacific Islander health issues with the National Council of Asian Pacific Islander Physicians, Asian & Pacific Islander American Health Forum, Association of Asian Pacific

Community Health Organizations, and ATW Health Solutions. He helped draft and led community advocacy for Executive Order 13125, which first established the White House Initiative on Asian Americans and Pacific Islanders in 1989. Bau has worked as interim executive director of the California Pan-Ethnic Health Network, program director at The California Endowment, policy director at the Asian & Pacific Islander American Health Forum, and immigration and civil rights attorney at the San Francisco Lawyers' Committee for Civil Rights. He was a founder of the Northern California Coalition on Immigrant and Refugee Rights and Services and has been a consultant on immigration issues for the National Immigration Law Center, Immigrant Legal Resource Center, and several foundations.

Erika Blacksher, PhD is an ethicist and engagement scientist who studies questions of justice raised by US health inequalities and the potential of democratic deliberation to make health a shared value. Dr. Blacksher's current research is focused on health justice theory and intersectionality, as well as the science of democratic deliberation. She collaborates on numerous public deliberation initiatives and leads her own, HealthCommons, designed to convene people diverse in race, place, class, and political orientation to problem solve about shared health challenges. She has an MA and PhD from the University of Virginia's bioethics program and undergraduate degrees in philosophy and journalism from the University of Kansas. After completing her doctorate, she was a Robert Wood Johnson Foundation (RWJF) Health and Society Scholar at Columbia University; research scholar at The Hastings Center; tenured faculty in the Department of Bioethics and Humanities, University of Washington; and John B. Francis endowed chair at the Center for Practical Bioethics.

Stacy A. Bohlen (Sault Ste. Marie Tribe of Chippewa Indians) is a nationally and internationally recognized thought leader, expert, and activist in American Indian and Alaska Native (AI/AN) health equity, policy, advocacy, and systems transformation. Through visionary approaches to AI/AN health, Bohlen was part of the inaugural international Indigenous health leadership team that developed the Indigenous Determinants of Health. Her activism and leadership with the United Nations (UN) Permanent Forum on Indigenous Issues, the World Health Organization, and the UN Expert Mechanism on the Rights of Indigenous Peoples contributed to advancing the Indigenous Determinants of Health as a right of Indigenous Peoples globally. With a policy career spanning nearly four decades, Bohlen has dedicated the past 26 years to elevating the voice of the nation's Tribes to achieve systems change for Native health. She led the rebuilding of the nation's premier Native health organization. Her activism during the COVID-19 pandemic resulted in unprecedented public health infrastructure funding for the nation's Tribes, the development of culturally informed community practices, and vaccine acquisition for Tribal governments that led to AI/ANs becoming the group most vaccinated against COVID-19. Bohlen's vision and activism led to significant funding increases for Native health and public health, the permanent reauthorization of the Indian Health Care Improvement Act, Advance Appropriations for the Indian Health Service (IHS), strengthening the Special Diabetes Program for Indians, preserving and growing Good Health and Wellness in Indian Country funding, and establishing a national public health research and advocacy presence in Indian Country. She continues her activism as the founder and CEO of Sage Tribal, a Washington, DC–based consulting firm dedicated to advancing Tribal health.

Melissa Borja, PhD is an associate professor of American culture at the University of Michigan, where she directs the Asian/Pacific Islander American Studies Program. A historian of migration, religion, race, and politics, she is the author of *Follow the New Way: American Refugee Resettlement Policy and Hmong Religious Change*. She advised Princeton's Religion and Forced Migration Initiative, leads the Virulent Hate Project, and contributed research to Stop AAPI Hate.

Tyson H. Brown, PhD is a professor of sociology and medicine at Duke University and director of the Samuel DuBois Cook Center on Social Equity. As a medical sociologist, race scholar, and population health scientist, his research integrates innovative theoretical frameworks with advanced data science and statistical methods to examine the causes, consequences, and solutions to racial inequality across domains such as education, economics, housing, politics, and the criminal legal system. His work provides rigorous evidence on structural racism as a fundamental cause of health inequities and maps its geographic variation, with the aim of advancing knowledge, informing policy, and fostering equity. Dr. Brown's contributions have been recognized with awards from the American Sociological Association and Duke University, a fellowship at Oxford University, and collaborations with the National Academies. His leadership has included service on Duke's Faculty Senate, the Board of Directors of the Population Association of America, and editorial boards of leading journals.

Marshall H. Chin, MD, MPH is the Richard Parrillo family distinguished service professor of healthcare ethics in the Department of Medicine at the University of Chicago. He is a practicing general internist and health services researcher with extensive experience working with multi-stakeholder teams to advance health equity through interventions at individual, organizational, community, and policy levels. Dr. Chin codirects the RWJF Advancing Health Equity: Leading Care, Payment, and Systems Transformation program and codeveloped the Roadmap to Advance Health Equity. He applies ethical principles to reforms to advance health equity, discussions about a culture of equity, and what it means for health professionals to care and advocate for patients and communities. Dr. Chin received the Society of General Internal Medicine's 2024 Robert Glaser Award for outstanding contributions to research, education, leadership, and mentoring in generalism in medicine, and was elected to the National Academy of Medicine in 2017.

Ivory Clarke, MS is the vice president of strategic relationships at the Missouri Foundation for Health. She has spent more than a decade working to advance equity from multiple vantage points—the environment, education, and health—and brings to her roles a deep understanding and appreciation of the power of knowledge sharing, partnerships, and relationship building to advance equitable outcomes. Prior to joining the Missouri Foundation for Health, she served as both the director of the Culture of Health Program and the inaugural equity and inclusion officer at the National Academy of Medicine (NAM), where she led a multiyear collaborative to identify strategies for creating and sustaining equitable health nationwide and guided the design of an institutional framework to embed inclusion, diversity, equity, and antiracism into NAM's organizational strategy. Her work reflects a commitment to translating research and collaboration into partnerships that transform systems and create lasting opportunities for all communities to thrive.

Loretta Grey Cloud (Kul Wicasa Lakota & Hunkpati Dakota), also known as *A Wica Hde Pin Win* (She Brings the People Home Woman), is an enrolled member of the Crow Creek Sioux Tribe. Grey Cloud is a proud graduate of Tribal College University, Salish Kootenai College, receiving her BS in life science in 2015. She performed her postbaccalaureate research at the National Institute of Dental and Craniofacial Research, National Institutes of Health (NIH), where she studied proteases and tissue remodeling. She received a Public Health Training Certificate for American Indian Health Professionals from the Johns Hopkins Bloomberg School of Public Health in 2019 before working at the IHS headquarters in the Office of the Directors. Grey Cloud currently serves as the associate director of operations for the Center for Indigenous Health Great Plains Hub in Rapid City, South Dakota.

Robynn Cox, PhD, MA is an associate professor in the School of Public Policy at University of California (UC), Riverside and senior scholar at the Federal Reserve Bank of Minneapolis' Opportunity & Inclusive Growth Institute. Dr. Cox is an economist with expertise in understanding how policies and institutions impact inequality. She is particularly interested in the intersection of the criminal legal system and inequality. Specifically, her work focuses on the racial, economic, political, health, and social consequences of criminal legal system and related policies (e.g., mass incarceration). Her work has been supported by various organizations such as the National Bureau of Economic Research, Federal Reserve Bank of Minneapolis, National Institute on Aging, US Department of Agriculture, and Rutgers' Institute for the Study of Employee Ownership and Profit Sharing. Dr. Cox also serves as president of the National Economic Association and on the advisory committee for NAM's Culture of Health Program.

Maria Christina Crouch (Deg Hit'an & Coahuiltecan), PhD is a clinical–community psychologist and an assistant professor adjunct at the Yale School of Medicine in the Department of Psychiatry. Her clinical work and program of research are focused on the intersection of trauma-informed care, evidence-based practices, and practice-based evidence (Indigenous approaches) to address alcohol and drug misuse and related health impacts of social determinants among AI/AN communities from a cultural, strengths-based approach.

Angela Diaz, MD, PhD, MPH is the dean for global health, social justice, and human rights and the Jean C. and James W. Crystal professor in the Department of Pediatrics, Department of Environmental Medicine and Public Health, and the Department of Global Health and Health Systems Design at the Icahn School of Medicine at Mount Sinai. After earning her MD at Columbia University College of Physicians and Surgeons, she completed an MPH from Harvard University and a PhD in epidemiology from Columbia University. Dr. Diaz is a scientist with continuous NIH funding for over 25 years. She has been active in public policy and advocacy in the United States and has conducted many international health projects in Asia, Central and South America, Europe, and Africa. She is a frequent speaker at conferences throughout the country and around the world.

Chelsea Dorsey, MD is a professor of surgery in the Section of Vascular Surgery and Endovascular Therapy at the University of Chicago Medicine. She is associate dean for medical student academics and advancement at the Pritzker School of Medicine, and senior vice chair of faculty and educational affairs in the Department of Surgery. Dr. Dorsey is nationally recognized for her commitment to advancing diversity in medicine, equitable access, and inclusive practices in surgical environments. Her research focuses on workforce diversity, optimizing resources for diverse learners, and structural interventions to improve health outcomes for underserved and underresourced Americans.

Abigail Echo-Hawk, MA is a national leader in public health research and the decolonization of data. She is revolutionizing the integration of Indigenous knowledge within public health systems and reshaping how governments, institutions, and medical professionals approach health for AI/AN peoples. Echo-Hawk's groundbreaking research and tireless advocacy around violence against Indigenous women have spurred policy changes across all levels of government. As a leading voice in the missing and murdered Indigenous women and girls (MMIWG) crisis, she coauthored a report that brought national attention to the data issues and the staggering number of MMIWG cases in 71 urban cities across the United States. Echo-Hawk has served on several scientific research committees, including for the National Academies of Sciences, Engineering, and Medicine, which oversaw the development of a framework for an equitable distribution of the COVID-19 vaccine. A proud citizen of the Pawnee Nation of Oklahoma,

Echo-Hawk is the executive vice president of the Seattle Indian Health Board and director of its research division, the Urban Indian Health Institute. Through these roles, she continues to champion Indigenous health, using her platform to inspire and drive meaningful change.

Wendy Ellis, DrPH, MPH is an assistant professor in global health and the founding director of the Center for Community Resilience at the Milken Institute School of Public Health at George Washington University. In 2024, she was appointed the inaugural director of the Institute for Racial, Ethnic, and Socioeconomic Equity at George Washington University. Her community-based research seeks to improve the health of marginalized populations by enabling cross-sectoral partners to align policy, program, and practice to address adverse childhood experiences in the context of adverse community environments—or as Dr. Ellis has coined it, "The Pair of ACEs." Her Pair of ACEs framing and community resilience framework have been adopted by local health departments and initiatives and incorporated into systems change initiatives and local, state, and federal policy.

Laufou Jacob Fitisemanu Jr., MPH is an educator and advocate with ancestral roots in Sāmoa, Hawaiʻi, Hong Kong, and Korea. He studies, works, and lives at the intersection of public health policy, clinical practice, and community advancement. A former city council member, presidential commissioner, and cofounder of the Utah Pacific Islander Health Coalition, he has developed and led health programs and initiatives for over a decade in government and private health sectors. He lives with his wife and two daughters in West Valley City, Utah, where he currently serves in the state House of Representatives.

Gilbert C. Gee, PhD is a professor and chair of the Department of Community Health Sciences at the Fielding School of Public Health at the University of California, Los Angeles (UCLA). His research focuses on health inequities using a multilevel and life course perspective.

Emily A. Haozous (Chiricahua Fort Sill Apache), PhD, RN is a nurse and research scientist at the Pacific Institute for Research and Evaluation's Southwest Center, based in Albuquerque, New Mexico. Dr. Haozous conducts community-based and community-guided research and evaluation in collaboration with Native American partners, including urban Tribal centers, reservation-based Tribal organizations, and Tribal governments. Her work focuses on issues of access to care, health equity, cancer and non-cancer pain management, cultural tailoring, and national trends in premature mortality. Dr. Haozous humbly conducts research in recognition of the generations that came before her and with the desire to build a better world for those generations yet to come. She has a clinical background in oncology, hospice, and palliative care nursing. Dr. Haozous received her undergraduate degree in music from UC Santa Cruz, and her master's and PhD in nursing from Yale University.

Nadia Islam, PhD is a professor and the director of translational research partnerships in the Department of Population Health at the New York University (NYU) Grossman School of Medicine. She is also the associate director for NYU's Clinical Translational Science Institute. Her rigorous research program, marked by a collaborative approach involving multiple clinical and community partners, focuses on developing culturally relevant community–clinical linkage models to promote health equity in disadvantaged communities. She is the principal investigator of several NIH- and Centers for Disease Control and Prevention–funded initiatives evaluating the impact of community health worker interventions on chronic disease management and prevention in diverse populations. Dr. Islam codirects the NYU–City University of New York Prevention Research Center and most recently, is leading a new national initiative to support community engagement in diabetes equity research. She is a medical sociologist with a PhD in sociomedical sciences from Columbia University. Her work has been featured in the *New England Journal of Medicine*, *JAMA*, *American Journal of Public Health*, and numerous other peer-reviewed journals.

Benjamin A. Jacuk (Dena'ina & Sugpiaq), ThM, MDiv is an enrolled citizen of the Kenaitze Indian Tribe. Benjamin is a graduate of Princeton Theological Seminary, where he received his MDiv and ThM. He now serves as the director of Indigenous research at the Alaska Native Heritage Center and works with ecclesial, federal, and academic institutions—such as the Roman Catholic Church, Princeton, and the Office of Army Cemeteries—to help uncover the history of assimilative boarding schools within North America. His research has also led to the return of thousands of pieces of material culture back to Alaska and is passionate about helping make a future for not only his two children, but all Alaska Native peoples.

Michelle Johnson-Jennings (Choctaw), PhD is a distinguished American Indian clinical health psychologist specializing in harm reduction, addiction research, and chronic disease prevention. She serves as a full professor, clinical health psychologist, and co-executive director for the Indigenous Wellness Research Institute, as well as director of the Indigenous Environmental Health and Land-Based Healing Division. Her pioneering work has advanced culturally responsive, community-driven health interventions, particularly for Indigenous women and children, integrating traditional practices with modern health strategies. She has codesigned land-based healing interventions that incorporate narrative reactive therapy, transforming trauma into love and hope. Her leadership in culturally specific frameworks—such as the Relationship-Centered Decision-Making Framework, Indigenous love-based research, and Indigenous land-based healing—has redefined Indigenous health approaches globally. Dr. Johnson-Jennings has secured international funding supporting groundbreaking interventions in obesity, addiction, and HIV prevention. As a founding scientific director for multiple Indigenous health and research centers, she has fostered global collaborations across First Nations, Māori, and AI/AN communities. Since 2011, she has been a dedicated Indigenous scientific mentor for NIH programs, shaping the future of Indigenous health research through culturally grounded, community-led solutions to health disparities.

Niaz Kasravi, PhD is a national expert and advocate on criminal justice, social justice, and racial justice with over 20 years of experience leading campaigns across the United States—including on police accountability, racial profiling, and death penalty abolition. She is the founder and director of the Avalan Institute for Applied Research, a research, advocacy, and training firm. She previously served as director of the Criminal Justice Program at the National Association for the Advancement of Colored People (NAACP) and as an associate for Amnesty International USA's Domestic Human Rights Program. Dr. Kasravi holds a PhD in criminology, law, and society from UC Irvine. In 2000, through a National Science Foundation grant, she traveled to Iran to work with Nobel Peace Prize laureate Shirin Ebadi on women's rights and justice reform in that country.

Tina Kauh, PhD, MS joined RWJF in 2012. As a senior program officer within the Research-Evaluation-Learning Unit, she develops new research and evaluation programs, supports the development of foundation strategy, evaluates the implementation and outcomes of RWJF-funded programming, and disseminates key learnings. Her work focuses on supporting the well-being of invisibilized communities and advancing research practices and policies related to the disaggregation of demographic characteristics that are critical for improving the outcomes of marginalized communities. Dr. Kauh is an expert in developmental psychology and program evaluation, having earned a PhD in human development and family studies from Pennsylvania State University with a doctoral minor in Statistics and a BA in psychology from Wellesley College. She has authored numerous research reports, peer-reviewed articles, and book chapters on data equity and child health and well-being.

Micere Keels, PhD is a professor in the Department of Comparative Human Development at the University of Chicago. She is the founding director of the Trauma Responsive Educational Practices Project, which is a research-translation and research–practice partnership that works to integrate mental health promotion interventions into educational systems and institutions. Dr. Keels is also the director and producer of *The Fight for Black Lives*, a health equity documentary film that chronicles the ways that racial stress and the American health care system disadvantage the health of Black Americans. Her research focuses on understanding how race, ethnicity, and poverty structure the supports and challenges that children and youth experience. She is particularly invested in systems-change interventions that can narrow intergenerational inequities.

Allison Kelliher (Dene/Koyukon Athabascan), MD, also known as *Maanoyeedlakkon* (Mother of Daylight), is an enrolled citizen of the Nome Eskimo Community and follows her mother's *Dena* (Koyukon Athabascan) family line from the Upper Innoko River. She is board certified in family and integrative medicine and has practiced in IHS, Tribal, urban, and private practice settings. She holds a BS from the University of Alaska Fairbanks, an MD from the University of Washington School of Medicine, and completed the Alaska Family Medicine residency in 2009. She started learning techniques as a child and completed apprenticeships with Alaska Native Tribal doctors. Her practice includes osteopathy, acupuncture, botanicals, healing touch, and ceremony. Themes in Dr. Kelliher's work include ethical and effective integration of Indigenous healing into clinical practice and relating the health of Indigenous Peoples to planetary health. She is affiliated with the University of North Dakota School of Medicine and Health Sciences as an adjunct associate professor.

Nadia Kim, PhD is the George Sumey Jr. professor in the liberal arts at Texas A&M University in the Department of Sociology. Her research focuses on race and citizenship hierarchies concerning Korean/Asian Americans and South Koreans, nativist racism in Los Angeles, environmental (in)justice, immigrant women, comparative racialization, and race theory. Throughout her work, Kim's approach centers (neo)imperialism, transnationality, and intersectionality. She is the author of multiple award-winning books, including *Imperial Citizens: Koreans and Race from Seoul to LA* and *Refusing Death: Immigrant Women and the Fight for Environmental Justice in LA*. She was also the lead editor of *Disciplinary Futures: Sociology in Conversation with American, Ethnic, and Indigenous Studies*. Long involved in social movements, Dr. Kim and/or her work has appeared on public radio and in *The Washington Post, The Boston Globe, The Chronicle of Higher Education, Red Table Talk, NYLON Magazine, The Korea Times,* and more.

Stephen Long is originally from Anchorage, Alaska and has a BA in marketing from the University of Alaska Anchorage. He has a strong interest in medical equity, especially for underserved rural populations, along with healing modalities such as the use of plant-based medicine, somatic therapy, and community support for mental and physical well-being.

Lenny López, MD, MPH, MDiv is a professor of medicine and chief of hospital medicine at the UC San Francisco's San Francisco Veterans Affairs Medical Center. He currently serves as co-editor-in-chief of the *Journal of General Internal Medicine*. Dr. López is active in health services research on health care disparities and the social determinants of health of chronic diseases that particularly impact older adults, such as cardiovascular disease. He has also focused on cultural factors unique to Latinx populations and has published on the intersection of acculturation, literacy, language and communication barriers, education status, and the experience of discrimination in everyday life among Latinos in the United States.

Julie Morita, MD is president and CEO of The Joyce Foundation, overseeing the charitable distribution of $65 million annually from assets of $1.3 billion. Before joining The Joyce Foundation, Julie was executive vice president of RWJF for five years and served in many capacities at the Chicago Department of Public Health for two decades, overseeing the public health needs of city's nearly three million residents. Julie has served as an advisor to the White House, US Department of Health and Human Services, Centers for Disease Control and Prevention, and numerous state and local public health agencies and is a member of NAM, the American Academy of Pediatrics, and the National Foundation for Infectious Diseases Board of Directors.

Velma McBride Murry, PhD, MS is the Lois Autrey Betts chair in education and development and serves as codirector of the Vanderbilt Institute for Clinical and Translational Research, Community Engagement Research Core. She is a distinguished university professor in health policy at the Vanderbilt School of Medicine and in human and organizational development at Vanderbilt's Peabody College and previously served as associate provost for research and innovation. Elected to NAM in 2020, she also serves on the NIH National Advisory Mental Health Research Council and related National Academies committees. Her research examines the significance of context on the everyday life experiences of Black families and their children, with a focus on how documented structural challenges and stressors cascade through families to influence parenting, family functioning, quality of life, and health. This work informed two randomized controlled trials—Strong African American Families and Pathways for African American Success—which prevent health compromising behaviors and foster protective processes that strengthen caregivers and youth well-being.

Melanie Nadeau (Turtle Mountain Band of Chippewa Indians), PhD, MPH, also known as Dr. Mel, completed both her MPH in community health education with a concentration in health disparities and her PhD in social/behavioral epidemiology at the University of Minnesota School of Public Health. Dr. Mel is a community-led scholar and has worked for more than 20 years on various research and evaluation projects within the American Indian community. She has successfully engaged a multitude of Tribal health stakeholders from across the nation and is dedicated to improving the health and well-being of Native communities. Dr. Mel currently serves as vice chair and associate professor for the Department of Indigenous Health at the University of North Dakota School of Medicine & Health Sciences.

LeiLani Nishime, PhD is a professor of communication at the University of Washington. She has written about multiracial Asian Americans, visual culture, and science fiction. Her current work centers on race and the environment and racialized technologies. She is the author of over 30 book chapters and articles in journals such as the *Journal of Asian American Studies, Journal of Cinema and Media Studies, Critical Studies in Media*

Communication, Quarterly Journal of Speech, and *Communication Theory.* She is the author of *Undercover Asian: Multiracial Asian Americans in Visual Culture* and coeditor of *East Main Street, Global Asian American Popular Culture,* and *Racial Ecologies.* She serves as an associate director of the Center for Communication, Difference, and Equity at the University of Washington, and coedits the Environmental Communication, Power, and Culture series for UC Press.

Paul M. Ong, PhD, MUP is a research professor at the UCLA Luskin School of Public Affairs with affiliation with the Asian American Studies Center and Institute of the Environment and Sustainability and is the director of the Center for Neighborhood Knowledge. His research focuses on racial, economic, environmental, and spatial inequalities.

José A. Pagán, PhD is a professor and chair of the Department of Public Health Policy and Management in the School of Global Public Health at NYU. He is also chair of the board of directors of NYC Health + Hospitals. He is a health economist and health services researcher who has led research, implementation, and evaluation projects on the redesign of health care delivery and payment systems.

Yvette C. Paulino, PhD is an Indigenous CHamoru of Guam in Micronesia. She is dean and professor of the Margaret P. Hattori-Uchima School of Health at the University of Guam, where she has led research in the Pacific on the epidemiology and public health of areca nut and betel quid chewing, including oral precancer screening of chewers, the effects of chewing on the oral microbiome and in liver cancer development, and a betel quid cessation program. Her recent efforts are focused on the Guma' Tinemtom (House of Wisdom) which features the Micronesia Data Laboratory and serves as a training ground for research transformation sustainability at the University of Guam.

Eliseo J. Pérez-Stable, MD was the director of the National Institute on Minority Health and Health Disparities at NIH. As director, he leveraged his personal history and passion for public health to help define a national agenda focused on improving minority health and reducing health disparities for all people, overseeing the institute's $535 million annual budget in 2024. Dr. Pérez-Stable began his work researching and supporting the health of underrepresented groups as a professor of medicine at UC San Francisco in the 1980s and served as chief and director of its Division of General Internal Medicine. Widely recognized as a leader in Latino health care and disparities research, he has published over 350 peer-reviewed papers and is committed to advancing knowledge in population science and promoting interventions to improve health.

Alonzo Plough, PhD, MPH joined RWJF as chief science officer and vice president of Research-Evaluation-Learning in 2014. He is responsible for aligning the foundation's work with the best evidence from research and practice on improving health equity and incorporating program evaluations into organizational learning. He also oversees the two grant-making portfolios focused on innovation and emerging issues: Ideas for an Equitable Future and Global Ideas for US Solutions. Dr. Plough has been a national leader in public health practice for over 25 years, serving as director of emergency preparedness and response at the Los Angeles County Department of Public Health, director and health officer for the Seattle and King County Department of Public Health, and director of public health for Boston. He started out as an academic researcher and was a professor in graduate programs at Boston University, Tufts, and Harvard. He is currently a clinical professor of population health at the University of Washington School of Public Health. Dr. Plough has published an extensive body of peer-reviewed research and is an author or editor of 8 books, the most recent being *Necessary Conversations: Understanding Racism as a Barrier to Achieving Health Equity*.

Dwayne Proctor, PhD has spent over 20 years working to ensure that Americans are healthy and thriving by implementing sustainable, systemic changes, prioritizing input from those most affected by disparities. He is president and CEO of the Missouri Foundation for Health, which addresses health equity issues across the state, including women's health, food justice, firearm violence, and infant health and vitality. He coauthored a piece published in *Health Affairs* that defined systemic and structural racism and approaches to dismantle it. Dr. Proctor is the board chair for the NAACP Foundation and the National Committee for Responsive Philanthropy. He serves on NAM's Leadership Consortium, which mobilizes resources in digital health and value-based incentives to improve systems with culture, inclusion, and equity in mind. Dr. Proctor was recently appointed to the Commission on Investment Imperatives for a Healthy Nation, which will identify transformative actions to make high-quality health care accessible for everyone.

Jen'nan G. Read, PhD is a professor of sociology at Duke University. She is a Carnegie Scholar whose expertise lies in the assimilation experiences of US Arabs and Muslims and on the social determinants of US health disparities. Her most recent work disaggregates ethnic groups classified by the US Census as non-Hispanic white and demonstrates considerable diversity in health outcomes when groups such as Arab Americans and Eastern Europeans are isolated from the generic "white" category. She has published widely on these topics, including a book and numerous peer-reviewed journal articles. Dr. Read spent her childhood in Libya and Egypt before returning to the United States at the age of 14. She graduated summa cum laude from Midwestern State University as student body president, received her PhD in sociology from the University of Texas at Austin, and held a two-year postdoctoral fellowship at Rice University in the James Baker Institute for Public Policy and Department of Sociology.

Anna Ricklin, MHS is a passionate advocate for healthy communities. She currently serves as the inaugural health in all policies manager for the Fairfax County Health Department in Virginia, where she acts as a health ambassador across county agencies. In this role, Ricklin promotes the integration of public health objectives into county plans, policies, and building projects. Formerly, she managed the American Planning Association's Planning and Community Health Center, where she directed applied research and place-based initiatives to advance healthy planning practice. Ricklin began her career at the Baltimore City Department of Transportation, which built her expertise in health impact assessment, active transportation planning, and cross-sector collaboration. She studied anthropology as an undergraduate and holds an MHS from the Johns Hopkins Bloomberg School of Public Health. She lives with her husband and two young daughters in Falls Church, Virginia.

José E. Rodríguez, MD is the associate vice president for health sciences workforce excellence and a tenured professor in the Department of Family and Preventive Medicine at University of Utah Health. For most of his career, Dr. Rodríguez has provided primary care for underserved minority communities. His main area of scholarship has been focused on underrepresented minority faculty in academic medicine. Dr. Rodríguez founded the Center for Underrepresented Minorities in Academic Medicine at Florida State University. He has produced leading scholarship highlighting the disparities in academic medicine for minority faculty. Currently, he and his team are funded by the Society of Teachers of Family Medicine and the American Board of Family Medicine to direct the Leadership through Scholarship Fellowship at the Society of Teachers of Family Medicine, focused on teaching academic skills to early-career family medicine faculty that are underrepresented in medicine. He is associate editor at *Annals of Family Medicine* and president of the Family Physicians Inquiries Network.

Muniba Saleem, PhD is an associate professor in the Department of Communication at UC Santa Barbara and an adjunct faculty associate in the Institute for Social Research at the University of Michigan. Her research examines how media affects interpersonal and intergroup relations between racial, ethnic, and religious groups using social scientific methods.

Mienah Zulfacar Sharif, PhD, MPH is an assistant professor in the Division of Community Health Sciences in the School of Public Health at UC Berkeley. Her research takes life course and international perspectives to examine the impacts of state-sanctioned violence on multiple indicators of health and well-being. Her work is guided by Public Health Critical Race Praxis and she prioritizes community-led research.

Brinda Sivaramakrishnan, MPH is a research associate at the Johns Hopkins Center for Indigenous Health and PhD candidate in the University of North Dakota Indigenous Health program. She holds a BA/BS in environmental studies and biological sciences and an MPH in forced migration and health. Brinda was born in New Delhi, India and her ancestral home is Tamil Nadu, India. Previously, she served as an epidemiologist for the Urban Indian Health Institute Diabetes Care and Outcomes Audit and researcher on the Washington State Tribal Food Sovereignty Survey during COVID-19.

Maile Tauali'i, PhD, MPH is a collaborative investigator for Hawaii Permanente Medical Group. Her work focuses on the utility and validity of health information for racial minorities and eliminating health disparities, specifically for Indigenous Peoples. In 2015, Dr. Tauali'i established the world's first global Indigenous MPH degree program and was awarded the University of Hawai'i Board of Regents' Excellence in Teaching Award. Prior work includes establishing the Urban Indian Health Institute, housed at the Seattle Indian Health Board. Her federal experiences include serving as a member of the National Advisory Committee on Racial, Ethnic, and Other Populations at the US Census Bureau from 2013 to 2019 and a member of the PhenX Working Group on Social Determinants of Health in 2020. She and her husband, five children, and three dogs live on a 7-acre food forest with their 'ohana, who aim to feed the community traditional, plant-based food from the land.

Tipiziwin Tolman (Sihasapa & Hunkpapȟa Lakȟota; Wičhiyena & Tizaptaŋna Dakȟota), MEd is an enrolled member of the Standing Rock Sioux Tribe and a descendant of the Spirit Lake Dakota of North Dakota. She is from the Pretends Eagle, Yellow Lodge, and Half Skunk families of Standing Rock, and the Young and Longie families of Spirit Lake. Tolman is a PhD candidate in the Cultural Studies and Social Thought in Education program at Washington State University. She holds a BS in Native American studies from Sitting Bull College and an MEd in Indigenous language revitalization from the University of Victoria. A certified elementary educator in Washington State, Tolman's research and praxis center on Lakota and Dakota language pedagogy, literacy, and the intergenerational teachings embedded in her great-grandparents' winter count. She is also co-owner of Haípažaža Pȟežuta, a business dedicated to traditional Indigenous plant-based wellness.

Antonia M. Villarruel, PhD, RN is a professor and Margaret Bond Simon dean of nursing at the University of Pennsylvania. Dr. Villarruel has extensive research and practice experience with Latino populations, community-engaged research, and health equity.

Donald Warne (Pine Ridge Oglala Lakota Tribe), MD, MPH is codirector of the Center for Indigenous Health and professor at the Bloomberg School of Public Health at Johns Hopkins University. Dr. Warne comes from a long line of traditional healers and medicine men. He received his MD from the Stanford University School of Medicine in 1995 and his MPH from the Harvard School of Public Health in 2002. He has work experience as a primary care physician with the Gila River Health Care Corporation; staff clinician with NIH; Indian Legal Program faculty at the Sandra Day O'Connor College of

Law at Arizona State University; executive director of the Great Plains Tribal Chairmen's Health Board; and chair of the Department of Indigenous Health and associate dean of the School of Medicine & Health Sciences at the University of North Dakota.

Steven H. Woolf, MD, MPH is a professor of family medicine and population health at Virginia Commonwealth University, where he is director emeritus of the Center on Society and Health and holds the C. Kenneth and Dianne Wright distinguished chair in population health and health equity. He has expertise in social epidemiology, and his research has focused on the factors that contribute to trends in population health and health inequities, including disparities in health outcomes across racial and ethnic groups. Dr. Woolf has focused on raising awareness among the public and policymakers about the social, economic, and environmental conditions that shape health and perpetuate inequities. He received his MD from Emory University and his MPH from Johns Hopkins University. Dr. Woolf was elected to the Institute of Medicine (now NAM) in 2001.

Matt Wray, PhD, MA is a professor and chair of sociology at Temple University. He earned his BA at the University of Michigan and MA and PhD from UC Berkeley. Wray was a RWJF Health and Society Scholar at Harvard University from 2006 to 2008 and a postdoctoral fellow at the Smithsonian National Museum of American History from 2000 to 2001. Trained as both a historian and social scientist, Dr. Wray's research combines expertise in the sociology of culture, race and ethnicity, and health and illness (with a focus on suicide and self-destruction). His research has long aimed to bring attention to the social, economic, and political marginalization of poor rural whites in the United States, beginning with the 1996 publication of his book *White Trash: Race and Class in America*. In 2023, Dr. Wray was awarded Temple University's Great Teacher Award, the university's highest teaching honor, for mentoring graduate and undergraduate students.

Ruth Enid Zambrana, PhD, MSW is a distinguished university professor at the University of Maryland in the Harriet Tubman Department of Women, Gender and Sexuality Studies, a cofounding director of the Consortium on Race, Gender and Ethnicity, and has a secondary appointment as a professor of family medicine at the University of Maryland Baltimore School of Medicine. As a medical sociologist, her scholarship applies a critical intersectional lens to structural racism, Hispanic ethnicity, and gender inequities in population health and higher education trajectories. She has published widely on health inequity in her major field concentrations: women's health, maternal and child health, socioeconomic life course impacts on health, and mental well-being of historically underrepresented minorities. She is the recipient of numerous awards, including the 2021 American Public Health Association Lyndon Haviland Public Health Mentoring Award and the 2023 John P. McGovern Endowed Lecturer Award from the University of Houston College of Liberal Arts and Social Sciences.

Index

Page numbers followed by *b*, *f*, and *t* indicate boxes, figures, and tables, respectively. Numbers followed by *n* indicate notes.

A

A magazine, 94*t*
AAPIs. *See* Asian American and Pacific Islanders
Aboriginal peoples, 212
ACA (Affordable Care Act), 21, 22*b*, 28, 65
access to health care
    actionable solutions to advance health equity, 289*t*
        for Asian Americans, 76
        for Latinos, 151–152, 153*t*, 154–155
    for AI/ANs, 27–29
    for Asian Americans, 64–65, 76
    for Black people, 108
    case studies, 150–151
    chronic health conditions and, 144–146
    for gay youth, 150–151
    for Latino populations, 139–146, 150–152, 153*t*, 154–155
    for NH/PIs, 229, 230*t*
    poverty and, 144–146, 263
    for undocumented immigrants, 64–65
    across US-affiliated Pacific Islands, 229, 230*t*
    for white people, 262–264
accidents, 255–256, 256*f*
accuracy, 38
Act 20: The Export Services Incentives Act, 174*t*
Act 22: The Individual Investor Act, 174*t*
Administration for Native Americans, 233
adolescent health, 150–151, 256
advocacy
    for Asian Americans during COVID-19, 71–74, 72*t*
    proposed solutions for change, 77
affirmative action, 133, 172*t*, 174*t*, 252
Affordable Care Act (ACA), 21, 22*b*, 28, 65, 139, 263, 265, 266
Affordable Care Act (ACA) Marketplace, 64, 65
Afghanistan, people from (Afghans), 50, 173*t*
AFQT (Armed Forces Qualification Test), 107
African Americans
    enslavement of, 97–98, 185, 245
    health occupations, 139, 140*t*
    homelessness/houselessness rate, 227
    racial and ethnic category, 5, 12, 286
    See also Black Americans; Black people
Afro-Caribbeans, 131, 138, 142–143, 145–146
    See also Caribbeans
Afro-Latino people, 134–137, 170*t*
    See also Latino populations
Age of (European) Exploration, 217

aggregation fallacy, 52, 59
AHA (American Heart Association), 34
Aid to Families with Dependent Children, 262
AIDS, 219
Al-Fayoume, Wadea, 185
Alabama
    anti-Asian racism, 58
    life expectancy and mortality, 255–257, 256*f*, 257*f*
    medical costs, 263
Alaska
    colonization of, 15–16, 16*b*
    federally recognized Tribes, 12
Alaska Native Claims Settlement Act (ANCSA), 12, 16*b*, 17
Alaska Native Corporations, 12
Alaska Natives
    historic considerations, 15–17
    historic timeline, 16*b*
    homelessness/houselessness rate, 227
    Indigenous peoples, 12
    priorities, 35
    village corporations, 17
    See also American Indians and Alaska Natives (AI/AN)
Alaska Statehood Act, 16*b*, 17
Aleut peoples, 16
Aleutian Islands, 16
Alexander VI, 15
Algeria, 179
Alien Land Laws (California), 58, 92*t*
Aluli, Noa Emmett, 217–218
Alzheimer's disease, 106
Amazigh, 180
Amerasia, 93*t*
American (term), 13
American Association of Medical Colleges, 31–32
American Citizens for Justice, 94*t*
American Community Survey, 181
American diet, 217
American Heart Association (AHA), 34
American Indian (term), 12–13
American Indian Higher Education Consortium, 31
American Indian Religious Freedom Act, 21, 22*b*
American Indians and Alaska Natives (AI/AN)
    access to quality health care, 27–29
    actionable solutions for, 34–39, 285, 296*t*–297*t*
    barriers that impact Native health, 26–33
    citizenship, 19–20
    court cases, 21, 22*b*
    cultural considerations, 21–26

cultural differences, 32–33
data sovereignty, 26
dropout rates, 31
economic infrastructure, 37
economic initiatives, 37–38
economic system, 32
education of, 29–32
    actionable solutions for, 38–39, 297t
    boarding schools, 19, 20f, 22b, 30
    reservation schools, 30
educational initiatives, 38
enrolled Tribal members, 12
enslavement of, 14–17
and environment, 25
federal policy eras, 17–21
federal trust responsibility, 17, 18
federally recognized Tribes, 12
financial systems, 32–33
health care workforce development, 31–32
health inequities, 284
health system actionable solutions, 36–37
health system initiatives, 35–37
history of systemic racism towards, 13–21
    Alaska timeline, 16b
    colonization timeline, 14b
    major laws and court cases timeline, 22b
homelessness/houselessness rate, 227
legislation affecting, 21, 22b
life expectancy, 259f
oral histories, 13–14
organizing framework, 21–26
politicization of, 12
population definition, 11–13
poverty, 37, 135
priorities, 35
racial and ethnic category, 5, 12, 286
reservation system, 248–249
sacred sites, 25–26
schools for, 38
social determinants of health, 35
state-recognized Tribes, 12
systemic racism and health of, 11–47
terminology for, 12–13, 13f
traditional medicine, 25–26
underrepresentation of, 170t
wealth concepts, 32
workforce development, 29–32
American Medical Association (AMA), 108
American polygeny, 98
American Recovery and Reinvestment Act, 72t
American Samoa, 211–213, 214f, 215
    actionable solutions for, 297t
    catalysts for change to reduce disparities and improve health equity, 236
    health care access, 229, 230t
    household income, 228
    military enlistment rates, 219–220
American Samoa Natives, 222t
American South, 248, 250
ancestral foods, 217
ancestral lands, 227
ANCSA (Alaska Native Claims Settlement Act), 12, 16b, 17
Angel Island, 92t
anti-Semitism, 246
    See also racism
Aotearoa (New Zealand), 211, 212, 217b, 219–221, 226
Apache Wars, 14b
APEN (Asian Pacific Environmental Network), 68–69
API (Asian or Pacific Islander), 221–223, 222b
APIA Vote, 95t
Appalachia, 255–256, 259–260, 263
apprenticeships, 235
Arab American Screenwriters, 195
Arab League, 180
Arab–Israeli conflict, 183, 184
Arabs/Arab Americans
    definition of, 179–180
    history of anti-Arab racism against, 95t, 182–184
    identity of, 182–183
    media representation of, 185, 190–192
    See also Middle Eastern and North African (MENA) Americans
architecture, 219
Argentines, 130t, 135
Arizona, 31, 135, 171t
Arizona v United States, 133
Armed Forces Qualification Test (AFQT), 107
Aryan supremacy, 251
ASIAN! (Asian Sisters for Ideas in Action Now!), 95t
Asian American and Pacific Islanders (AAPIs)
    racial and ethnic category, 222t, 223, 286
    See also Native Hawaiian and Pacific Islanders; Pacific Islanders
Asian American Feminist Antibodies: Care in the time of Coronavirus online zine, 72t
Asian American Feminist Collective, 72t
Asian American Movement, 73, 93t
Asian American Pacific Islander Nurses Association, 95t
Asian American Policy Review, 94t
Asian American studies, 93t
Asian Americans
    age-adjusted death rates, 223
    aggregation fallacy, 52, 59
    anti-Asian racism, 49–91
        case studies, 67–74
        fundamental challenges, 50–54
        history of, 92t–96t, 174t
        history of research on, 55

across systems, 54–66, 54f, 66–67
youth harassment, 70–71
community mobilization and advocacy
during COVID-19, 71–74, 72t
history of, 71–73, 92t–96t
COVID-19 death rate, 225b
data infrastructure, 74–75
definition of, 50, 222t
disaggregated from NH/PIs, 221–224, 224b
disease-related violence against, 70–71
earnings, 60–61
ethnic groups, 52, 53t
health care, 64–66
health care access, 64–65, 229
health care costs, 66
health inequities, 49–91, 54f, 284
health occupations, 63, 65, 139, 140t
history of research on, 55
homelessness/houselessness rate, 227
invisibility of, 52–54
life expectancy, 257, 259f
media representations, 62–63, 76
median household wealth, 136
median income, 61
model minority myth, 5, 51–52, 61, 66
per capita income, 60
perpetual foreigner stereotype, 50–51
population, 223–224
poverty rates, 135
proposed solutions for change, 74–77
racial and ethnic category, 5, 286
research agenda, 74–75
terminology, 223
wealth, 61
youth, 70–71
Asian Americans Advancing Justice, 72t, 94t
Asian and Pacific Islander American Health Forum, 94t
Asian Left Forum, 95t
Asian or Pacific Islander (API), 221–223, 222t
Asian/Pacific American Heritage Month, 94t
Asian Pacific American Labor Alliance, AFL-CIO, 95t
Asian Pacific Americans, 223
Asian Pacific Environmental Network (APEN), 68–69
Asian Pacific Islander American Institute for Congressional Studies, 95t
Asian refugees, 59–60
Asian Revolutionary Circle, 95t
Asians and Pacific Islanders for Community Empowerment (API FORCE), 95t
AsianWeek, 93t
Asiatic Zone, 57, 188
Assimilation Era, 14b, 17, 18–20
Association for Asian American Studies, 93t, 95t
Association of American Indian Physicians, 29
Association of Asian Pacific Community Health Organizations, 94t, 229
Assyrians, 180, 188–189
asthma, 67–68, 144–145, 150–151
atomic bomb testing, 220
Auckland Islands (Maungahuka), 217b
Australasia, 211, 212f
Australia, 15, 226

B

Baclayon, Keoki Kīkaha Pai, 233
Bahrain, 179
Bangladeshis, 49, 53t, 61
banks, 32, 37
Banks, Joseph, 217
Beef (Netflix), 62
best practices, 6
Bhutan, 60
BIA (Bureau of Indian Affairs), 19
Biden, Joe, 70, 197
Biden administration, 65
BIE (Bureau of Indian Education), 30–31, 38
The Big Aiiieeeee!, 93t
Bikini, 220
birth control experimentation, 133, 172t
birthright citizenship, 92t, 169t
Bismarck Archipelago, 211
Black Americans
cognitive impairment among, 106–108
health inequities, 97
Jim Crow laws against, 250
racial and ethnic category, 5, 12
See also Black people
Black Codes, 111
Black Elk, 32
Black Freedom movement, 251–252
Black Hills, 25, 26
Black Panthers, 73
Black people, 97–127
adverse childhood experiences, 100
anti-Black racism, 73, 98–99
criminal legal systems, 104–108
health care systems, 108–111
health effects, 99–101, 111–114
history of, 51, 251
place-based systems, 101–104
racism-related stress, 100
cancer, 108–109
chronic health conditions, 145–146
enslavement of, 97–98, 185, 245
health care for, 97–98
health disparities, 97, 98–99, 104–105
health inequities, 284
health occupations, 109, 139, 140t
homelessness/houselessness rate, 227
incarcerated, 105, 106–107, 113

infant mortality, 109–111
life expectancy, 100, 257, 258f, 259f
maternal health, 104–105
maternal mortality, 109–111
median household wealth, 136
mortality rates, 256–257, 257f
place-based economic repair(ations) for, 111, 112–113
place-based systems and, 101–103
poverty rates, 135
slave health deficit, 97–98
stress, racism-related, 100
underrepresentation of, 170t
urban ghettos, 248–249
youth suicide, 101–103
See also Black Americans
Black Power, 51
Black–Korean Alliance, 94t
Boarding School Era, 14b
boarding schools, 19, 20f, 22b, 30
Bollywood, 63
Bracero Agreement, 171t
Bracero Program, 171t
brain drain, 60
Brazilians, 129
breadfruit, 217
breast cancer, 108
Bridges, Khiara, 108
Bright, Leina'ala, 233
Broadway, 94t
Bronx Community College, 149
brown peril fears, 50–52
Brown v Board of Education, 172t, 251
BTS, 63
bubonic plague, 70
Bureau of Indian Affairs (BIA), 19, 22b
Bureau of Indian Education (BIE), 30–31, 38
Burlington, Vermont, 185
Burmese, 53t

C

California
  Alien Land Laws, 58, 92t
  Asian Americans in, 56, 60–61
  Chinese Americans in, 68
  COVID-19 death rate, 225b
  death rates, 225b, 255
  earnings, 60–61
  federally recognized Tribes, 12
  Latino populations in, 135, 136–137, 141
  Proposition 187, 133
California Commission on Asian Pacific Islander Affairs, 77
California Gold Rush, 56
California Health Interview Survey, 181
California Sterilization Law, 171t
Cambodians, 51, 53t, 59–61, 69
Canada, 13, 19, 35
cancer
  disparities in white people, 255–256, 256f
  racial disparities, 108–109
  racial inequities, 68
capital, 32, 37
capitalism, 32, 252, 259–260
  racial, 265
cardiovascular disease, 145
Caribbeans, 14b, 131, 135
Carlisle Indian Industrial School, 19, 20f
Caroline Islands, 211
Carson, California, 68–69
categorization, 247
  See also data categorization
Caucasians, 50, 188
Cecil G. Sheps Center for Health Services Research (University of North Carolina), 113
2030 Census, 197
Centers for Disease Control and Prevention (CDC)
  Health Disparities and Inequities Report, 98
  Social Vulnerability Index, 144
Centers for Medicare and Medicaid Services (CMS), 66
Central Americans
  access to health resources, 145–146
  child health, 144
  diasporic movements, 131, 156
  discrimination against, 136–137
  education and employment of, 138–139
  ethnic group, 135
  health care for, 142–143
  history, law and policy intersections, 133–134
Central Intelligence Agency (CIA), 60
cerebrovascular diseases, 255–256, 256f
Chae Chan Ping v United States, 92t
Chaldeans, 180
Chamorros, 232
CHamoru, 217b, 218–219, 235–236
CHamoru Studies Program, 235
Chan is Missing (1982), 94t
Chang, Calvin, 225b
Chavez, Cesar, 93t
Cherokee, 18
Cherokee Nation, 22b
Chicago, Illinois, 113
Chickasaw, 18
Chief Huråo Academy, 235–236
childcare, 152t
children
  boarding schools for, 19, 20f
  of first-generation parents, 146–147
  health inequities, 143–144
  hidden victims, 194

INDEX | 329

Indian Child Welfare Act, 21, 22b
infant mortality, 109–111
poverty rates, 143–144
residential schools for, 19
Children's Health Insurance Program (CHIP)
  eligibility, 64
  Latino dependence on, 143–144
  per capita expenditures, 27, 28t
  untapped benefits, 262
  across US-affiliated Pacific Islands, 230t
Chile, 130t, 212
Chin, Vincent, 94t
China, 96t
"China virus" language, 67, 70, 72t
Chinatown (New York City), 93t
The Chinese American, 92t
Chinese American Citizens Alliance, 92t
Chinese Americans
  ethnic group, 52, 53t
  health inequities, 68
  racism toward
    hate crimes, 70
    history of, 50, 58, 69, 92t–93t
    history of research on, 55
    in media coverage, 64
    scapegoating, 56–57
  resistance, 222t
Chinese Equal Rights League, 92t
Chinese Exclusion Act, 55, 56–57, 63, 92t, 188, 286
Chinese immigrants, 56–57, 64
#Chinesevirus, 70
CHIP. *See* Children's Health Insurance Program
Choctaw, 18
Christians, 14b, 15, 16, 180, 188
chronic health conditions
  case study, 150–151
  effects of, 284
  and health care access, 144–146
  in Latino populations, 144–146, 150–151
  in white people, 255–256, 256f
chronic obstructive pulmonary disease (COPD), 145
Chuuk, 222t
citizenship
  barriers to, 50, 75
  birthright, 92t, 169t
  vs. lawful permanent residency, 215
  vs. nationality, 215
  naturalized, 75, 92t, 247n
  tri-citizenship, 12
Civil Liberties Act, 57, 92t
Civil Rights Acts, 133, 172t, 174t, 251, 259
civil rights law, 292–293
Civil Rights Movement, 21, 51, 111, 189, 251–252
Civil War, 111, 247–248, 250

clash of civilizations mindset, 183
Clean Air Act, 55
climate change, 232
Climate Change Model of Indigenous Resilience, 21–23, 24f
Clinton, Bill, 95t
CLS. *See* criminal legal system
CNMI. *See* Commonwealth of the Northern Mariana Islands
coal heritage campaign, 260
coconut haustorium, 217
Code of Indian Offenses, 18–19, 21, 22b
COFA nations. *See* Compact of Free Association
cognitive impairment, 104–105
Cold War, 93t
college students, 169t
Colombians, 130t, 135
colonialism, 59, 60, 169t, 250
colonization
  of Alaska, 15–17, 16b
  definition of, 169t
  history of, 14–17, 14b, 16b, 245
  impacts of, 219–221, 295–296
  settler, 15
Colorado, 135
colorblind racial ideology, 252
colorism, 169t
Columbus, Christopher, 12–13, 14–15, 14b
Comity Agreement, 16,16b
Commission to the Five Civilized Tribes (Dawes Commission), 19
Committee to Free Chol Soo Lee, 94t
Commonwealth of Nations, 212
Commonwealth of the Northern Mariana Islands (CNMI), 211, 214f
  actionable solutions to advance health equity, 297t
  catalysts for change, 236
  health care access, 229, 230t
communications
  anti-Asian racism in, 62–64, 76
  proposed solutions for change, 76
  See also media coverage
community-based adolescent health, 150
community college, 152t
community health centers (CHCs), 153t
community mobilization
  among Asian Americans during COVID-19, 71–74, 72t
  proposed solutions for change, 77
community public health clinics, 150–151
community voices, 5
Comoros, 180
Compact of Free Association (COFA) nations, 212, 215, 222t

actionable solutions to advance health equity, 297t
catalysts for change, 236
conceptual framework, 3, 3f
Congressional Asian Pacific American Caucus, 95t
Connecticut, 135
conservation, 218–219
Cook, James, 216
Cook Expedition, 217
Cook Islands, 211, 212
Coptic Christians, 180
Costa Ricans, 130t
costs
  of living, 228, 228b, 260
  medical, 263
court cases, major
  affecting AI/AN peoples, 21, 22b
  affecting Latino populations, 171t–174t
Courts of Indian Offenses, 22b
COVID-19
  anti-Asian racism and, 67, 69–74
  community mobilizing and advocacy and, 71–74
  data disaggregation, 225b
  death rates, 225b
  disease-related violence, 70–71
  employment and, 138
  in media, 63
  medical debt due to, 141
  mortality from, 62
  pandemic, 49, 60, 96t
  poverty and, 143–144
COVID-19 Hate Crimes Act, 70, 72t, 73, 96t
Creek, 18
criminal legal system (CLS)
  actionable solutions to advance health equity, 293
  and MENA inequities, 192–194
  place-based economic repair(ations) in, 112–113
  and racial cognitive impairment disparities, 106–108
  and racial maternal health disparities, 104–105
  racial profiling, 187, 192–193
  See also legal system
criminalization of trauma, 105
critical race theory, 266, 267
Cuban Adjustment Act, 134, 172t
Cuban Refugee Program, 134, 172t
Cubans/Cuban Americans, 156
  chronic health conditions, 145
  employment of, 139
  history of, 133–134, 171t, 172t
  poverty rates, 135

socioeconomic and educational profile, 130t, 135
cultural differences, 32–33
cultural genocide, 15, 16, 220–221, 231
cultural health, 28
cultural perspective, 28
cultural racism, 62
cultural wisdom, 235
current context, 182–187
cyberbullying, 70

D

DACA (Deferred Action for Childhood Arrivals), 75, 174t, 295
data categorization
  actionable solutions to advance health equity, 287
  racial and ethnic categories, 5, 12, 214–215, 221, 222t, 249–253, 285–286
  racial domination process, 247
data collection
  actionable solutions to advance health equity, 285–287, 297t
  case studies, 224b, 225b
  disaggregated, 221–224, 297t
    case studies, 224b, 225b
    and health intervention, 224, 225b
  and health intervention, 224, 225b
  Indigenous data sovereignty, 26
  local-level identifiers in, 197
  masking in, 223, 224b
  MENA identifiers in, 197, 198–199
  NHPI Data Policy Lab, 225b
  Tribal data sovereignty, 297t
  visibility and representation in, 214–215
data invisibility, 186–187
Dawes Act, 18–19, 20, 22b
Dawes Commission (Commission to the Five Civilized Tribes), 19
decolonization, 230–231
Deferred Action for Childhood Arrivals (DACA), 75, 174t, 295
dehumanization, 16
DEI (diversity, equity, and inclusion), 1, 252
dementia, 106–107
Department of Homeland Security, 57, 192–193, 197
diabetes, Type 2, 224, 225b
Directive 15 (OMB), 197
discrimination
  anti-Black, 108
  anti-immigrant, 136–137
  anti-Latino, 136–137, 251
  anti-MENA, 194
  and cognitive impairment, 106
  COVID-related, 71

in health care, 108
legal, 247–248
pathways for, 4
racial or ethnic, 56–57, 106, 247–248
disease-related violence, 70–71
disenfranchisement, 219–221
District of Columbia, 65
diversity, equity, and inclusion (DEI), 1, 252
Djibouti, 180
Doctrine of Discovery (*Inter Caetera*), 15, 18
Dominican Republic, 14–15
Dominicans, 130*t*, 145, 150–151
Dotbuster gang, 94*t*
drinking water, 220
Du Bois, W. E. B., 97, 250

E

Earned Income Tax Credit (EITC), 262, 268, 291
East Coast Asian American Student Union, 93*t*
Easter Island (Rapa Nui), 211, 212, 219–221
ecology
    Integrated Indigenous-Ecological Model, 21, 23*f*
    medicinal plants, 233, 235
economic development, 37
economic infrastructure investments, 290
economic justice, 153
economic migrants, 173*t*
economic system
    actionable solutions for AI/AN peoples, 37–38
    actionable solutions to advance health equity, 288–291, 296*t*
    AI/AN initiatives, 37–38
    AI/AN peoples, 32–33
    anti-Asian racism in, 59–62
    case study, 228*b*
    economies disparities, 227–228, 228*b*
    extractive economy, 259–260
    gig economy, 260, 261
    Indigenous economies, 227–228
    Pacific Islands, 227–228
    place-based economic repair(ations), 111, 112–114
    proposed solutions for change for Asian Americans, 75–76
economically disadvantaged people, 170*t*
ecosystems, 34–35
Ecuador, 130*t*, 212
education
    actionable solutions to advance health equity, 291–292
    for AI/ANs, 38–39, 297*t*
    for Indigenous sovereignty, 297*t*
    for Latinos, 151–152, 152*t*, 153–154
    for NH/PIs, 297*t*
    of AI/ANs, 29–32, 38–39

American Indian history, 38
Asian American history, 73–74, 96*t*
boarding schools, 19, 20*f*, 22*b*, 30
and death rates, 255
Hawaiian Educational philosophy (Kumu Honua Mauli Ola), 234
of Latinos, 137–139, 140*t*, 141–142, 155
    actionable strategies for, 151–152, 152*t*, 153–154
    case studies, 148–149
low education–related health inequities, 137–139, 255, 257
    case studies, 148–149
    economic burden of, 143
nutrition, 229
of Pacific Islanders, 232–233, 234
parental, 169*t*
pathways to health disparities, 103–104
public, 103–104
racial disparities in, 103–104
reservation schools, 30
residential schools, 19
and rising Black youth suicide, 102–103
school system, 235–236
TEAACH Act (Illinois), 73–74, 96*t*
Tribal colleges, 31, 38, 297*t*
educational disparities, 103–104, 232–233, 234, 257–258
educationally disadvantaged people, 170*t*
Egypt, 179
EITC (Earned Income Tax Credit), 261, 268, 291
elders, 35
Emancipation Proclamation, 250
empire, 182–183
employment
    actionable solutions to advance health equity, 288–291
    actionable strategies for Latinos, 151–152, 152*t*–153*t*, 153–154, 155
    case studies, 146–148
    and death rates, 255
    of Latinos, 137–139, 155
        actionable strategies, 151–152, 152*t*–153*t*, 153–154, 155
        case studies, 146–148
    as lever of inequality, 137–139, 261
    workforce development, 29–32, 65, 155
Enewetak, 220
English, 250
English-only ordinances, 50–51
enslavement
    of Black people, 97–98, 185, 245
    of Indigenous peoples, 14–17
entertainment, 237
environmental justice, 67–69
environmental perspectives, 25
environmental racism, 67–69

Erikson, Leif, 14–15
Eskuelan Mañaina, 235–236
ethnic categories. *See* racial and ethnic categories
ethnic or racial discrimination, 56–57, 106, 247–248
Ethnic Studies, 93*t*
ethnoburbs, 67
eugenics, 251
Eugenics Board, 171*t*
Europe, 15
European Americans, 129
   white. *See* white people
European colonialism, 250
Everything Everywhere All at Once (2022), 62
evidence
   MENA health, 181–182
   See also data collection
Executive Order 9066 (1942), 57, 92*t*
Executive Order 11246 (1965), 172*t*
Executive Order 13125 (1999), 95*t*
Executive Order 13767 (2017), 174*t*
extractive economy, 259–260

F

FACES (Filipino/American Coalition for Environmental Solutions), 68–69
Far Right, 253
FAS (Freely Associated States), 219, 222*t*, 229, 230*t*
federal AI/AN policy eras, 17–21
Federal Deposit Insurance Corporation (FDIC), 32
federal Indian trust responsibility, 17, 18
Federal Refugee Resettlement Program, 173*t*
federally recognized Tribes, 12
Federated States of Micronesia (FSM), 211, 212, 215, 222*t*
Fiji, 211, 213, 226
Filipino-American Association, 92*t*
Filipino/American Coalition for Environmental Solutions (FACES), 68–69
Filipinos/Filipino Americans, 56
   COVID-19 mortality, 62
   ethnic group, 52, 53*t*
   health inequities, 67–69
   health outcomes, 58–59
   racism against
      case study, 68–69
      environmental, 68–69
      history of, 49, 51, 58, 92*t*–94*t*, 222*t*
      resistance, 222*t*
financial security, 224–226
financial systems, 32–33, 224–226
First Anglo-Powhatan War, 14*b*
first generation, 169*t*

First Nations, 13, 19
fishing, 234–235
Florida, 57, 135, 136–137, 141
Floyd, George, 3, 72*t*
Fong Yue Ting v United States, 92*t*
food stamps, 2–3, 262
football, 237
foreign-born immigrants, 169*t*
foreign policy, 182–185, 199, 294–295
foreigner, perpetual (stereotype), 50–51
former Soviet Union, 182–183
Fort Laramie Treaty, 26
France, 15, 220
Freely Associated States (FAS), 219, 222*t*, 229, 230*t*
French and Indian War, 14*b*
French Polynesia, 211, 219–221
FSM (Federated States of Micronesia), 211, 212, 215, 222*t*
funerary customs, 226
further research, policy, and programming, 198–199, 267–269
Futuna, 211

G

G. I. Bill, 252
Gadsden Purchase, 171*t*
Galápagos Islands, 212
Gaza, 184, 185, 198
Geary Act, 92*t*
gender-affirming care, 230
generational status, 169*t*
genocide
   cultural, 15, 16, 220–221, 231
   of Indigenous peoples, 11, 15, 16, 185, 245, 295–296
   linguistic, 220–221
Gentlemen's Agreement of 1907, 57
Georgia, 22*b*, 255–256, 256*f*, 263
German–Spanish Treaty, 213
Germany, 213, 251
Gidra, 93*t*
gig economy, 260, 261
Global South, 67–68
Gold Rush, 56
Graber, David, 32
Great Britain, 15, 213
Great Recession, 262
Great Sioux War, 14*b*
Great Society, 259
Grutter v Bollinger, 174*t*
Guam, 211–215, 214*f*, 218–219
   actionable solutions to advance health equity, 297*t*
   catalysts for change to advance health equity, 236

INDEX

CHamoru language and culture revitalization, 235–236
colonization, occupation, and disenfranchisement impacts, 219–221
economics, 228
health care access, 229, 230*t*
history of, 171*t*
homelessness, 227
household income, 228
military occupation of, 220
school system, 235–236
traditional healers, 228–229
Guamanians, 232
Guatemalans, 130*t*, 147–148, 173*t*
Gulf War, 189
gun control, 266, 269

H

Hā'ena ahupua'a (Hā'ena land division), 234–235
Hā'ena Community-Based Subsistence Fishing Area, 234–235
Haiti, 14–15
Haitians, 129
Hampton Institute, 19
Harlins, LaTasha, 94*t*
Hart–Cellar Act, 133, 134, 172*t*
Harvard University, 94*t*, 174*t*
Hassan, Ahmad, 188
hate crimes, 70, 96*t*, 185, 249
Hau'ofa, Epeli, 212
Hawai'i, 211–213, 214*f*, 215
   actionable solutions to advance health equity, 297*t*
   Asians in, 56
   catalysts for change to advance health equity, 236
   colonization, occupation, and disenfranchisement impacts, 219–221
   death rates, 255
   economic disparities, 228
   environmental racism, 67–68
   Hā'ena Community-Based Subsistence Fishing Area, 234–235
   health, wellness, and wisdom, 216
   health care access, 229, 230*t*
   health care facilities, 229
   homelessness, 227
   household income, 228
   life expectancy, 217
   literacy rate, 217*b*
   military occupation of, 220
   Nā Wai 'Ehā waters, 231
   notable achievements, 217*b*
   population decline, 219–220

traditional food and lifestyle restoration case studies, 218*b*
traditional healers, 228–229
traditional health and healing, 233
Hawaiian Educational philosophy, 234
Head Start, 147
health care
   access to care. *See* access to health care
   actionable solutions to advance health equity, 287–288, 289*t*, 296*t*
   considerations for action and further research, 269
   for Latinos, 151–152, 153*t*
   anti-Asian racism and, 64–66
   anti-Black discrimination in, 108
   for Asian Americans, 64–66
   barriers to care, 263
   for Black people, 108
   case studies, 150–151
   community-based adolescent care, 150–151
   cost of care, 66, 263
   culturally safe and appropriate care, 76–77
   for gay youth, 150–151
   Indigenous, 228–230, 235, 237
   lā'au lapa'au (curing medicine), 233
   for Latino populations, 139–143, 150–152, 153*t*
   native healers, 237
   traditional health and healing, 233
health care facilities, 230*t*
health care system
   actionable solutions to advance health equity
      for AI/AN people, 36–37
      for Asian Americans, 76–77
      for Latino people, 142–143
   AI/AN initiatives, 35–37
   anti-Black racism, 108–111
   and cancer continuum, 108–109
   Indian Health Service (IHS), Tribal health systems, and urban Indian health programs (I/T/U system), 12, 36
   and maternal and infant mortality, 109–111
   place-based economic repair(ations) in, 113–114
   political determinants of social inequality, 139–143
   across US-affiliated Pacific Islands, 230*t*
   and white health disparities, 262–264
health care teams, 142–143
health care workforce
   AI/AN, 29, 31–32
   Asian American, 63, 65, 140*t*
   Black, 109, 140*t*
   development of, 31–32, 65, 155
   health professionals, 29, 63
   Latino, 139, 140*t*, 142, 155

media representation of, 63
health disparities
  in Black people, 98–99, 108–109
    educational disparities and, 103–104
    maternal health disparities, 104–105
  in cancer, 108–109
  catalysts for change to reduce, 236
  considerations for action and further research, 267–269
  data invisibility, 186–187
  educational disparities and, 103–104
  epidemiology of, 253–267
  examples, 255–257
  labor and wages and, 259–261, 268
  maternal health disparities, 104–105
  in MENA Americans, 186–187
  in NH/PIs, 231, 236
  in pain management, 98
  root causes of, 257–267
  in white people
    considerations for action and further research, 267–269
    epidemiology of, 253–267
    examples, 255–257
    labor and wages and, 259–261, 268
    root causes, 257–267
    whiteness and, 264–267
Health Disparities and Inequities Report (CDC), 98
health equity, 1, 297
healthy immigrant effect, 136, 182
health inequities, 1, 297
  actionable solutions to advance health equity, 285–297
  in Asian Americans, 49–91, 54f, 70–71, 284
  in Black Americans, 97–98
  case studies, 67–74, 148–149
  catalysts for change to reduce, 236
  in children, 143–144
  conceptual model of, 282, 283f
  economic burden of, 143
  fundamental causes of, 258–259, 288
  intersecting systems of oppression and, 226–230
  in Latino populations, 143
  low education–related, 137–139, 255, 257
    case studies, 148–149
    economic burden of, 143
  marginalization and, 181, 187–194, 221–224
  in MENA Americans, 179–209, 246b
  mental health inequities
    in Asian Americans, 70–71
    in Muslim Americans, 194
  militarization and, 220
  in Muslim Americans, 194
  in NH/PIs, 231
  root causes, 282–284

slave health deficit, 97–98
systemic and structural racism and, 282, 283f
in white Americans, 245–280
health insurance
  anti-Asian racism and, 64
  disparities in cancer and, 109
  Latino children and, 143–144
  state-funded, 65
  uninsured Latinos, 141
  universal coverage, 153t, 154–155
  untapped benefits, 262
  among US-affiliated NH/PI jurisdictions, 229, 230t
health interventions, 224, 225b
Health Opportunities Pilot (University of North Carolina), 113
health professionals, 29, 63
  See also health care workforce
heart disease, 145, 255–256, 256f
He'eia Fishpond, 218b
hepatitis, 219
HHS. See US Department of Health and Human Services
Higher Education Act, 169t
Hilberg, Raul, 246
Hindoo Invasion, 51
Hirabayashi, Gordon, 57
Hispanic (term), 129, 131t
Hispanic Community Health Study/Study of Latinos, 136
Hispanic paradox, 136
Hispanics
  child health, 143–144
  chronic health conditions, 144–146
  ethnic group, 134–137
  health occupations, 139, 140t
  homelessness/houselessness rate, 227
  life expectancy, 259f
  racial and ethnic category, 5, 286
  socioeconomic and educational profile, 130t
  terminology, 129, 131t, 173t
  underrepresentation of, 170t
  See also Latino populations
Hispaniola, 14–15
historical context
  Alaska Native, 15–17, 16b
  American Indian
    in educational curricula, 38
    federal policy eras, 17–21
  Asian American
    in educational systems, 73–74, 96t
    racism and resistance, 92t–96t
  colonization, 14–17, 14b, 16b, 245
  federal AI/AN policy eras, 17–21
  Indigenous, 13–14, 14b
  intersections with law and policy, 132–134
  Mexican and Puerto Rican, 132–134

Middle Eastern and North African (MENA), 182–187
of racial and ethnic categories, 249–253
of structural racism, 182–187
of systemic racism in policy, 13–21, 14b
HIV, 237
Hmong Americans, 49, 53t, 58–61, 66, 69
Hollaback!, 72t
Hollywood Diversity Report, 190
Holocaust, 251
homelessness/houselessness, 227
Homestead Act, 18
homicide rates, 256
Hondurans, 130t
Hong Kong, 71
Hoʻoulu ʻĀina, 218b
hospitality industry workforce, 141
Hostage Crisis (Iran), 192–193
House of Representatives, 184
household characteristics, 144
houselessness, 227
housing, 108, 144, 219, 226–227

I

ʻĪao Stream, 231
IHS. *See* Indian Health Service
Illinois, 73–74, 96t, 135, 136–137
Illinois Department of Corrections, 113
immigrants
  access to care, 64–65
  anti-immigrant propaganda, 194
  anti-immigrant rhetoric, 185
  case studies, 147–148
  definition of, 169t
  discrimination against, 136–137, 251
  foreign born, 169t
  racialization of, 134–135, 188–190, 251
  unauthorized or undocumented, 64–65, 136–137, 147–148, 169t
Immigration Act of 1917, 57
Immigration Act of 1924 (Johnson-Reed Act), 92t, 171t
Immigration Act of 1965, 57, 59
Immigration Act of 1990, 134
Immigration and Nationality Act, 169t, 173t, 188–189
Immigration and Naturalization Service (INS), 133
immigration policy
  actionable solutions to advance health equity, 294–295
  history of, 133–134, 169t, 171t, 172t, 173t, 251
immigration quotas, 133–134, 172t, 188, 251
Immigration Reform and Control Act, 173t
imperialism, 59, 60, 182–183, 213

incarceration, 105, 106–107, 113
Indian (term), 12–13
Indian Americans, 50–52, 53t, 58, 61, 92t
Indian Appropriation Act, 22b
Indian Child Welfare Act, 21, 22b
Indian Citizenship Act (Snyder Act), 14b, 19–20, 22b
Indian Civil Rights Act, 22b
Indian Health Care Improvement Act, 21, 22b
Indian Health Service (IHS)
  Budget Formulation Committee (NIHB), 27, 35–36
  expenditures, 27, 28t
  funding, 27, 35–36, 296, 296t
  Indian Health Service (IHS), Tribal health systems, and urban Indian health programs (I/T/U system), 12, 36
  Purchased and Referred Care system, 28
Indian New Deal (Indian Reorganization Act), 20, 22b
Indian Relocation Act, 20, 22b
Indian Removal Act, 18, 22b
Indian Reorganization Act (Wheeler-Howard Act/Indian New Deal), 20, 22b
Indian Self-Determination and Education Assistance Act, 21, 22b
Indian Wars, 14b
Indigenous Central Americans, 131
Indigenous data sovereignty, 26
Indigenous Determinants of Health Working Group, 34
Indigenous diet, 217
Indigenous economies, 227–228
Indigenous Healers and Educators Regional Taskforce, 31
Indigenous healing, 235, 237
Indigenous health systems, 228–230
Indigenous language revitalization, 233, 235–236
Indigenous peoples
  actionable solutions to advance health equity, 296, 296t–297t
  Climate Change Model of Indigenous Resilience, 21–23, 24f
  definition of, 11, 170t
  economic systems, 32
  enslavement of, 14–17
  financial systems, 32–33
  genocide of, 11, 15, 16, 185, 245, 295–296
  health care, 228–230
  history of, 13–14, 14b
  homelessness/houselessness rate, 227
  Integrated Indigenous-Ecological Model, 21, 23f
  Mexicans, 170
  Pacific Islanders. *See* Pacific Islanders
  priorities, 35
  sacred sites, 26

terminology for, 12–13, 13f
United Nations Permanent Forum on Indigenous Issues, 226–227
See also American Indians and Alaska Natives (AI/AN); Native Hawaiian and Pacific Islanders (NH/PIs)
Indigenous sovereignty, 295–296, 296t–297t
individual population approach, 4–6
individualism, 252, 266
Indonesians, 53t
infant mortality
 Black, 109–111
 disaggregated rates, 224b
 health care system and, 109–111
 "It Takes a Village: Giving Our Babies the Best Chance" program, 224b
 Pacific Islander, 224b
 white rural rates, 256
information, 285–287
Instagram, 63
institutional racism, 151–155
 See also structural racism; systemic racism
institutional review boards (IRBs), Tribal, 26
Integrated Indigenous-Ecological Model, 21, 23f
Inter Caetera (Doctrine of Discovery), 15
intergenerational relationships, 35
intersectionality, 132, 137, 226–230
Inuits, 13
invisibility, 52–54
Iran, 189, 192–193
Iranians, 60, 188–189, 192–193
Iran–Iraq War, 189
Iraqi uprisings, 189
Iraqis, 179, 189
IRBs. See institutional review boards
Irish Americans, 183
Islamic State of Iraq and Syria (ISIS), 185
Islamophobia, 73, 184–186
Israel, 182–183, 184
Israeli–Palestinian conflict, 189
"It Takes a Village: Giving Our Babies the Best Chance" program, 224b
Itliong, Larry, 93t

J

Jackson, Robert, 57
Jackson, Sheldon, 16, 16b
Japan, 57, 213
Japanese American Citizens League, 92t
Japanese Americans
 community mobilization and advocacy during COVID-19, 73
 ethnic group, 52, 53t
 history of racism against, 50–51, 56–57, 92t
 mass incarceration of, 50–51, 57, 92t, 248–249
 resistance, 222t
Jetté, Jules, 16, 16b
Jews, 180, 246
Jim Crow laws, 97, 111, 185, 245, 248, 250, 286
John F. Kennedy airport, 95t
Johnson, Dwayne, 237
Johnson–Reed Act (Immigration Act of 1924), 92t, 171t
Johnson v McIntosh, 18
Joint Commission, 221
Jones–Shafroth Act, 133, 171t
Jordan, 179
Journal of Asian American Studies, 95t
justice
 actionable solutions to advance health equity, 292–293
 economic, 153
 environmental, 67–69
 injustice and policy barriers, 231–233

K

kahunas, 228–229
Kalākaua, 213, 217b
Kānaka Māoli, 212
Kansas City, Kansas, 185
Ke Kula 'o Samuel M. Kamakau Laboratory Public Charter School, 234
Kearny Street Workshop, 93t
Kentucky, 255–256, 256f
King, Rodney, 94t
King Philip's War, 14b
Kiribati, 211, 226
knowledge bearers, 35, 218–219
Kōkua Kalihi Valley Comprehensive Family Services, 218b
Korean American Coalition, 94t
Korean Americans, 52, 53t, 56, 69, 94t
Koreatown (Los Angeles), 94t
Korematsu, Fred, 57
Korematsu v United States, 57, 92t
Kosrae, 222t
Kula exchange, 217b
Kumu Honua Mauli Ola (Hawaiian Educational philosophy), 234
Kurds, 180
Kuwait, 179, 189

L

lā'au lapa'au (curing medicine), 233
labor
 actionable solutions to advance health equity, 288–291

considerations for action and further research, 268
proposed solutions for Asian Americans, 75–76
anti-Asian racism in, 59–62, 75–76
union membership, 153t, 260, 268
US history of, 73, 93t, 95t
and white health disparities, 259–261, 268
Lakota Nation, 26, 32
The Lancet Planetary Health, 34
land management, 35, 133, 227–228, 233, 296t
land ownership, 133, 227, 228
language
"China virus," 67, 70, 72t
Indigenous, revitalization of, 233, 235–236
Laotians, 51–52, 53t, 59–61, 69
Latine (term), 129, 131t
Latino (term), 129, 131t
Latino populations
actionable strategies for, 151–155, 152t–153t
case studies, 146–151
child health, 143–144
demographic shift, 156
discrimination against, 136–137, 251
economic burden of health inequities, 143
education and employment of, 137–139, 140t, 141–142
actionable strategies for, 151–152, 152t–153t, 153, 155
case studies, 146–149
educational profile, 130t, 134–136
ethnic group, 134–137
health care, 139–143
actionable strategies for, 151–152, 153t, 154–155
case studies, 150–151
health care access, 144–146
health inequities, 284
health insurance coverage, 141–142
health occupations, 139, 140t, 155
heterogeneity of, 132–137, 156
history, law and policy affecting, 132–134, 171t–174t, 251
homelessness/houselessness rate, 227
life course and well-being of, 129–168
life expectancy, 257
low-income, 143–144
median household wealth, 136
medical debt, 141
poverty rates, 143–144
projected increase, 129
self-identification, 129
social determinants of health (SDOH), 143–146
socioeconomic profile, 130t, 134–136
subgroups, 129
terminology, 129, 131t, 169t–170t

underrepresentation of, 170t
undocumented immigrants, 136–137, 147–148
unemployment, 141
uninsured, 141–142
See also Mexicans/Mexican Americans; Puerto Ricans
Latinx (term), 129, 131t
Lau v Nichols, 93t
law(s). *See* legislation
lawful permanent residents, 215
Lebanese Civil War, 189
Lebanese immigrants, 179, 188–189
Lee, Chol Soo, 94t
Lee, Wo, 56
legal system
actionable solutions to advance health equity, 292–293
anti-Asian racism in, 55–59, 75
anti-Black racism in, 104–105, 106–108
and health inequities, 55–59
proposed solutions for change, 75
structural racism in, 292–293
See also criminal legal system (CLS)
legislation
anti-DEI, 1
civil rights law, 251, 292–293
Jim Crow laws, 97, 111, 185, 245, 248, 250, 286
major laws affecting AI/AN peoples, 21, 22b
major laws affecting Latino populations, 132–134, 171t–174t
minimum-wage laws, 138–139, 260
leisure and hospitality industry workforce, 141
lesbian, gay, bisexual, transgender, queer, and questioning (LGBTQ+) populations, 150–151, 229–230, 252
Libya, 179
life expectancy, 216–217
Life's Essential 8, 37
lifestyle, traditional, 217–218, 218b
linguistic genocide, 220–221
literacy, 232
Little Mosque on the Prairie (CBC Television), 195
local-level MENA identifiers, 197
Lord Howe Island, 212
Los Angeles, California, 60, 70, 94t
Los Angeles County-USC Medical Center, 173t
Louisiana, 56, 58
lung cancer, 68, 109

M

Madrigal v Quilligan, 173t
Makua Pu'uhonua (Marine Refuge), 235
Mallapragada, Madhavi, 64
Mana Academy, 234

Manifest Destiny, 14b, 15, 18
Manu'a, 213
manufacturing, 260, 263
Māori, 212, 217b
Marathon oil refinery, 68
marginalization
  case studies, 146–151
  pathways of, 4, 181, 187–194, 221–224
  processes of, 246–253
Mariana Islands, 235
  See also Commonwealth of the Northern Mariana Islands (CNMI); Northern Mariana Islands
Marquesas Islands, 211
Marshall Islands, 211–212, 215, 218, 220, 222t
masking, 223
Massachusetts, 135
maternal health, 104–105, 108, 109–111
Maui, 231
Maungahuka (Auckland Islands), 217b
Mauritania, 180
media coverage, 195, 293–294
media representation
  of Asian Americans, 62–64, 69, 76
  of health professionals, 63
  key recommendations for, 293–294
  of MENA and Muslim individuals, 185, 190–192, 195
  proposed solutions for, 76
Medicaid
  actionable strategies to advance health equity
    for AI/ANs, 36
    for Latinos, 153t, 154–155
  availability across US-affiliated Pacific Islands, 229, 230t
  efforts to dismantle, 2–3, 65
  eligibility, 12, 64, 65, 139, 215, 263
  expansion of, 21, 28, 263, 264f, 269
  opposition to, 109, 265–266
  timeline, 22b
  Latino dependence on, 143–144
  per capita expenditures, 27, 28t
  untapped benefits, 262
medical abuse, 133, 172t
medical costs, 263
medical debt, 141, 263
Medicare
  AI/AN enrollments, 36
  availability across US-affiliated Pacific Islands, 230t
  legal system and, 55
  Part A eligibility, 139
  per capita expenditures, 27, 28t
medicinal plants, 233, 235
Melanesia, 211, 212f, 217b
MENA Arts Advocacy Coalition, 195
Mendez v Westminster, 133, 172t

mental health, 70–71, 102, 150, 194
meritocracy, 266
mestizo, 169t
Metis, 13
Mexican Repatriation Program, 171t
Mexican–American war, 133, 171t
Mexicans/Mexican Americans
  11th generation US citizen (case study), 148
  access to health resources, 145–146
  actionable strategies to advance health equity, 151–152, 152t–153t
  adolescent health, 150–151
  case studies, 146–148, 150
  child health, 144
  children of first-generation parents, 146–147
  chronic health conditions, 145
  discrimination against, 136–137
  education and employment of, 138–139, 142, 146–148
  ethnic group, 134–137
  health care, 141–142, 145, 150
  health insurance coverage, 141–142
  history of, 93t, 132–134, 171t, 172t
  Indigenous, 170t
  life course and well-being of, 129–131, 155–156
  mixed-race ancestry, 169t
  population, 129
  poverty rates, 135
  socioeconomic and educational profile, 130t, 134–136
México, 133, 171t
Michigan, 94t
Michigan Asian Pacific American Affairs Commission, 77
Micronesia, 211–213, 212f, 215, 226–228
Micronesian Islands Forum, 232
Middle Eastern and North African (MENA) Americans
  actionable opportunities to advance health equity, 181
  areas for further research, policy, and programming, 198–199
  areas for immediate intervention, 194–197
  criminal legal system and, 192–194
  data invisibility, 186–187
  discrimination against, 194
  evidence on, 181–182
  health disparities, 186–187
  health inequities, 187–194, 246b, 284
  history of racism toward, 51, 57, 182–187
  identifiers, 197, 198–199
  identity, 182–183
  local-level identifiers, 197
  marginalization, 187–194
  media representation of, 185, 190–192, 195
  misclassification as white, 6

policies that targeted, 192–194
racial and ethnic category, 5, 179, 189, 246b, 286
racialized origins, 188–190
structural inequities and health of, 179–209
terminology, 179–180
US Census category, 197, 198
US foreign policy and, 182–183
See also Arabs/Arab Americans
migrants, 169t
Migration and Refugee Assistance Act, 173t
military service, 219–220
Mills, Charles, 251–252
minimum wage, 138–139, 152t
minimum-wage laws, 138–139, 260
Miss Saigon, 94t
Mississippi, 255–256, 256f, 263
mixed-race ancestry, 169t
Mo (Netflix), 195
Moana Nui, 216
model minority myth or stereotype, 5, 51–52, 61, 66
Mody, Navroze, 94t
Moloka'i Diet, 217–218
Moloka'i Heart Study, 217–218
Morocco, 179
mortality rates, 255–257
motor vehicle accidents, 256, 256f, 263
Mount Rushmore, 26
Mount Sinai Adolescent Health Center (MSAHC), 150
multiculturalism, 252
multiracial people, 169t, 227
Muslim Ban, 51, 55, 58–59, 95t
Muslim Women's Test, 195
Muslims/Muslim Americans
anti-Muslim propaganda, 194
anti-Muslim racism, 73, 184
history of, 51, 57, 58–59, 95t
policies, 192–194
anti-Muslim violence, 185
categorization of, 180
criminal legal system and, 192–194
health outcomes, 58–59
media representation of, 190–192, 195
mental health inequities, 194
racial profiling of, 192–193
surveillance of, 193
Myanmar, 60

N

Nā Kumu Lā'au Lapa'au, 233
Nā Wai 'Ehā waters, 231
Namonuito, 227–228
National Academies of Sciences, Engineering, and Medicine (NASEM), 2
National Asian American Telecommunication Association (now Center for Asian American Media), 94t
National Asian Pacific American Women's Forum, 95t
National Center for American Indian Enterprise Development, 34
National Council of Asian Pacific Americans, 95t
National Football League, 237
National Health and Interview Survey (NHIS), 181
National Health Care Quality and Disparities Reports, 98
National Indian Health Board (NIHB), 27, 34, 35–36
National Institutes of Health, 98
National Korean American Service & Education Consortium, 95t
National Medical Association, 98
National Origins Quota Act, 188
national security, 192
National Security Entry-Exit Registration System (NSEERS), 192–193, 197
National Strategy to Advance Equity, Opportunity, and Justice for Asian American, Native Hawaiian, and Pacific Islander Communities, 96t
nationality, 215
Native American Pacific Islanders, 222t
Native American Programs Act, 222t
Native Americans, 222t
See also American Indians and Alaska Natives
Native BioData Consortium, 26
Native Hawaiian and Other Pacific Islander (NHOPI) category, 222t, 285–286
Native Hawaiian and Pacific Islanders (NH/PIs)
acronyms in common usage for, 221–223, 222t
actionable solutions to advance health equity, 296t–297t
catalysts for change, 236
age-adjusted death rates, 223
colonization, occupation, and disenfranchisement impacts, 219–221
COVID-19 death rate, 225b
definition of, 222t
disaggregated data, 221–224, 224b, 225b, 232, 297t
economic disparities, 228
education disparities, 232–233
employment–population ratio, 228
food insecurity, 226
health care access, 229, 230t
health disparities, 229–230
health inequities, 284
health insurance coverage, 229

homelessness/houselessness rate, 227
immigration statuses, 215
life expectancy, 216–217
median income, 228
multiracial, 215
population, 216f, 223
racial and ethnic category, 5, 12, 214–215, 221–223, 286
resistance, reformation, restoration, 230–231
suicide rates, 226
Type 2 diabetes, 224, 225b
underrepresentation of, 170t
See also Pacific Islanders
Native Hawaiians, 232
See also Native Hawaiian and Pacific Islanders (NH/PIs)
native healers, 237
Native health, 26–33
native languages, 220–221
natural resources, 220, 227–228
Naturalization Act, 247n
naturalized citizenship, 75, 92t, 188, 247n
Nauru, 211, 217
Nazi racial hygiene, 251
Nebraska, 263
neighborhood conditions, 101–102, 103–104
Neihardt, John, 32
neocolonialism, 60
neoliberalism, 252, 260
Nepali Americans, 53t, 61
Netherlands, 15
New Caledonia, 211, 219–221
New Deal, 259
New Guinea, 211
New Hebrides (Vanuatu), 211
New Jersey, 135
New Mexico, 135, 171t
New World, 15
New York (state), 135, 136–137, 148–149
New York City, New York, 60, 93t, 94t, 113
New York Police Department (NYPD), 193
New York Taxi Workers' Alliance, 95t
New York Times, 62
New Zealand (Aotearoa), 211, 212, 217b, 219–221, 226
NHIS (National Health and Interview Survey), 181
NHOPI (Native Hawaiian and Other Pacific Islander), 222t
NHPI Data Policy Lab, 225b
Nicaraguan Adjustment and Central American Relief Act, 174t
Nicaraguans, 130t
NIHB. *See* National Indian Health Board
9/11 attacks, 57, 95t, 189–190, 192–193
Niue, 211, 212
Nixon administration, 21

Norfolk Island, 212
North America, 15
North American Free Trade Agreement, 260
Northern Europeans, 250
Northern Guam Lens Aquifer, 220
Northern Mariana Islands, 212, 213, 227, 228–229
NSEERS (National Security Entry-Exit Registration System), 192–193, 197
nuclear weapons testing, 220
Nulato, 16
Nuremberg Trials, 251
nutrition education, 229

O

O'ahu, 218b
Oak Creek, Wisconsin, 185
Obeidi-Alsultany Test, 195
obesity disparities, 112, 256
occupation impacts, 219–221
Oceania, 211–214, 212f
    ancestral foods, 217
    catalysts for change to reduce disparities and improve health equity, 236
    climate change, 232
    colonization, occupation, and disenfranchisement impacts, 219–221
    costs of living, 228, 228b
    economic system, 227–228
    health, wellness, and wisdom, 216–219
    health care access, 228–230
    Indigenous economies, 227–228
    key facts, 213b
    militarization of, 220
    reconnections, 236–237
    resistance, reformation, restoration, 230–231
    revitalization and restoration impacts, 233–236
    suicide rates, 226
    wealth and income, 224–226, 228
Oceanic diet, 217
Office of Management and Budget (OMB)
    definition of Asians, 50
    definition of white people, 246b
    Directive 15, 197
    Policy Directive 15, 4, 15, 173t, 189
    Race and Ethnic Standards for Federal Statistics, 4
    racial and ethnic categories, 5, 12, 214–215, 221, 222t, 249–253, 285–286
    terminology, 129, 131t, 179–180, 215, 221, 222t
Ohai, Levon, 233
Ohio, 74
Okinawans, 56
Oklahoma, 18
older adults, 71

INDEX | 341

Oman, 179
OMB. *See* Office of Management and Budget
Operation Wetback, 172*t*
opportunity structures, 284–285
oppression pathways, 4, 226–230
Organic Act, 16*b*
"other" category, 52–54
Ozawa, Takao, 92*t*
Ozawa v United States, 50, 92*t*

P

Pacific Association for Radiation Survivors, 220
Pacific Confederacy, 213
Pacific Island Health Officers' Association, 232
Pacific Islanders, 211–244
    age-adjusted death rates, 223
    British colonization of, 15
    case study, 228*b*
    catalysts for change to reduce disparities and improve health equity, 236
    colonization, occupation, and disenfranchisement impacts, 219–221
    disaggregation of, 221–224, 224*b*, 225*b*, 232, 285–286, 297*t*
    economic disparities, 227–228, 228*b*
    education disparities, 232–233, 234
    financial security, 224–226
    health care, 228–229
    health disparities and inequities, 231
    immigrants, 57
    Indigenous knowledge of, 218–219
    infant mortality rates, 224*b*
    injustice and policy barrier impacts, 231–233
    Medicaid eligibility, 215
    military representation, 219–220
    notable achievements, 216–217, 217*b*
    oppression and inequities, 226–230
    poverty, 224–226
    racial and ethnic category, 221–223
    reconnections, 236–237
    resistance, reformation, restoration, 230–231
    revitalization and restoration impacts, 233–236
    suicide rate, 226
    terminology, 223
    visibility and representation in data, 214–215
    youth suicide rate, 226
    See also Asian American and Pacific Islanders; Native Hawaiian and Pacific Islanders
Pacific Islands Forum, 232
Pacific Ocean
    islands, 211–214, 212*f*
    sea level rise, 232
    US political relationships in, 213–214, 214*f*
    See also Oceania; Pacific Islanders
Pacific War, 213–214
Paepae o He'eia, 218*b*
paid leave, 152*t*
pain management, 98
Pakistanis, 50, 53*t*
Palau, 211, 212, 215, 219, 222*t*
Palestinians/Palestinian Americans, 179, 183, 185, 188–189
Panamanians, 130*t*, 135
parental education status, 169*t*
Pell Grants, 169*t*
People's CORE, 94*t*
perpetual foreigner stereotype, 50–51
Persian Gulf, 182–183
Personal Responsibility and Work Opportunity Act, 173*t*, 260
Peruvians, 130*t*
Pettersen, William, 62
Philippines, immigrants from. *See* Filipinos
Phillips 66 oil refinery, 68
physicians, 29, 109
    See also health care workforce; health professionals
Pillars Fund, 195
Pitcairn Island, 212
place-based economic repair(ations), 111, 112–114
place-based systems, 101–104
plants, medicinal, 233, 235
Pohnpei, 222*t*
Poles, 173*t*
policy
    areas for further research, policy, and programming, 198–199
    federal AI/AN eras, 17–21
    history and law intersections, 132–134
    history of systemic racism in, 13–21, 14*b*
Policy Directive 15 (OMB), 4, 15, 173*t*, 189
political determinants of health, 132, 170*t*
Polynesia, 211, 212*f*, 213
Polynesian Confederacy, 213
Poor People's Campaign, 261
Population Control Law 116, 171*t*
Portugal, 15
poverty
    and death rates, 255–256
    deep, 261
    definition of, 224–226
    economic initiatives for, 37
    and health care access, 143–146, 263
    and health disparities, 103–104, 255–257
    measures of, 33
Presidential Memorandum Condemning and Combating Racism, Xenophobia, and Intolerance Against Asian Americans and Pacific Islanders in the United States, 72*t*

President's Advisory Commission, 77
pretextual stops, 196
Preventing Maternal Deaths Act, 108
preventive care, 144
primary care, 144
    See also health care
private health systems, 36
programs, 198–199
propaganda, 194
proportionate universalism, 267–268
Proposition 187 (California), 133
prostate cancer, 108, 109
prostratin, 219
public education, 103–104
public health systems, 36
    See also health care system
Public Law No. 102-450, 94t
Pueblo peoples, 170t
Puerto Ricans
    access to health care, 145–146, 150–151
    actionable strategies to advance health equity, 151–152, 152t–153t
    adolescent, 150–151
    birth control experimentation, 172t
    case studies, 146–149, 150–151
    chronic health conditions, 144–145, 150–151
    citizenship, 133, 171t
    education and employment of, 138–139, 146–148, 153
    ethnic group, 134–137
    female sterilization, 171t
    health care for, 142–143, 150–151
    health insurance coverage, 141–142
    history, law and policy, 132–134, 171t, 172t
    life course and well-being of, 129–131, 155–156
    mixed-race ancestry, 169t
    population, 129, 130t
    poverty rates, 135
    socioeconomic and educational profile, 130t, 135–136
    US citizen (case study), 148–149
Puntan, 219

Q

Qatar, 179
quality health care. See health care
Queen's Medical Center (Hawai'i), 229

R

race, 12
Race and Ethnic Standards for Federal Statistics (OMB), 4
racial and ethnic categories, 5, 12, 214–215, 221, 222t, 285–286
    construction of, 249–253
"other" category, 52–54
    social determinants of health (SDOH), 144
racial capitalism, 265
racial discrimination, 56–57, 106, 247–248
racial disparities
    in cancer, 108–109
    in cognitive impairment, 106–108
    educational disparities and, 103–104
    in educational opportunity, 103–104
    health disparities, 98–99, 103–104
    in maternal and infant mortality, 109–111
    in maternal health, 104–105
    in obesity, 112
    in pain management, 98
racial domination, 246–253
racial profiling, 187, 192–193, 196–197
racial segregation, 248
    See also segregation
racialization, 134–135, 169t, 188–190
racialized violence, 185, 249
    See also hate crimes
racism
    anti-Asian, 49–91
        case studies, 67–74
        fundamental challenges, 50–54
        history of, 92t–96t, 174t
        history of research on, 55
        across systems, 54–66, 54f, 66–67
        youth harassment, 70–71
    anti-Black, 73, 98–99
        and health, 103–104
        health effects, 99–101, 111–114
        and maternal and infant mortality, 109–111
        and maternal health, 104–105
        and rising Black youth suicide, 101–103
    anti-Muslim, 73, 184
        history of, 51, 57, 95t
        opportunities for dismantling, 181, 194–197
        policies, 192–194
    cultural, 62
    environmental, 67–69
    history of, 14b, 15
    institutional. See also structural racism; systemic racism
        dismantling, with systemic changes, 151–155
    internalized, 52
    legalization of, 57
    pathways for, 4
    structural. See also systemic racism
        and Asian American health inequities, 49–91, 54f
        and Black people's health, 97, 98–101
        case studies, 67–74
        conceptual model of, 282, 283f
        cross-cutting solutions to advance health equity, 281–307

current context, 182–187
definition of, 170*t*
health effects, 1, 297
historical context, 182–187
impact on health inequities, 282, 283*f*
and MENA health inequities, 179–209
opportunities for dismantling, 181, 194–197
systemic. *See* systemic racism
racism-related stress, 100
Radiation Exposure Compensation Act, 220
Ramy, 195
Rapa Nui (Easter Island), 211, 212, 219–221
Reagan administration, 173*t*
reconnections, 236–237
Reconstruction Era, 111, 245, 248, 250, 286
redlining, 100–102, 252
reformation, 230–231
Refugee Act of 1980, 59–60, 173*t*
refugees, 51, 59–60, 172*t*, 185
Removal Era, 14*b*, 17, 18
Reorganization Era, 14*b*, 17, 20
replacement theory, 253
Report of the Secretary's Task Force on Black and Minority Health, 2
research areas, 198–199, 267–269
reservation schools, 30
reservation system, 248
residential schools, 19
residential segregation, 111, 285
resistance, 92*t*–96*t*, 222*t*, 230–231
restoration, 218*b*, 230–231, 233–236
revitalization, 233–236
Riz Test, 195
Robert Wood Johnson Foundation, 66
Roman Catholic Church, 16
Rongelap, 220
Roosevelt, Franklin D. (FDR), 57
Runit Island, 220
rural America, 256, 262–263
rural health penalty, 256
Russia, 15–16, 16*b*
Russian Orthodox Church, 16

S

Sablan, Joaquin Flores, 227
sacred sites, 25–26
safety net programs, 2–3, 261–262, 268, 288–291
Saguaro cactus, 35
Saipan, 227
Sakhi for South Asian Women/Domestic Workers Committee/Domestic Violence Project, 95*t*
Salvadorans, 130*t*, 146–147, 173*t*
Samoa, 211–215
Samoans
college attainment rates, 232

COVID-19 death rate, 225*b*
notable achievements, 217*b*, 237
suicide rates, 226
traditional diet, 217
traditional homes, 219
San Francisco, California, 60, 70, 92*t*, 93*t*
San Francisco State College, 93*t*
San Francisco Unified School District, 93*t*
Saudi Arabia, 179, 189
school system, 235–236
scientist–community partnerships, 287
SDOH. *See* social determinants of health
sea level rise, 232
seclusion, 248–249
second-generation college students, 169*t*
Section 503 (1973), 172*t*
Secure Communities Program, 174*t*
segregation
and cognitive impairment, 106
health effects, 111, 112–113, 114
Jim Crow, 97, 111, 185, 245, 248, 250, 286
residential, 111, 285
Self-Determination Era, 14*b*, 17, 21, 27
Seminole, 18
Seminole Nation v United States, 17
settler colonialism, 169*t*
settler colonization, 15
Sikh Coalition, 95*t*
Sikhs, 50–51, 57, 185
simultaneity, 137
slave health deficit, 97–98
slave trade, transatlantic, 97–98
Snares Islands (Tini Heke), 217*b*
Snyder Act (Indian Citizenship Act), 14*b*, 19–20, 22*b*
social categorization, 247
social class, 255
social determinants of health (SDOH), 1, 132, 137
actionable strategies that address, 151–152, 153*t*, 154–155
AI/AN, 35
definition of, 170*t*
indicators, 144
intersections, 143–146
Latino, 143–146, 151–152, 153*t*, 154–155
racial disparities, 108
social factors, 144
white, 253–255
social determinants of mental health, 102
social media, 70
social programs, 265, 266
See also safety net programs
Social Vulnerability Index, 144
Society Islands, 211
socioecological model, 253, 254*f*
socioeconomic status, 144–145, 257–259
Solomon Islands, 211, 226

Somalia, 180
South Americans, 129, 133–134, 135, 145, 156
South Asian Americans, 50–51, 57, 70, 94t, 95t
South Asian Americans Leading Together (SAALT), 50–51, 95t
South Asian Lesbian and Gay Association, 95t
South Asians, 61
South Carolina, 255
South Dakota, 26
South West Asian and North African (SWANA) Americans, 51
  See also Middle Eastern and North African (MENA) Americans
Southeast Asia, 61
Southeast Asia Resource Action Center, 93t
Southeast Asian Americans, 55, 68
sovereignty, 26, 295–296, 296t–297t
Soviet Union, former, 182–183
Spain, 14b, 15, 171t, 213
Spanish immigrants, 129, 130t, 135
Spanish–American war, 133, 171t
state-funded health insurance, 65
state-recognized Tribes, 12
Statistical Policy Directive No. 15, 4, 15, 173t, 189
stereotypes
  model minority, 5, 51–52, 61, 66
  perpetual foreigner, 50–51
sterilization, 133, 171t, 173t, 251
Stone Age, 237
Stop AAPI Hate, 72t, 96t
stress, 99–101, 255, 284
stress-coping model, 106
structural racism
  cross-cutting solutions to advance health equity, 281–307
  definition of, 170t
  health inequities due to, 1, 297
  in Asian Americans, 49–91, 54f
  in Black people, 97, 98–101
  case studies, 67–74
  conceptual model of, 282, 283f
  current context, 182–187
  in MENA Americans, 179–209
  historical context, 182–187
  opportunities for dismantling, 181, 194–197
  See also systemic racism
structural solutions, 282–285, 283f
Student for Fair Admissions v President & Fellows of Harvard College, 174t
student loan debt, 152t
students, 169t
subsistence fishing, 234–235
substance misuse, 256, 263
Sudan, 180
suicide, 101–103, 226, 256, 263
Superfund sites, 25

Supplemental Security Income, 262
surfing, 237
surveillance, 193
Sustain Hawai'i, 233
sustainability, 218–219
Syrians, 179, 188–189
systemic changes
  conceptual model for solutions, 282–285, 283f
  dismantling pathways of institutional racism with, 151–155
systemic racism
  and American Indian and Alaska Natives, 11–47
  and Asian Americans, 49–91
  and Black youth suicide, 101–103
  and cancer continuum, 108–109
  and cognitive impairment, 106–108
  criminal legal
    and cognitive impairment, 106–108
    and maternal health, 104–105
  definition of, 1
  health care
    and cancer continuum, 108–109
    and maternal and infant mortality, 109–111
  health effects, 1–9, 99–101, 103–104, 111–114
  and health inequities
    conceptual model of, 282, 283f
    marginalization pathways, 187–194
  history of, 13–21, 14b
  marginalization flows, 187–194
  and maternal and infant mortality, 109–111
  and maternal health, 104–105
  and MENA Americans, 187–194
  need for discussion on, 2–3
  place-based
    and Black youth suicide, 101–103
    and health, 103–104
  place-based economic repair(ations) for, 111, 112–113
  in policy, 13–21, 14b
  See also structural racism
systems, 4
systems approach, 4

T

Taino, 14–15
Taiwanese, 53t
TANF (Temporary Assistance for Needy Families), 262
Tape family, 92t
Tape v Hurley, 92t
taro poi, 217
taxes, 266
  See also Earned Income Tax Credit (EITC)
Tea Party, 253

INDEX | 345

TEAACH Act (Illinois), 73–74, 96t
Temporary Assistance for Needy Families (TANF), 262
temporary protected status, 134
Temporary Protection Act, 134, 173t
Tennessee, 255–256, 256f
Termination Era, 14b, 17, 20–21
terminology
　acronyms in common usage, 221–223, 222t
　for Indigenous peoples, 12–13, 13f
　for Latino populations, 129, 131t, 169t–170t
　for MENA populations, 179–180
　for Pacific Islanders, 223
terrorization, 249, 250
　See also hate crimes
Texas, 58, 135, 136–137, 141
Thai, 53t
Thind, Bhagat Singh, 50, 92t
TikTok, 63
Tini Heke (Snares Islands), 217b
Tlaib, Rashida, 184
Tokelau, 211, 212
Tonga, 211, 213–214, 226, 232, 237
Torres Strait Islands, 212
traditional food and lifestyle, 217–218, 218b, 230–231
traditional healers, 228–229, 233, 235
traditional knowledge, 34–35, 235
traditional medicine, 25–26, 233, 235
traditional stewardship, 227–228, 233
traditionally and historically underrepresented people, 170t
Trail of Tears, 18
transatlantic slave trade, 97–98
Transfer Act, 22b
transportation, 144
trauma, 105
treaties, major, 22b, 171t–174t
Treaty of Cession, 16b
Treaty of Guadalupe Hidalgo, 171t
Treaty of Paris, 171t
tri-citizenship, 12
Tribal colleges, 31, 38, 297t
Tribal data sovereignty, 297t
Tribal health systems, 12, 36
Tribal IRBs, 26
Tribal Nations, 12, 20, 36
Tribal sovereignty, 26
TRIO programs, 169t
Trump, Donald, 69, 70, 185
Trump administration, 65, 71, 95t
Trust Territory of the Pacific Islands, 212, 214, 214f
Tuamotu Islands, 211
Tunisia, 179
Turkish immigrants, 188–189
Turtle Island, 32
Tutuila, 213
Tuvalu, 211
Twitter, 70
Type 2 diabetes, 224, 225b

U

Ulithi, 227–228
unauthorized/undocumented immigrants, 64–65, 136–137, 147–148, 169t
unemployment insurance, 262
Unequal Treatment: Confronting Racial and Ethnic Disparities in Health Care (NASEM), 2
Ungan peoples, 16
United Arab Emirates, 179
United Farm Workers, 73, 93t
United Nations Permanent Forum on Indigenous Issues (UNPFII), 30–31, 34, 226–227
United Territories of Pacific Islanders Alliance Washington (UTOPIA-Washington), 229–230
universal coverage, 153t
universalism, proportionate, 267–268
University of California, Berkeley, 93t
University of California, Los Angeles (UCLA), 93t, 225b
University of California, Santa Barbara, 95t
University of Guam, 235
University of Hawai'i, 217
University of New Mexico, 30–31
University of North Carolina, 113
University of Southern California (USC) Medical Center, 173t
UNPFII (United Nations Permanent Forum on Indigenous Issues), 30–31, 34
urban Indian health programs, 12, 36
US Border Patrol, 172t
US Census
　2030 Census, 197
　actionable solutions to advance health equity, 286
　American Community Survey, 181
　definition of Asians, 50
　definition of Hispanic, 129, 131t, 173t
　definition of Latino, 129, 131t
　definition of multiracial people, 169t
　definition of white, 246b, 247
　MENA categories, 197, 198, 246b
US Commission on Civil Rights, 94t
US Constitution, 111, 247–248
　14th Amendment, 56
　　Equal Protection Clause, 172t, 247–248
　Article VI, Clause 2, 18
US Department of Health, Education, and Welfare, 22b

US Department of Health and Human Services (HHS), 22b, 36, 98
US Department of the Interior, 19, 22b
US Department of War, 16
US Preventive Services Task Force, 36–37
US Supreme Court
  Johnson v McIntosh, 18
  Seminole Nation v United States, 17
  United States v Thind, 92t
  United States v Wong Kim Ark, 92t
  Yick Wo v Hopkins, 56
USA PATRIOT Act, 57, 193–194, 295
Utah Department of Health, 224b
UTOPIA-Washington (United Territories of Pacific Islanders Alliance Washington), 229–230
Utrik, 220
Uvea (Wallis), 211

V

value systems, 224–226
Vanuatu (New Hebrides), 211, 219, 226
Venezuelans, 130t, 135
Vespucci, Amerigo, 13
Veterans Health Administration, 27, 28t
Vietnam, 51
Vietnam War, 59, 60
Vietnamese Americans, 52, 53t, 59–62, 69
violence
  disease-related, 70–71
  racialized, 185, 249. See also hate crimes
voting, 75
voting rights, 20
Voting Rights Act, 21, 93t, 221

W

Wacquant, Loïc, 246
wages
  considerations for action and further research, 268
  minimum wage, 138–139, 152t
  minimum-wage laws, 138–139, 260
  wage theft, 138–139
  and white health disparities, 259–261, 268
Waiehu Stream, 231
Waiheʻe River, 231
Waikapū Stream, 231
war in Gaza, 185, 198
War on Poverty, 259
War on Terror, 73, 95t, 193, 194
Watsonville, California race riots, 51
Wayne County, Michigan, 186–187
wealth, 32
weathering, 100

West Virginia, 255–256, 256f
Western Europeans, 15
Western Samoa. See Samoa
Wheeler–Howard Act (Indian Reorganization Act), 20, 22b
white health advantage, 255, 256–257
White House Initiative on Asian Americans, Native Hawaiians, and Pacific Islanders, 77, 95t, 236
white people
  Appalachians, 255–256, 259–260
  death rates, 255
  definition of, 246b
  health disparities, 253–267
    considerations for action and further research, 267–269
    examples, 255–257
    health care system and, 262–264
    labor and wages and, 259–261
    root causes, 257–259
    social safety net and, 261–262
  health inequities, 245–280
  health occupations, 139, 140t
  heterogeneity of, 245–246
  homelessness/houselessness, 227
  life expectancy, 255–256, 256f, 257, 258f, 259f
  marginalization processes, 246–253
  medical debt, 263
  MENA category, 188
  mortality rates, 255–257, 256f, 257f
  racial and ethnic category, 5, 12, 189, 249–253, 286
  racial domination processes, 246–253
  racial resentment, 251–252
white race advantage, 135
white supremacy, 14b, 15, 245, 246–249, 251–253
white trash stigma, 265
whiteness, 246–247, 249–253, 264–267
whiteness studies, 266–267
whole-person care, 151
Wi-Fi, 32, 37
Williams, David, 111
Wo, Yick, 56
women
  health disparities, 104–105, 108, 109–111
  reproductive health rights, 133, 171t, 172t
women's work, 56
Wong Chin Foo, 92t
Wong Kim Ark, 92t
Worcester v Georgia, 22b
workforce development, 29–32, 65, 155
World Health Organization, 229
World War I, 213
World War II, 57, 92t, 213–214, 248
Wyoming, 31

Y

Yap, 222*t*, 227–228
Yasui, Minoru, 57
yellow face, 63
yellow peril fears, 50–52
Yellow Power movement, 93*t*
Yemeni Civil War, 189
Yemenis, 179, 189
Yick Wo v Hopkins, 92*t*
yo'âmtes, 228–229, 235

Yolk magazine, 95*t*
youth
    Deferred Action for Childhood Arrivals (DACA), 75, 174*t*, 295
    mental health inequities, 70–71
    suicide rates, 101–103, 226
Yutu, 227

Z

Zoroastrians, 180